Obstetric Anesthesia

Craig M. Palmer, MD
Professor of Anesthesiology
University of Arizona
Tucson, Arizona

Robert D'Angelo, MD
Professor, Obstetric and Gynecologic Anesthesia
Wake Forest University School of Medicine
Winston-Salem, North Carolina

Michael J. Paech, FANZCA
Winthrop Professor and Chair of Obstetric Anaesthesia
School of Medicine and Pharmacology
The University of Western Australia
Perth, Australia

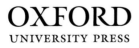

OXFORD
UNIVERSITY PRESS

OXFORD
UNIVERSITY PRESS

Oxford University Press, Inc., publishes works that further
Oxford University's objective of excellence
in research, scholarship, and education.

Oxford New York
Auckland Cape Town Dar es Salaam Hong Kong Karachi
Kuala Lumpur Madrid Melbourne Mexico City Nairobi
New Delhi Shanghai Taipei Toronto

With offices in

Argentina Austria Brazil Chile Czech Republic France Greece
Guatemala Hungary Italy Japan Poland Portugal Singapore
South Korea Switzerland Thailand Turkey Ukraine Vietnam

Copyright © 2011 by Oxford University Press, Inc.

Published by Oxford University Press, Inc.
198 Madison Avenue, New York, New York 10016

www.oup.com

Palmer, Craig M., author.
Obstetric anesthesia / Craig M. Palmer, Robert D'Angelo, Michael J. Paech
p. ; cm.
Includes bibliographical references and index.
ISBN 978-0-19-973380-4
1. Anesthesia in obstetrics. 2. Analgesia. I. D'Angelo, Robert, author.
II. Paech, Michael J., author. III. Title.
[DNLM: 1. Anesthesia, Obstetrical. 2. Analgesia, Obstetrical. 3. Gynecologic Surgical
Procedures—methods. WO 450]
RG732.P36   2011
617.9'682—dc22
2010050965

9 8 7 6 5 4 3 2 1

Printed in the United States of America
on acid-free paper

Contents

Preface

Obstetric anesthesia is a rapidly expanding, constantly evolving field; some years ago we saw a need for a practical guide to patient care and management—one that could be consulted quickly (and often) to outline a concrete course of clinical management, covering how to manage specific patients in specific situations. What drug to give, how to give it, how much to give, and when to stop and try something different. Our goal has been to provide anesthesiologists and anesthetists, both in training and in practice, with that practical reference.

Our first attempt to provide such a reference met many of these objectives, but in one area fell far below our vision. In 2002 we published the *Handbook of Obstetric Anesthesia* with a different publisher, who had their own vision for the text, and while the information and style of the *Handbook* were what we envisioned, its physical form was not. Rather than being a pocket-sized, inexpensive, "ready reference," it was a larger, hardcover text. While visually appealing, it was more at home on a bookshelf than in the pocket of a scrub suit or on an anesthesia cart.

With our new partnership with Oxford University Press, we have at last achieved what we set out to do 10 years ago. We have worked diligently to make the information easy to use—when possible, we have tried to distill essential information into tables, charts, diagrams, and flowcharts that can be quickly accessed and applied. We have used bullet points to highlight key points of management, and the essential background, rationale, and science behind clinical decision making. This is not intended to be an exhaustive reference textbook, although the readings and references at the end of each chapter do provide additional background and the basis for further study.

Of course, there is usually more than one means to an end, but where our experience has shown one approach works best, we've advocated it. Where there are equally viable options, we've tried to present each, with the advantages and disadvantages of alternative approaches.

All three of us have dedicated our careers to the anesthetic care of obstetric patients, as have our contributors. We care for these patients and deal with these problems every day. *Obstetric Anesthesia* draws on our experience and study to tell you what we do, how we do it, and why.

Craig M. Palmer, MD
Robert D'Angelo, MD
Michael J. Paech, FANZCA

Contributors

Valerie A. Arkoosh, MD, MPH
Professor of Clinical Anesthesiology and Critical Care
Professor of Clinical Obstetrics and Gynecology
University of Pennsylvania School of Medicine
Philadelphia, PA

Emily Baird, MD, PhD
Assistant Professor of Clinical Anesthesiology and Critical Care
University of Pennsylvania School of Medicine
Philadelphia, PA

Laura S. Dean, MD
Assistant Professor, Obstetric & Gynecologic Anesthesia
Wake Forest University School of Medicine
Winston-Salem, NC

Kenneth E. Nelson, MD
Associate Professor, Obstetric & Gynecologic Anesthesia
Wake Forest University School of Medicine
Winston-Salem, NC

Medge D. Owen, MD
Professor, Obstetric & Gynecologic Anesthesia
Wake Forest University School of Medicine
Winston-Salem, NC

John A. Thomas, MD
Associate Professor, Obstetric & Gynecologic Anesthesia
Wake Forest University School of Medicine
Winston-Salem, NC

Abbreviations

Ach	acetylcholine
ACOG	American College of Obstetricians and Gynecologists
AMPA	α-amino-3-hydroxy-5-4-isoxazolepropionic acid
ASA	American Society of Anesthesiologists
BP	blood pressure
bpm	beats per minute
CNS	central nervous system
CPD	cephalopelvic disproportion
CS	cesarean section
CSEA	combined spinal-epidural anesthesia
CSF	cerebrospinal fluid
DIC	disseminated intravascular coagulation
EA	epidural anesthesia
EBP	epidural blood patch
ECG	electrocardiogram
ECV	external cephalic version
EGA	estimated gestational age
FHR	fetal heart rate
FRC	functional residual capacity
GA	general anesthesia
HOCM	hypertrophic obstructive cardiomyopathy
ICP	intracranial pressure
IM	intramuscular
IU	international units
IUGR	intrauterine growth retardation
IV	intravenous
IVC	inferior vena cava
IVH	intraventricular hemorrhage

LA	local anesthetic
LBW	low birth weight
LMA	laryngeal mask airway
LMWH	low molecular weight heparin
LOR	loss of resistance
MAC	minimum alveolar concentration
mcg	microgram
MLK	myosin light-chain kinase
MMR	maternal mortality ratio
NMDA	N-methyl-D-asparate
NSAIDs	nonsteroidal anti-inflammatory drugs
NYHA	New York Heart Association
PCEA	patient-controlled epidural anesthesia
PCIA	patient-controlled intravenous analgesia
PDPH	post-dural puncture headache
PE	pulmonary embolism
PIH	pregnancy-induced hypertension
ppm	parts per million
PPV	positive-pressure ventilation
PTL	preterm labor
PVR	pulmonary vascular resistance
RDS	respiratory distress syndrome
SA	spinal anesthesia
SVC	superior vena cava
SVR	systemic vascular resistance
TPA	tissue plasminogen activator
UFH	unfractionated heparin
UPP	uterine perfusion pressure
WDR	wide dynamic range

Chapter 1

Neuroanatomy and Neurophysiology

Craig M. Palmer, MD

Introduction

The practice of obstetric anesthesia, more than any other subspecialty area within current anesthetic practice, is rooted in regional anesthesia techniques, primarily neuraxial blockade. In recent decades, our understanding of the structure and function of the nervous system, at every level (particularly at the cellular and molecular level), has been advancing rapidly. Just as understanding the physiology of pregnancy is essential to providing care during the peripartum interval, understanding the basics of neuroanatomy and neurophysiology is central to optimizing use of regional anesthetic techniques in this population.

Neuroanatomy

Afferent Neural Pathways

Peripheral Pathways

The peripheral neural pathways associated with labor sensation were first described by Head in 1893; more recent work, notably by Cleland and Bonica, clarified our understanding.

- Neurons carrying sensation from the first stage of labor (i.e., the onset of contractions through complete cervical dilation) travel with the lumbar sympathetics and enter the spinal cord between the T_{10} and L_1 levels (Figure 1.1).

- Sensation from the second stage of labor (from complete cervical dilation through delivery of the infant) travels peripherally via the pudendal nerve and enters the spinal cord at the S_2 through S_4 levels.
- The cell bodies of these primary afferent neurons lie in the dorsal root ganglion, and send their projections into the spinal cord through the dorsal root entry zone.

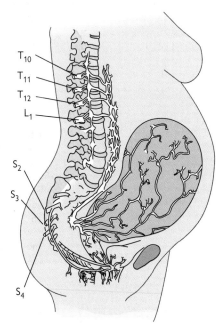

Figure 1.1 Peripheral neural pathways associated with labor sensation. Sensation from the first stage of labor is carried by neurons that travel with the lumbar sympathetic plexus and enter the spinal cord between levels T_{10} to L_1. Sensation from distention of the perineum (largely during the second stage of labor) enters the spinal cord between S_2 through S_4, traveling peripherally via the pudendal nerve. Reprinted with permission from Brown DL. Spinal, epidural and caudal anesthesia: anatomy, physiology, and technique, pp. 181–201. In: Chestnut DH, *Obstetric Anesthesia, Principles and Practice*. 1994, Elsevier.

In addition to the anatomic separation of the pathways of the first and second stages of labor, the peripheral neurons of these pathways are also morphologically distinct. Peripheral neurons can be characterized on the basis of their size and degree of myelination (Table 1.1).

- Type C fibers predominate in the first stage of labor; these small fibers are poorly myelinated, and their conduction velocity is quite slow.
  - These primary afferents synapse not at one single point or on a single secondary neuron, but branch widely with multiple synaptic connections—not only at the level of entry to the cord, but also one or two levels above and below the level of entry. This diffuse branching contributes to the poorly localized nature of sensation associated with the first stage.
- During the second stage of labor (distention of the perineum), larger type Aδ fibers dominate. These neurons are significantly larger in diameter and better myelinated, do not branch as widely, and have more rapid conduction velocities.

> The anatomic and morphologic distinctions between the first- and second-stage neural pathways have clear clinical correlates. First-stage labor pain results from uterine contractions and cervical dilation; it is cramping and visceral in nature, diffuse and poorly localized. Sensation of the second stage is primarily due to perineal distention and is more localized, due mainly to less branching of synaptic connections and the faster conduction velocity in the sacral pathways. Parturients tend to feel this sensation in their perineum rather than in their abdomen. This more discrete sensation gives rise to the parturient's ability to sense "the urge to push" and to know when delivery is imminent.

It is important to realize that these two types of sensation are not mutually exclusive: pain associated with the first stage of labor does not stop miraculously with the entry into the second stage of labor, but it is often superseded by pain resulting from distention of the perineum due to descent of the fetal head. Dependent on the progression of a woman's labor, sensation typically ascribed to the second stage may be significant during the first stage of labor if the fetal station (the level of the fetal head within the maternal pelvis) is changing rapidly. Generally speaking, however, sensations traveling via the

Table 1.1 Classification of Peripheral Nerve Fibers

Fiber	Myelinated	Fiber diameter (microns)	Conduction velocity (m/sec)	Function	Resistance to local anesthetic blockade
A-alpha	Yes	12–20	70–120	Innervation of skeletal muscles Proprioception	++++
-beta	Yes	5–12	30–70	Tactile sensory receptors (touch, pressure)	+++
-gamma	Yes	3–6	15–30	Skeleton muscle tone	+++
-delta	Yes	2–5	12–30	Stabbing pain Touch Temperature	++
B	Yes	<3	3–15	Preganglionic autonomic fibers	+
C	No	0.3–1.3	0.5–2	Burning and aching pain Touch Temperature Pruritus	+

Adapted from: Voulgaropoulos, D. and Palmer, C.M. (1996) Local Anesthetic Pharmacology. In: Prys-Roberts C, Brown BR Jr. and Nunn JF (eds). *International Practice of Anaesthesia*. Butterworth-Heinemann, Oxford.

sacral nerve roots do not become significant until labor is well advanced.

Central Pathways

Labor sensation also follows well-defined pathways *after* entry to the central nervous system; the first synapse in the afferent sensory pathway occurs in the dorsal gray matter of the spinal cord.

- Histologically, several (ten) distinct zones are found in the gray matter, commonly referred to as *Rexed's lamina*. These zones are distinct because of variations in the cell type and neuronal connections within each, reflecting differences in information processing and function.
  - Lamina I is the most superficial and dorsal of these lamina in the spinal cord.
  - Laminae I through V are most important in discussion of afferent sensory information associated with labor (Figure 1.2).

The initial synapse may be located in any of the lamina between I and V, but current understanding of these pathways focuses on laminae II and V.

- Most of the primary afferent neurons synapse initially in the more superficial lamina (I and II).

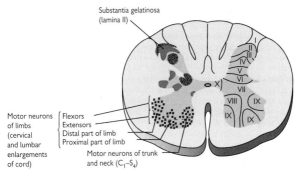

Substantia gelatinosa (lamina II)

Motor neurons of limbs (cervical and lumbar enlargements of cord)
{ Flexors
Extensors
Distal part of limb
Proximal part of limb }

Motor neurons of trunk and neck (C_1–S_4)

Figure 1.2 Diagrammatic cross section of the spinal cord illustrating Rexed's lamina of the gray matter. Most primary afferent neurons associated with labor sensation synapse initially between laminas II through V. Lamina II is also referred to as the *substantia gelatinosa*, and is the primary synaptic site of most sensory afferent fibers entering at the T_{10} to L_1 levels (i.e., the first stage of labor). The ventral lamina are associated primarily with motor neurons. Modified from Watson C. Basic Human Neuroanatomy. 1995, Lippincott Williams & Wilkins.

- Primary afferent neurons branch widely, synapsing on multiple secondary neurons not only at the level of entry to the cord, but also one to two levels higher and lower.
- Lamina II is also referred to as the *substantia gelatinosa*, and is a primary synaptic site for most sensory afferent fibers entering at the T_{10} to L_1 levels.

In order for primary afferent input to reach the level of conscious sensation, second- or higher-order neurons must project cephalad to the primary sensory cortex.

- Neurons within lamina V known as "wide dynamic range" (or WDR) neurons play an important role in the initial processing of afferent input. These WDR neurons receive afferent projections from large numbers of other neurons at the same and nearby levels of the cord.
- These afferent projections may be from primary afferent neurons, but can also be from local "interneurons," which project short distances between a few lamina, or levels within the gray matter.

The WDR neurons play one of the initial roles in processing the input they receive from these multiple synapses; their name derives from the wide range in the *rate* of depolarization characteristic of these neurons.

- With minimal input, their rate of firing is very low; with greater input, they are capable of firing action potentials in great bursts (Figure 1.3).
- Through this variability in firing rate, these spinal WDR neurons modulate input to higher levels of the CNS.

Projections from the dorsal gray matter cross to the contralateral ventral white matter of the cord, and then travel cephalad via the spinothalamic tract (Figure 1.4). The next synapse occurs, appropriately enough, in the thalamus.

- Neurons located in the thalamus project at last to the primary sensory cortex, and the parturient becomes aware she is having a contraction.

Descending Pathways

In addition to the afferent pathways described above, descending pathways within the central nervous system play an active role in the processing of nociceptive information (Figure 1.5).

- These descending pathways originate in the primary sensory cortex, and project caudally to the midbrain, synapsing on neurons in the periaquaductal gray matter.

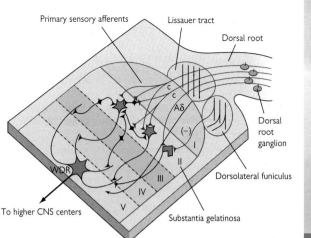

Figure 1.3 Diagrammatic cross section of the dorsal nerve root entry zone of the spinal cord. Wide dynamic range (WDR) neurons are located in deeper levels of the gray matter, receiving synaptic connections and input from many other neurons and projecting centrally. The dorsolateral funiculus carries a descending pathway. Primary afferent neurons may send branches to spinal levels above and below their level of entry to the cord via Lissauer's tract. Interneurons project between lamina and levels of the gray matter. A wide variety of both excitatory and inhibitory synaptic connections are possible.

- These neurons in turn project to the medulla, to the rostral ventral nuclei.
- Neurons with cell bodies lying in these nuclei project to the spinal cord via the dorsilateral funiculus to synapse within the dorsal gray matter of the spinal cord.

It is not clear at present exactly what activates this descending pathway *in vivo*, but it is effective. Studies in animals have shown that electrical stimulation of the periaquaductal gray matter and the rostral ventral nuclei not only produces analgesia in animals (implied by behavioral criteria), but also inhibits output of lamina V (WDR) neurons in the afferent (ascending) pathway.

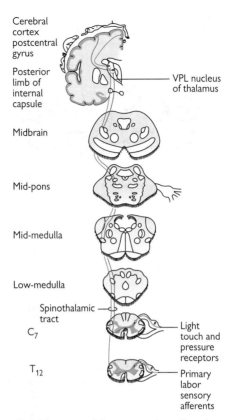

Cerebral
cortex
postcentral
gyrus

Posterior
limb of
internal
capsule

VPL nucleus
of thalamus

Midbrain

Mid-pons

Mid-medulla

Low-medulla

Spinothalamic
tract

C_7

Light
touch and
pressure
receptors

T_{12}

Primary
labor
sensory
afferents

Figure 1.4 Cephalad extension of labor sensory pathways. Secondary neurons whose cell bodies lie in the dorsal gray matter of the spinal cord project via the spinothalamic tract to the thalamus. Another synapse occurs in the pathway before projection to the primary sensory cortex. Modified from Palmer C. Spinal Neuroanatomy and Neuropharmacology. In: Seminars in Anesthesia, Perioperative Medicine and Pain. Vol. 19, No. 1., 2000, Elsevier.

Neuropharmacology

Neuraxial Medications

Local Anesthetics

Local anesthetics have been the mainstay of regional anesthesia in obstetrics for decades, and will likely continue in this role for decades to come.

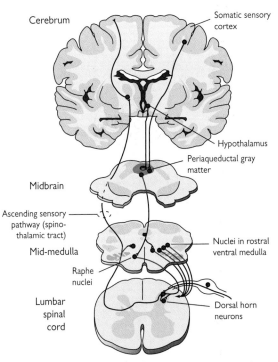

Figure 1.5 Descending inhibitory pathway. Neurons with cell bodies in the sensory cortex project caudally, synapsing in the periaqueductal gray matter of the midbrain. Another synapse occurs in the medulla before the pathway terminates in the gray matter of the dorsal lumbar spinal cord. Modified from Palmer C. Spinal Neuroanatomy and Neuropharmacology. In: Seminars in Anesthesia, Perioperative Medicine and Pain. Vol. 19, No. 1., 2000, Elsevier.

Structural Characteristics

All local anesthetics share certain structural characteristics.

- All have an aromatic ring at one end; all have a hydrocarbon chain of varying length and composition in the middle; and all have an amine group (-NH₂) at the other end.

The aromatic ring and hydrocarbon chain are nonpolar, but the amine group may reversibly bind a free proton (H⁺) to acquire a positive charge and allow the molecule to become polar (Figure 1.6).

- The protonation of local anesthetics is a physical characteristic that can be described in terms of pK$_a$; when local anesthetics are placed in

Esters

Chloroprocaine

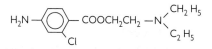

Amides

Bupivacaine

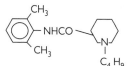

Ropivacaine

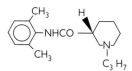

Lidocaine

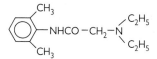

Figure 1.6 Representative chemical structures of commonly used local anesthetics. All local anesthetics have an aromatic ring at one end, an intermediate hydrocarbon chain linkage, and an amine group at the other end. The intermediate linkage may be either an ester (-COO) or an amide (-NH).

aqueous solution, the pK_a is the pH at which the charged (polar) and uncharged (nonpolar) forms are present at equal concentrations.

• Decreasing the pH (increasing the free H^+ concentration) will increase the proportion of molecules in the charged or polar state; increasing the pH (decreasing the free H^+ concentration) will have the opposite effect.

• Both the charged and uncharged forms of the molecule are necessary for the clinical effects of local anesthetics.

Site of Action

The sodium channel of the neuronal cell membrane Local anesthetics reversibly bind to sodium channels in the neuronal cell membrane, altering the ion permeability and decreasing the excitability of the neuron. The sodium channel is a large transmembrane protein with four repeating "domains."

- *In vivo*, the channel forms a donut-shaped ring with a central pore. In the resting state, the pore is closed and the channel is inactive.
- In response to depolarization of the neuronal membrane, the channel undergoes a conformational change that opens the pore and allows the passage of sodium ions.
- Local anesthetics reversibly bind to the intracellular surface of the sodium channel in its resting state and prevent the conformational change.
- It is the polar, protonated form of the local anesthetic molecule that is able to bind to the channel.

> The idea that cell membrane receptors can mediate drug effects was first postulated in the 1800s, but only recently has substantial progress been made in the area of receptor pharmacology.

To reach its site of action, the local anesthetic must diffuse across at least two nonpolar barriers (Figure 1.7):

- The lipid-bilayer of the neuronal membrane
- The overlying epineurium

> Local anesthetics diffuse across these nonpolar membranes much more readily in their nonpolar, uncharged form. However, the pK_as of all the clinically used local anesthetics are above physiologic pH of 7.4; *in vivo*, equilibrium favors the protonated, charged form of the molecule, slowing penetration to the site of action. Raising the pH shifts the equilibrium to favor the uncharged state, and speeds the clinical onset of the block. This is the physiochemical basis for the addition of bicarbonate to epidural local anesthetics to speed their action.

Clinical Use

It has long been maintained that the smaller the diameter and the more poorly myelinated the neuron, the more susceptible it is to local

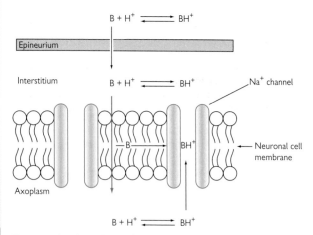

$$B + H^+ \rightleftharpoons BH^+$$

Epineurium

Interstitium $\quad B + H^+ \rightleftharpoons BH^+ \quad$ Na$^+$ channel

—B——→ BH$^+$ ← Neuronal cell
membrane

Axoplasm

$$B + H^+ \rightleftharpoons BH^+$$

Figure 1.7 Local anesthetic diffusion from epidural space to site of
action at the sodium channel on the intracellular surface of the neuronal cell
membrane. "B" represents the local anesthetic molecule (i.e., bupivacaine).
Modified from Santos AC, Pederson H, and Finster M. Local anesthetics. In:
Obstetric Anesthesia, Principles and Practice (ed. Chestnut DH) p. 202-228,
1994, Elsevier.

anesthetic block. Some recent *in vitro* investigations have called
into question this traditional understanding. What is still quite
clear clinically is that nerve fibers transmitting labor sensation are
susceptible to effective block at very low concentrations of local
anesthetics.

- The fibers transmitting first-stage sensation, felt to be mainly type C
  fibers, are readily blocked with very low concentrations of
  local anesthetics. Whether this susceptibility is the result of inherent properties of the neuron, or the result of other factors affecting
  drug distribution and binding *in vivo*, is less important than clinical
  effect.
- The fibers innervating the perineum, mainly type Aδ fibers, generally require a higher local anesthetic concentration for effective
  blockade and pain relief.
- Both types can be readily blocked with concentrations of local
  anesthetics, which should have minimal effect on large motor fibers
  to not only the lower extremities, but also to the musculature of
  the pelvic floor.

Maintaining muscular tone of the pelvic muscles may play an important role in the progress of labor by guiding the descent and rotation of the fetal head as it traverses the pelvic outlet. This "differential blockade" explains the ability to eliminate nociception (pain) without completely eliminating awareness of labor; the sensation of "pressure" associated with contractions is carried mainly via larger Aβ fibers, which are relatively resistant to blockade.

Other Adjuncts

Other adjuncts that can be used for neuraxial regional anesthesia appear to exert their effects through specific receptor populations in the neural pathways described above.

Our current understanding of neurotransmission indicates:

- The primary neurotransmitter between first-order type C afferent neurons and second-order neurons appears to be an excitatory amino acid neurotransmitter, probably **glutamate**. Glutamate acts primarily at non-NMDA (α-amino-3-hydroxy-5-4-isoxazolepropionic acid, or AMPA) receptors on the postsynaptic membrane.

- A second major neurotransmitter appears to be **norepinephrine**, a catecholamine (monoamine) with an affinity for α-2 adrenergic receptors. Norepinephrine is released by descending inhibitory pathways terminating in the dorsal grey matter of the spinal cord (Figure 1.8).

- **Substance P** appears to be another relevant neurotransmitter, acting primarily on neurokinin receptors. It may also be released synaptically by these neurons as a facilitative neurotransmitter, but it appears to function only to augment the postsynaptic response.

- **Acetylcholine** is also important, apparently in the descending inhibitory pathway. Muscarinic (cholinergic) receptors are found in the gray matter of the dorsal horn of the spinal cord.

Application or release of norepinephrine at this level of the spinal cord increases the level of acetylcholine (Ach) in spinal cord interstitial fluid, at the same time as it produces analgesia. Evidence indicates that acetylcholine is most likely released by locally projecting interneurons to act on second- or higher-order (WDR) neurons in the primary afferent pathway.

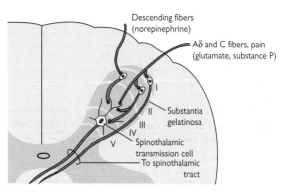

Descending fibers
(norepinephrine)

Aδ and C fibers, pain
(glutamate, substance P)

I

II — Substantia
gelatinosa

III

IV

V — Spinothalamic
transmission cell

To spinothalamic
tract

Figure 1.8 Neurotransmitters in the dorsal horn. Descending inhibitory pathways release norepinephrine, which is excitatory and acts primarily on locally projecting neurons in the gray matter. These neurons in turn release acetylcholine, which is inhibitory, at synapses with neurons of the afferent sensory pathway projecting cephalad via the spinothalamic tract. Neurotransmitters released by primary afferent neurons include glutamate and substance P. Reprinted from *Seminars in Anesthesia, Perioperative Medicine and Pain*, Vol. 19 Issue no. 1, Palmer C, Neuroanatomy and Neuropharmacology: An Obstetric Anesthesia Perspective, pp. 10–17, Copyright (2000), with permission from Elsevier.

Opioids

Almost all neuraxially administered opioids are analgesic.

Site of Action

Like local anesthetics, opioids also exert their influence via specific receptor populations. There are at least 3 types of opioid receptors in the human central nervous system: mu, kappa, and delta.

In 1975, enkephalins, a form of endogenous opioid, were isolated and characterized. By the late 1970s, autoradiographic mapping of the central nervous system had revealed opioid receptor distribution. High concentrations of mu receptors were found in the substantia gelatinosa (lamina II) of the spinal cord and the periaquaductal gray matter of the midbrain.

The initial synapse of many of the primary afferents associated with labor occurs in the substantia gelatinosa (lamina II), particularly for the first stage of labor.

- Opioid receptors are concentrated on the terminals of type C, but not Aδ neurons (Figure 1.9).
- To a lesser extent, they are also found on the surface of post-synaptic second-order neurons.
- About 75% of opioid receptors are on the presynaptic C fiber terminals.

Presynaptically, opioid agonists result in decreased release of neurotransmitters by the primary afferent. Postsynaptically, receptor activation decreases excitability of the postsynaptic membrane.

Spinal or epidural opioids are much more effective analgesics during the first stage of labor, where C fiber input predominates. Though not completely ineffective during the second stage, the lack of presynaptic inhibition on the Aδ fibers, which dominate the second stage, significantly reduces opioid efficacy. Like the substantia gelatinosa, the periacquaductal gray matter of the midbrain has a very high concentration of opiate receptors, and is an important synaptic junction of the descending inhibitory pathway discussed above. In animals, injection of an opioid such as morphine in the midbrain substantially inhibits spinal nociceptive reflexes.

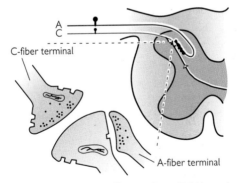

Figure 1.9 Primary synapses in the afferent pathway. Opioid receptors (the small squares in the neural cell membranes) are located presynaptically on Type C fibers and on postsynaptic membranes, but not on presynaptic Type A-delta fibers. Reprinted from *Seminars in Anesthesia, Perioperative Medicine and Pain, Vol. 19 Issue no. 1*, Palmer C, Neuroanatomy and Neuropharmacology: An Obstetric Anesthesia Perspective, pp. 10–17, Copyright (2000), with permission from Elsevier.

- Both effects are mediated by membrane-bound G protein, and result from an increase in K^+ permeability.

Clinical Use

When injected in the epidural or intrathecal space, very small quantities of virtually all opioids provide significant analgesia.

- While opioids can be injected alone, they are usually combined with local anesthetics, and significantly augment analgesia at very low doses.
- Exceeding the necessary dose required for analgesia usually only increases the incidence of side effects.

Specific clinical application of individual opioids is generally driven by differences in duration, speed of onset, and potency.

- Duration of an opioid is usually inversely proportional to lipid solubility; highly lipid-soluble opioids tend to have a shorter duration of action.
- Speed of onset is usually proportional to lipid solubility, and inversely proportional to water solubility.

Table 1.2 Comparative Properties of Neuraxial Opioids			
Opioid	Lipid Solubility	Speed of Onset	Duration
Morphine	Low	Slow	Long
Fentanyl	High	Fast	Short
Sufentanil	Very High	Very fast	Very short
Meperidine	Moderate	Intermediate	Intermediate

α-2 Adrenergic Agonists: Epinephrine

The analgesic effects of spinal epinephrine have long been known, and for decades epinephrine has been used with local anesthetics for surgical anesthesia, via both the epidural and intrathecal routes, to prolong the duration of the block. The reason usually advanced for this prolongation has been epinephrine's action as a local vasoconstrictor, slowing the uptake (and therefore metabolism) of the local anesthetic. With the characterization of α-2 adrenergic receptor populations in the superficial lamina of the spinal cord, an alternative and possibly more plausible explanation is epinephrine's ability to activate spinal α-2 adrenergic receptors on afferent neurons.

- The descending inhibitory pathway described above terminates in lamina II of the dorsal gray matter, the substantia gelatinosa.

- Receptors for norepinephrine are located both presynaptically and postsynaptically on primary afferent neurons and secondary neurons, respectively.
- Norepinephrine release from the descending neurons inhibits transmission in the primary afferent pathway.
- While significant α-2 agonist binding occurs on dorsal root ganglion cells, which suggests the presynaptic action, the most profound inhibitory effect occurs within the substantia gelatinosa, indicating a postsynaptic effect.
- The result is selective inhibition of C and A-δ fiber evoked activity in the WDR neurons of lamina V.

Clinical Use

Epinephrine added to both intrathecal and epidural local anesthetics augments the resulting block, not only in terms of duration but also intensity.

- Very small doses (+/− 10 mcg) of epinephrine have been shown to augment some intrathecal local anesthetics.
- When used with epidural local anesthetics, epinephrine dose is greater (though still usually 5 mcg/ml or less), which may indicate greater mechanism of action via vasoconstriction.
- The effect of epinephrine is most apparent when used with short-acting local anesthetics.

Other α-2 Adrenergic Agonists: Clonidine

Among other α-2 adrenergics, only clonidine has been systematically investigated and used as a labor analgesic in humans.

- Like epinephrine, neuraxial clonidine results in significant analgesia. It causes major dose-related side effects, notably decreased blood pressure, decreased heart rate, and sedation.
- While the effectiveness of intrathecal and epidural clonidine for labor analgesia is apparent, these side effects have so far prevented widespread clinical utilization. It is not currently recommended for routine clinical use in obstetrics.

Anticholinergics: Neostigmine

Neostigmine is the only anticholinesterase that has been systematically investigated as a neuraxial labor analgesic in humans to date. Presumably, neostigmine exerts its effect within the descending inhibitory pathway, preventing the breakdown of acetylcholine. Like clonidine, its effectiveness as an analgesic has been overshadowed by an unacceptable side effect profile:

- Even when used in very low doses in combination with opioids and local anesthetics, the incidence of nausea and vomiting has proven unacceptable.

It is not clear whether other anticholinesterases will eventually prove to have fewer side effects and be safe for use in humans.

Further Reading

1. Carr DB, Cousins MJ. Spinal route of analgesia: opioids and future options. In: Cousins MJ, Bridenbaugh PO, eds. *Neural Blockade in Clinical Anesthesia and Management of Pain.* Philadelphia: Lippincott-Raven; 1998:915-941.

2. Cleland, JGP. Paravertebral anesthesia in obstetrics. *Surg Gynecol Obstet.*1933; 57;51-62.

3. Collins JG, Kitahata LM, Matsumoto M, *et al.* Spinally administered epinephrine suppresses noxiously evoked activity of WDR neurons in the dorsal horn of the spinal cord. *Anesthesiology.* 1984;60:269-275.

4. Detweiler DJ, Eisenach JC, Tong C, *et al.* A cholinergic interaction in alpha 2 adrenoreceptor mediated antinociception in sheep. *J Pharmacol Exp Ther.* 1993;265: 536-542.

5. Gordh T Jr, Jansson I, Hartvig P, *et al.* Interactions between noradrenergic and cholinergic mechanisms involved in spinal nociceptive processing. *Acta Anaesthiol Scand.* 1989;33:39-47.

6. Klimscha W, Tong C, Eisenach JC. Intrathecal α2-adrenergic agonists stimulate acetylcholine and norepinephrine release from the spinal cord dorsal horn in sheep. An in vivo microdialysis study. *Anesthesiology.* 1997;87:110-116.

7. Lui SS, McDonald SB. Current issues in spinal anesthesia. *Anesthesiology.* 2001;94:888-906.

8. Paech MJ, Pavy TJG, Orlikowski CEP, *et al.* Patient-controlled epidural analgesia in labor: the addition of clonidine to bupivacaine-fentanyl. *Reg Anesth Pain Med.* 2000;25:34-40.

9. Purves D, Augustine GJ, Fitzpatrick D, *et al.* eds. *Neuroscience.* Sunderland, MA: Sinauer Associates; 1997.

10. Sabbe MB, Yaksh TL. Pharmacology of spinal opioids. *J Pain Symptom Manage.* 1990;5:191-203.

11. Stamford JA. Descending control of pain. *Br J Anaesth.* 1995;75:217-227.

12. Strichartz GR, Berde CB. Local anesthetics. In: Miller RD, ed. *Miller's Anesthesia.* Philadelphia: Elsevier; 2005:573-603.

13. Sukara S, Sumi M, Morimoto N, Saito Y. The addition of epinephrine increases the intensity of sensory block during epidural anesthesia with lidocaine. *Reg Anesth Pain Med.* 1999;24:541-546.

Chapter 2

Anatomic and Physiologic Changes of Pregnancy

Laura S. Dean, MD
Robert D'Angelo, MD

Introduction

Profound physiologic and mechanical changes occur during pregnancy. Unique alterations allow for the development of a growing fetus, and prepare the parturient for the demands of labor and delivery. Anesthesia providers must recognize the anesthetic implications of this altered physiology in order to care for patients throughout the puerperium, as well as during non-obstetric surgery. Many physiologic adaptations occur during the first trimester, making recognition of pregnancy in women of childbearing age imperative.

Cardiovascular

Hemodynamics

- Cardiovascular parameters are altered progressively throughout pregnancy (Table 2.1).

Table 2.1 **Cardiovascular Adaptations at Term Gestation**	
Parameter	Change
Cardiac Output	↑ 20%–50%
Stroke Volume	↑ 30%
Heart Rate	↑ 20%
Systemic Vascular Resistance	↓ 30%
Mean Arterial Pressure**	↓ 20%
Plasma Volume	↑ 10–50%
Oxygen Consumption†	↑ 50%

** Mean arterial blood pressure will fall as a result of a decrease in systemic vascular resistance despite the increase in cardiac output.
† Cardiac oxygen consumption increases in parallel with cardiac output throughout labor.

- Beginning as early as 4–8 weeks gestation and plateauing between 16–24 weeks, these alterations become further dependent on changes in the parturient's position, as aortocaval compression worsens beyond 20 weeks gestation.
- Systemic vascular resistance decreases as a result of increased circulating estrogen and progesterone.
- This decrease in systemic tone results in reduced afterload and preload, triggering a reflex increase in heart rate.
- Volume restoring mechanisms cause release of angiotensin and aldosterone to elevate blood volume.
- Cardiac output increases, with contributions from both stroke volume and heart rate.
- The increased cardiac output is redistributed to meet the demands of the growing fetus and altered maternal physiology (Table 2.2).
- Increased left ventricular wall thickness and ventricular cavity accommodate the elevated cardiac output. Despite remodeling, contractility is probably unchanged.

Table 2.2 **Redistribution of Blood Flow During Pregnancy**	
Organ	Increase in Blood Flow
Uterus	800 ml/min
Skin	300–400 ml/min
Renal	400 ml/min
Breasts	200 ml/min
Overall Increase During Pregnancy	1.5–2 liters/min

- It is crucial to recognize the normal changes in the cardiac exam that occur during pregnancy (Table 2.3).

At the time of delivery, hemodynamic alterations are further exaggerated. During uterine contractions, 300–500 ml of blood is autotransfused into the systemic circulation from the intervillous circulation, causing a surge in stroke volume. Cardiac output increases during labor, peaks immediately after delivery, and does not return to prepregnancy values until a month or so after delivery (Table 2.4). This should be a time of vigilance in patients with cardiac valvular lesions. In general, hemodynamics return to prepregnancy baseline during the first 6 months postpartum.

Blood Volume

A 40%–50% increase in blood volume during pregnancy meets the metabolic demands of the enlarging uterus and growing fetus. This relative hypervolemia is crucial for protecting the mother and fetus from hemorrhage at delivery, and from the deleterious effects of decreased venous return in the supine position.

- The mechanisms accounting for the increase in blood volume are multifactorial.
- Progesterone relaxes venous smooth muscle, thus increasing venous capacitance. The increase in blood volume may be a response to fill this increased vascular capacity.
- Estrogen and progesterone are also thought to directly mediate an increase in hepatic renin production, which triggers enhanced secretion of aldosterone. The resultant retention of sodium allows for the increase in total body water.
- As early as the first trimester, increased renin and angiotensin diminish the pressor response to angiotensin during pregnancy. In contrast, response to norepinephrine infusions is unchanged.

Table 2.3 Cardiac Exam During Pregnancy*

- Occasional S_4
- Accentuated and Split S_1
- 90% have Systolic Ejection Murmur
- Normal S_2
- 20% have Diastolic Flow Murmur
- 80% have S_3 Heart Sound

* Flow murmurs correlate with the increase in blood volume rather than the alteration in the cardiac output. A pericardial effusion (9%) may cause isoelectric T waves and ST changes on the electrocardiogram.

Table 2.4 Percent Change in Cardiac Output During Puerperium

Stage	Change from Baseline
Prepregnancy CO	Baseline
Term	↑ 50%
Stage 1 Labor	↑ 75%
Stage 2 Labor	↑ 110%
Immediately Following Delivery	↑ 160%
1 Hour After Delivery	↑ 90%
2 Days After Delivery	↑ 45%
2 Weeks After Delivery	↑ 10%

Aortocaval Compression

A symptomatic reduction in cardiac output in the supine position occurs in up to 15% of parturients, and is referred to as the *supine hypotensive syndrome*. Although supine hypotension is classically described beyond 20 weeks gestation, partial or complete compression can occur before this time.

Manifestations of supine hypotensive syndrome include:

• Dizziness
• Nausea
• Maternal hypotension
• Shortness of breath
• Tachycardia
• Fetal distress

Compression of the inferior vena cava by the enlarged uterus reduces venous return and can result in profound hypotension. Abdominal aortic compression further compromises uterine blood flow. If aortocaval compression is suspected in a hypotensive patient, the compressed inferior vena cava may act like two pieces of wet glass that resist separation. Neuraxial or general anesthesia will exaggerate these hemodynamic effects. Alleviating the compression and restoring adequate venous return are paramount.

Treatment consists of:

• Ensuring left uterine displacement
• Elevation of the legs (not Trendelenburg positioning)
• Fluid administration
• Vasopressor administration

It is important to recognize that the standard 15-degree lateral tilt that is vital for the obstetric patient may not be adequate to relieve aortocaval compression in all parturients. The lateral decubitus position, or even the knee chest position, may be necessary to alleviate maternal hypotension or fetal heart rate decelerations.

Pulmonary

Numerous physiologic and mechanical pulmonary adaptations occur during pregnancy, as summarized in Table 2.5. Anatomic changes in the airway and chest wall with anesthetic implications (especially during general anesthesia and attempted tracheal intubation) include:

- Venous engorgement and edema of the oropharynx, nasopharynx and larynx

Table 2.5 Pulmonary Physiologic Changes at Term Gestation

Parameter	Change During Pregnancy
Respiratory Rate	↑10%*
Tidal Volume	↑40%
Expiratory Reserve Volume	↓ 20%
Residual Volume	↓ 20%
Functional Residual Capacity	↓ 12%–25%**
Vital Capacity	No change***
Total Lung Capacity	Very minimal to no change
O_2 Consumption	↑ 40%†
Minute Ventilation	↑ 40%–50%
Diaphragm Excursion	Increased
FEV1 and FEV1/F VC	No change‡
Basal Metabolic Rate	↑ 14%

* Early in the first trimester, hyperventilation is stimulated by a progesterone-mediated hypersensitivity of respiratory centers to CO_2.

** The decrease in FRC results from reduced ERV and RV and may result in airway closure during tidal breathing in as many as 50% of term parturients in the supine position.

*** Despite elevation of the diaphragm by the enlarging uterus there is no change in vital capacity because of the simultaneous increase in chest wall diameter.

† The increase in cardiac output is greater than the increase in oxygen consumption so the AVO_2 difference in early pregnancy is decreased. As cardiac output plateaus and the metabolism of the fetus and growing uterus further increases O_2 consumption the AVO_2 difference approaches pre-pregnancy levels.

‡ There are no documented changes in airway flow or diffusion capacity.

- Vocal cord edema resulting in hoarseness
- Redundant soft tissue in the mouth, neck and chest
- Enlarged breast tissue
- Increased chest circumference 5–7 cm in both anterior posterior and transverse diameters

Acid–Base Physiology in Pregnancy

- Hyperventilation induces a slight respiratory alkalosis.
- Decrease in $PaCO_2$ leads to slightly increased PaO_2 in early pregnancy.
- Renal compensation decreases plasma HCO_3 allowing for a near normal pH.
- Although respiratory alkalosis shifts the oxyhemoglobin dissociation curve to the left, 2,3-DPG production rises 30% above nonpregnant levels and shifts the curve back to the right.
- P50 is increased from 26.7 to 30.4, aiding oxygen delivery to the fetus.
- The increase in minute ventilation, cardiac output and blood volume, along with a fall in alveolar dead space, contribute to a negligible arterial to end tidal CO_2 difference at term.
- Arterial blood gas values seen in nonpregnant and pregnant patients are listed in Table 2.6.

- These pulmonary changes have important implications for the parturient undergoing general anesthesia for cesarean delivery (see also Chapter 4).
- Hyperventilation should be avoided, as hypocarbia can lead to uterine vasoconstriction and decreased placental blood flow. Alkalosis will also shift hemoglobin oxygen dissociation curve to the left, decreasing release of O_2 to fetus.

Table 2.6 Arterial Blood Gas Results in Normal Pregnancy

Parameter	Pregnant	Nonpregnant
$PaCO_2$	26–32 mmHg	40 mmHg
PaO_2	92–106 mmHg	100 mmHg
Supine PaO_2	101→94 mmHg	100 mmHg
HCO_3	16–21 meq/l	24 meq/l
pH	7.405–7.44	7.40

Gastrointestinal

A number of physiologic changes impact the gastrointestinal system during pregnancy, labor, and delivery.

- The stomach is displaced and rotated cephalad by the increasingly gravid uterus.
- Progesterone diminishes lower esophageal sphincter tone by relaxing smooth muscle.
- The gravid uterus increases gastric pressure and elevates the lower esophagus into the thorax in many women. Consequently, many parturients experience pyrosis, or heartburn, due to gastroesophageal reflux.
- Gastric emptying is not altered during gestation but is likely slowed during labor. Opioid analgesics further delay emptying, regardless of the route of administration.
- Gastric acid secretion is probably not altered in pregnancy.

> The obstetric patient poses unique challenges for the conduct of general anesthesia: the likelihood of difficult mask ventilation and failed intubation is higher than normal at a time when aspiration is also more likely to occur. Aspiration prophylaxis to reduce the chance of pneumonitis should be strongly considered (see Chapter 4).
>
> - All pregnant women should be considered to have full stomachs regardless of NPO status, secondary to delayed stomach emptying during labor.
> - Oral intake of solids should be strongly discouraged during labor, despite calls by some groups for more liberalized policies. Both the American College of Obstetricians and Gynecologists and the American Society of Anesthesiologists support only the oral intake of modest amounts of clear liquids during labor.

Renal

Increased vascular and interstitial volumes result in slightly enlarged kidneys. The pelvis, calyces and ureters are dilated by the smooth muscle relaxation effects of progesterone and probably by the mechanical effects of the gravid uterus.

Additional changes associated with pregnancy include:

- Renal plasma flow and glomerular filtration increase early in the first trimester. These changes precede the increase in plasma volume, suggesting hormonal mechanisms.
- BUN and creatinine are lowered as GFR and renal plasma flow increase (Table 2.7). Even mild elevations in plasma levels should be investigated for evidence of renal disease.
- Glucosuria, independent of blood sugar concentration, is noted soon after conception. The renal tubules are likely unable to accept the increased filtered load of glucose accompanying the increase in GFR.
- Uric acid tubular reabsorption declines, so that plasma uric acid concentration increases in the third trimester.
- Plasma osmolality decreases early in pregnancy as water is retained in excess of sodium. The osmotic threshold for thirst declines, prompting fluid intake to contribute to the decline in osmolality.

Hepatic and Gallbladder

The diagnosis of liver disease in pregnancy is confounded by the normal changes that occur in liver function studies during gestation.

- Bilirubin, AST, ALT and LDH all increase to high normal.
- Alkaline phosphatase increases 2–4 times normal due to placental production.
- Plasma cholinesterase levels decline 20%–30% by term pregnancy. However, the simultaneous increase in volume of distribution likely counters any clinically significant prolongation of neuromuscular blockade from succinylcholine.

Table 2.7 Renal Hemodynamics Associated with Pregnancy (Listed as Change from Prepregnancy Values)

Parameter	First Trimester	Third Trimester
RPF	↑ 75%–85%	↑ 50%
GFR	↑ 50%	↑ 50%
Filtration Fraction – RPF/GFR	↓	↔
Creatinine	WNL	↓ 0.4–0.6 mg/dl
BUN	8–9 mg/dl	7–8 mg/dl

The incidence of gallbladder disease increases with pregnancy. Cholecystokinin release is decreased, which leads to a reduced contractile response. This change is probably mediated by increased progesterone levels, leading to a sluggish milieu with propensity for gallstone formation.

Glucose Metabolism

Although insulin secretion rises during gestation, parturients exhibit a relative insulin resistance. Circulating placental hormones (particularly human placental lactogen, or HPL) likely mediate this insulin resistance, decreasing peripheral sensitivity to insulin.

- Carbohydrate loads result in higher plasma glucose levels than in nonpregnant patients, allowing for placental transfer of glucose to the fetus.
- Shortly after delivery of the fetus and placenta, insulin sensitivity returns to baseline.
- Insulin should be administered cautiously prior to delivery because of the propensity for hypoglycemia immediately postpartum.

> Insulin does not cross the placenta, so the fetus is responsible for secreting its own insulin in response to glucose loads. The fetus of a hyperglycemic mother may become profoundly hypoglycemic after delivery when it no longer receives a glucose load, but still has elevated circulating levels of insulin.

Thyroid

Although there is an elevation of total serum thyroxin during gestation, and the thyroid gland is often noted to be enlarged, a euthyroid clinical state is maintained throughout pregnancy.

Hematologic

Enhanced renal erythropoietin production increases red blood cell volume. However, plasma volume increase is proportionately greater than the red cell volume increases, resulting in a relative hemodilutional anemia (Table 2.8).

Table 2.8 Physiologic Anemia of Pregnancy	
Parameter	Level During Pregnancy
Blood Volume	↑ 45%
Plasma Volume	↑ 55%
Red Cell Volume	↑ 30%
Hemoglobin	11.6 mg/dl
Hematocrit	33.5 mg/dl

Other blood elements are similarly affected by pregnancy.

- Platelet aggregation and turnover are accelerated during gestation, but platelet count remains unchanged or falls slightly with no apparent clinical effect.
- Clotting mechanisms are activated, with an elevated serum concentration of fibrinogen and all clotting factors except XI and XIII. Although this hypercoagulable state may be a protective mechanism to allow hemostasis after delivery, embolic complications remain a leading cause of morbidity and mortality during pregnancy.
- Leukocytosis peaks postpartum, with an increase in polymorphonuclear leukocytes (PMNL). However, PMNL function is likely impaired during gestation, contributing to increased risk of infection.

Neurologic

Parturients in general have an elevated pain threshold due to increased endogenous enkephalins and endorphins.

- Pregnant patients require approximately one-third less local anesthetic for regional anesthesia. Several explanations for this increased sensitivity to local anesthetics have been suggested (Table 2.9). It is well documented that pregnant women have elevated CSF progesterone levels and this elevation likely alters neuronal structure and allows for an enhanced local anesthetic effect. Most experts favor this as the most likely explanation for reduced anesthetic requirements.

Uterus

The nongravid uterus is about 5 cm x 6 cm in size and increases to 25 cm x 30 cm by term gestation.

Table 2.9 Theories for Increased Local Anesthetic Sensitivity during Pregnancy
Decreased epidural space secondary to epidural venous engorgement
Increased abdominal pressure enhancing transdural spread of local anesthetics
Exaggerated lumbar lordosis allowing increased cephalad spread of local anesthetic
Progesterone-enhanced sensitivity of nerves to local anesthetics

- Uterine blood flow increases from 50 ml/min to 500–800 ml/min at term. Uterine vessels are maximally vasodilated. The fraction of cardiac output to the uterus increases from 3%–4% in the nonpregnant state to 12% or more at term.
- Uterine perfusion is not autoregulated; a significant decrease in systemic blood pressure will result in impaired uteroplacental blood flow. Uterine contractions result in decreased placental perfusion and can lead to fetal compromise.

Further Reading

1. Blechner JN. Maternal–fetal acid-base physiology. *Clin Obstet Gynecol.* 1993;36: 3-12.
2. Clapp JF 3rd, Seaward BL, Sleamaker RH, *et al.* Maternal physiologic adaptations to early human pregnancy. *Am J Obstet Gynecol.* 1988;159:1456-1460.
3. Clapp JF III, Capeless E. Cardiovascular function before, during and after the first and subsequent pregnancies. *Am J Cardiology.* 1997;80: 1469-1473.
4. Dafnis E, Sabatini S. Effect of pregnancy on renal function. Physiology and pathophysiology. *Am J Med Sci.*1992;303:184-205.
5. Datta S, Hurley RJ, Naulty JS, *et al.* Plasma and cerebrospinal fluid progesterone concentration in pregnant and nonpregnant women. *Anesth Analg.* 1986;65: 950-954.
6. Duvekot JJ, Cheriex EC, Pieters FA, *et al.* Early pregnancy changes in hemodynamics and volume homeostasis are consecutive adjustments triggered by a primary fall in systemic vascular tone. *Am J Obstet Gynecol.* 1993;169:1382-1392.
7. Lund CJ, Donovan JC. Blood volume during pregnancy: Significance of plasma and red cell volumes. *Am J Obstet Gynecol.* 1967;98: 394-403.
8. Gaiser R. Physiologic Changes of Pregnancy. In Chestnut DH, Polley LS, Tsen LC, Wong CA, eds. *Chestnut's Obstetric Anesthesia Principles and Practice* (4th Ed.) Philadelphia, PA: Mosby Elsevier; 2009:15-36.

9. Weinberger SE, Weiss ST, Cohen WR, et al. Pregnancy and the lung. *Am Rev Respir Dis.* 1980;121:559-581.

10. Wong CA, McCarthy RJ, Fitzgerald PC, et al. Gastric emptying of water in obese pregnant women at term. *Anesth Analg.* 2007;105: 751-755.

Chapter 3

Pain Relief for Labor and Delivery

Robert D'Angelo, MD
John A. Thomas, MD
Michael J. Paech, FANZCA

Introduction

Contemporary regional analgesic techniques provide rapid, almost complete analgesia while minimizing risk to the mother and fetus. Paralleling the increase in the use of regional anesthesia during the past three decades, the incidence of anesthesia related maternal mortality has decreased dramatically. U.S. statistics suggest that the use of regional analgesia for labor increased from less than 20% in 1981 to more than 65% today.

Epidural Analgesia

Advantages

Continuous epidural techniques allow analgesia to be maintained for prolonged periods of time; the presence of the catheter also allows the quality of the analgesia to be varied should conditions change, or instrumental or operative delivery be required. In addition, epidural analgesia has a low incidence of side effects and reduces the need for general anesthesia in high-risk patients.

Disadvantages

The major disadvantage of epidural analgesia is primarily related to increased manpower requirements. Providing epidural analgesia in obstetrics is relatively labor intensive:

- It takes approximately 20 minutes to induce each anesthetic.
- As many as 30% of epidural catheters require manipulation for intravenous cannulation or inadequate analgesia.
- Nearly 10% of epidural catheters will require replacement.
- Most labor suites are not situated near the main operating suite.

Anesthesia services must balance efficient use of manpower with patient safety and satisfaction. This chapter focuses on an evidence-based approach to providing labor analgesia while accomplishing these goals.

Indications

As noted in a joint statement by the American Society of Anesthesiologists and the American College of Obstetricians and Gynecologists, "There is no other circumstance when it is considered acceptable for a person to experience severe pain, amenable to safe intervention, while under a physician's care."

Contemporary obstetric anesthesia practice dictates that any parturient requesting pain relief during any phase of labor, and irrespective of cervical dilatation, is a candidate for epidural analgesia. This assumes an epidural service exists at that institution, and that the patient has no contraindications to regional anesthesia.

Contraindications

Although absolute contraindications to neuraxial blockade are rare, a number of relative contraindications occur that may preclude the use of regional anesthesia (Table 3.1). When relative contraindications exist, the risk of a complication occurring must be weighed against the benefits of the regional anesthetic, on a case-by-case basis.

Preparation

Prior to placement of the epidural catheter or induction of epidural analgesia for labor, a focused history and physical exam should

| Table 3.1 **Contraindications to Regional Anesthesia** | |
Absolute	*Relative**
Patient Refusal or the Inability to Cooperate	Mild Coagulopathy
Localized Infection at the Insertion Site	Severe Maternal Cardiac Disease such as Eisenmenger Syndrome or Aortic Stenosis
Septic shock	
Severe Coagulopathy	Neurologic Disease (e.g., Spina Bifida)
Uncorrected Hypovolemia	Severe Fetal Depression

* The risk of a complication occurring must be weighed against the benefits of the regional anesthetic on a case-by-case basis.

be performed. This should include an explanation of risks and benefits of the procedure, and informed consent obtained (verbal or written). Other essential steps include:

- Obtaining laboratory tests when appropriate: for example, a platelet count if a patient is preeclamptic (see Chapter 7) or a partial thromboplastin time for a patient on IV heparin (see also Chapter 6).
- To assure that an obstetrician is available for an obstetric emergency.
- Intravenous access should be established.
- Administer 250–500 ml of a non-dextrose containing balanced salt solution before epidural placement, if time allows.

Drugs and equipment for resuscitation should be immediately available to treat hypotension, seizures, or cardiac arrest. The American Society of Anesthesiologists has published Guidelines for Regional Anesthesia in Obstetrics (Table 3.2).

Equipment

Disposable epidural kits generally include sterile preparatory solutions, anesthetic and needles for local infiltration, a sterile drape, an epidural needle, a syringe for loss of resistance, saline, and an epidural catheter. In addition, recommended equipment includes:

- A winged Tuohy type needle, with a 9 cm barrel marked into 1 cm increments for catheter insertion; the markings help determine the depth from the patient's skin to the epidural space.
- An epidural catheter that is clearly marked along the distal 20 cm in 1 cm increments, to assist with determining the amount of catheter

Table 3.2 Guidelines for Regional Anesthesia in Obstetrics*

1. Appropriate resuscitation equipment and drugs must be immediately available including: oxygen, suction, equipment to maintain an airway and perform endotracheal intubation, ability to provide positive pressure ventilation, and ability to perform advanced cardiac life support.
2. Regional anesthesia should be initiated by, or under the medical direction of, a physician with appropriate privileges.
3. Regional anesthesia should not be initiated until the patient is examined by a qualified individual, and the obstetrician with the knowledge of maternal and fetal status and the progress of labor approves of the labor anesthetic and is readily available to supervise labor and manage any complications that may arise.
4. An intravenous infusion should be established and maintained throughout the regional anesthetic.
5. The parturient's vital signs and fetal heart rate should be monitored.
6. Regional anesthesia for cesarean section requires that the Standards for Basic Anesthetic Monitoring be applied, and that the obstetrician be immediately available.
7. Qualified personnel, other than the attending anesthesiologist, should be immediately available for newborn resuscitation.
8. The anesthesia care provider should remain readily available during the regional anesthetic to manage anesthetic complications until the post-anesthesia condition is stable.
9. The Standards for Post-Anesthesia Care should be applied.
10. A physician should be available to manage complications and provide CPR for patients receiving post-anesthesia care.

* Adapted from the guidelines approved by the ASA House of Delegates on Oct 12, 1988 and amended on Oct 17, 2007.

that remains within the epidural space after removal of the epidural needle.

- Multiport catheters (closed tip and with 3 lateral holes at 0.5, 1.0, and 1.5 cm from the distal tip) reduce the incidence of inadequate analgesia compared to single-orifice catheters. Flexible wire-reinforced epidural catheters reduce the incidence of intravenous cannulation.
- A clear sterile drape to assist with landmark and midline identification, especially during difficult epidural placement.

Technique

A recommended technique for continuous lumbar epidural analgesia is outlined in Table 3.3.

Table 3.3 Recommended Technique for Lumbar Epidural Analgesia

- Sitting position: Cross-legged, or with feet supported and knees bent, to allow as much flexion of the lumbar spine as possible.
- Sterile prep and drape any interspace between L_2 and S_1 (L_{3-4}, L_{4-5}, or L_5–S_1 preferred)
- LOR with saline, cephalad-directed needle bevel
- Midline approach
- Once the epidural space is identified, insert the epidural catheter 4–6 cm
- If aspiration negative, test catheter for spinal or intravenous placement with either single or double Lidocaine test dose:
  - <u>Single test dose:</u> 1.5% Lidocaine 45 mg + Epi 15 mcg (3 ml). If negative, administer 15 ml (5 + 5 + 5 ml) 0.0625%–0.125% Bupivacaine + Fentanyl 2 mcg/ml to initiate labor analgesia
  - <u>double test dose:</u> *2% Lidocaine 40 mg (2 ml) followed in 5 min if negative by 2% Lidocaine 100 mg (5 ml) followed in 1 min if negative by 2% Lidocaine 60 mg (3 ml to total 200 mg)
- Adequate analgesia: Begin infusion of 0.0625%–0.125% Bupivacaine + Fentanyl 2 mcg/ml for maintenance
- For PCEA, use the following initial settings:
  - Basal rate   6–12 ml/h
  - Bolus dose   5–6 ml
  - Lockout   8–12 min
  - Hourly limit   20–30 ml
- For continuous infusion analgesia, begin infusion at 10 to 14 ml/h
- Inadequate analgesia: If pain persists 15 min after Lidocaine administration, pull catheter so 3–4 cm remains within the epidural space and administer additional local anesthetic (2% Lidocaine 100 mg); if pain relieved, begin maintenance as above
- Persistent inadequate analgesia: If pain persists after 5 min, remove and replace epidural catheter.

* The double Lidocaine test dose is recommended to test the adequacy of the epidural catheter in patients at high risk of requiring a cesarean section.
LOR = loss of resistance; PCEA = patient controlled epidural analgesia.

Positioning and Choice of Interspace

The patient may be positioned in either the lateral decubitus or sitting position during epidural catheter placement. Each anesthesia provider will develop a personal preference; however, they must become adept at epidural catheter insertion with the patient in the lateral position, because emergency clinical scenarios such as a prolapsed cord may necessitate lateral positioning should a regional anesthetic be required. The primary advantage of the sitting position is easier identification of midline, especially in obese patients. In contrast, the lateral decubitus position may be more comfortable for the patient, especially during the late phases of labor.

Recommendations that Facilitate Placement

- With either position, ask the patient to either place her elbows on her knees while reaching around her abdomen, or over a pillow placed over the abdomen; both maneuvers will reduce lumbar lordosis.
- Sitting "Indian Style" (ankles crossed and the knees fully abducted) facilitates the elbow on knee position.
- If the patient cannot assume this position, placing her feet on a stool with knees raised and flexed, rather than dangling off the bed, is a reasonable alternative.
- Although textbooks often recommend the interspace that is easiest to palpate, between the L_2 spinous process and the sacrum, it is best to avoid the L_2–L_3 interspace to reduce the likelihood of spinal cord damage. The spinal cord ends at L_2 in 4% of the population and up to 25% of procedures occur one interspace higher than predicted.

Loss of Resistance and Needle Advancement

A loss of resistance (LOR) technique is recommended to locate the epidural space; the use of air or saline for LOR remains controversial. As long as injection of significant volumes of air into the epidural space is avoided (i.e., inject 1–4 ml or less), either air or saline can be used safely and effectively for LOR to identify the epidural space. Most clinicians currently advocate the use of saline: saline better expands the epidural space, facilitating catheter insertion, and theoretically reduces the incidence of intravenous cannulation and inadequate analgesia. Saline is also incompressible and may be preferential when teaching/learning the LOR technique.

Advantages of air LOR include a "better feel," easier identification of accidental dural puncture (clear fluid is identified), and the extra step of opening a vial of saline is avoided. In contrast to saline, air causes an almost immediate headache if injected intrathecally, and theoretically prevents diffusion of local anesthetic to all nerve roots.

There are two common techniques for epidural needle advancement, an intermittent LOR technique and a continuous LOR technique (Figure 3.1a and 3.1b).

Intermittent Technique

- A "winged" epidural needle is recommended.
- Grasp the wings between the thumbs and index fingers while pressing the middle fingers of each hand against the needle shaft near the insertion site to prevent excess movement.

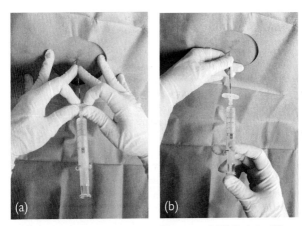

Figure 3.1 (a) The "Intermittent Loss of Resistance (LOR) Technique" for epidural catheter placement is pictured. With this technique, the wings of the epidural needle are grasped between the thumb and index finger of each hand, while the middle fingers are pressed against the needle shaft near the insertion site to prevent excess movement. The needle is advanced a short distance (1–2 mm), then LOR is ascertained by depressing the plunger with either hand. (b) The "Continuous LOR Technique" is demonstrated in this picture. The thumb and index finger of the nondominant hand firmly secure the epidural needle near the insertion site, while the back of the hand is placed against the patient's back to prevent excess movement. Continuous pressure is then applied to the syringe with the dominant hand as the needle is slowly and continuously advanced.

- Advance the needle a short distance (1–2 mm), stop, and check for LOR by depressing the syringe plunger with one hand while securing the needle with the other hand.
- Repeat until LOR is achieved.

Continuous Technique

- Ensure that the back of the hand is pressed onto the patient's back to prevent excess movement.
- Secure the epidural needle near the patient's back with the thumb and index finger of the nondominant hand.
- Apply continuous pressure to the syringe plunger with the dominant hand as the needle is slowly but continuously advanced until LOR is achieved.

With either technique, depression of the plunger will be met with resistance while the epidural needle is in either the interspinous ligament or the ligamentum flavum. When the epidural needle bevel passes through the ligamentum flavum into the epidural space, gentle pressure will easily depress the plunger, which defines "loss of resistance."

Bevel Direction

It has been suggested that inserting the epidural needle with bevel facing vertically, rather than horizontally (in relation to the long axis of the back) significantly reduces the incidence of headache in cases of accidental dural puncture. However, after vertical insertion the epidural needle is usually rotated cephalad to facilitate midline epidural catheter insertion. Since rotation of the epidural needle may in itself increase the likelihood of dural puncture, it is generally recommended to avoid the extra step of needle rotation. Cautiously approaching the epidural space and inserting the epidural needle using a horizontal, cephalad orientation minimizes the incidence of unintended dural puncture.

Epidural Catheter Insertion (Table 3.3)

Insert the epidural catheter 5–6 cm into the epidural space if possible.

- Catheters inserted >6 cm increase the risk of intravenous cannulation.
- Catheters inserted <5 cm are more likely to become dislodged during prolonged labors, especially in obese patients.
- If using a catheter reinforced with a wire coil, hold the catheter during insertion so that the coils do not generate right or left rotational force which could theoretically facilitate lateral insertion.
- Remove and replace epidural catheters associated with a persistent paresthesia (see also intravenous cannulation section).
- When withdrawing an epidural catheter for any reason during the procedure, remove the epidural catheter and needle as one unit, since pulling the epidural catheter through the epidural needle can shear the catheter tip.
- Should a portion of epidural catheter shear during removal, inform the patient. Surgical removal is rarely warranted unless there are persistent neurological symptoms.

Epidural Catheter Testing

After securing the catheter, place the patient in the semilateral position to avoid aortocaval compression, and carefully aspirate the epidural catheter. If negative for cerebrospinal fluid (CSF) or blood, the catheter should be further tested to rule out accidental intrathecal or intravenous placement.

- The purpose of a test dose is to produce early signs of toxicity but not produce a high spinal block, seizures or cardiopulmonary arrest.
- If a test dose containing local anesthetic is administered, the patient should be monitored for motor block (signs of intrathecal placement) and symptoms such as tinnitus or perioral numbness (signs of intravenous placement).
- In addition, some patients may develop a "glassy-eyed look" and will not be able to communicate effectively for 2–3 minutes after an intravenous injection.

Several epidural test solutions have been proposed and are outlined in Table 3.4. The most commonly used test dose is a 3 ml solution 1.5% lidocaine 45 mg plus epinephrine 15 mcg, as a single test to rule out both intrathecal and intravenous catheter placement. Regardless of test dose, it is important to:

- Monitor maternal heart rate after administration
- Administer test doses between contractions, since painful contractions increase maternal heart rate
- Wait at least 5 minutes before assessing motor block

The double test dose is an attractive alternative, because it avoids the pitfalls associated with epinephrine. It is particularly suited for use in patients at high risk of urgent operative delivery.

Table 3.4 Epidural Test Doses
Double Test Dose:
2% Lidocaine 40 mg (2 ml) IT test followed in 3–5 minutes, if negative, by 2% Lidocaine 100 mg (5 ml) IV Test
Single Test Doses:
1.5% Lidocaine 45 mg + Epi 15 mcg (3 ml)
2% Chloroprocaine 60 mg + Epi 15 mcg (3 ml)
0.25% Bupivacaine 7.5 mg + Epi 15 mcg (3 ml)
Others:
Isoproterenol 5 mg
Fentanyl 100 mcg
Doppler Detection of Air 1–2 ml

- The primary benefit is that lidocaine can produce good labor analgesia within 7–10 min when the catheter is sited properly.
- When using the double test dose, 2% plain lidocaine 2 ml (40 mg) serves as an intrathecal test, followed in 5 min by a 5 ml (100 mg) dose to rule out intravenous cannulation.

Regardless of the specific test dose chosen, carefully testing each epidural catheter may reduce maternal and fetal risk, and is therefore recommended.

Intrathecal Catheter

Significant motor block and complete pain relief within 5 min of the test dose suggest an intrathecal cannulation. Should this occur, the catheter can either be removed and replaced at another interspace, or left in place and used as a spinal catheter (see continuous spinal analgesia).

Intravenous Catheter

If an intravenous catheter is detected by either aspiration or the test dose, withdraw the catheter in 1 cm increments while gently aspirating until blood can no longer be aspirated. If the catheter tip rests 3 cm or more within the epidural space (which is likely in 50% of intravenous cannulations), adequate analgesia will still be successfully produced in > 90% of cases. The remaining 50% of intravenous catheters, that have < 3 cm remaining within the epidural space at the point that blood can no longer be aspirated, should be removed and replaced.

Establishing a Block

Once a negative test dose is confirmed, local anesthetic should be administered incrementally to obtain a T_{10}–T_8 sensory block.

- 10–15 ml of dilute local anesthetic plus opioid is usually required, whether or not the lidocaine plus epinephrine test dose was administered.
- If the double test dose was administered, an additional 3 ml of 2% lidocaine to total 200 mg will produce a dense sensory block and some degree of motor block.

Epidural Catheter Management

Approximately 20%–30% of patients experience inadequate epidural analgesia. Maldistribution of local anesthetic has been postulated as a possible explanation, and may have a variety of causes.

- The catheter may deviate from midline during insertion, leading to a maldistribution of local anesthetic within the epidural space.

- Septa within the epidural space may prevent uniform distribution of local anesthetic.
- The use of air for loss of resistance may introduce bubbles that impede complete spread of local anesthetic.
- Previous surgery, or even previous epidural anesthetics, may create scar tissue or other mechanical obstructions that inhibit complete spread of the local anesthetic.

Regardless of the cause, these epidural catheters should be withdrawn until adequate analgesia is established, or replaced. The following technique is recommended as an aggressive approach to epidural catheter management, so that within 20 minutes of epidural catheter insertion the patient is either comfortable or the epidural catheter is replaced:

- If pain persists 15 min after the test dose, withdraw the catheter so that 3–4 cm remains within the epidural space, and administer additional local anesthetic.
- If not comfortable within 5 minutes, remove and replace the epidural catheter.

This approach improves overall efficiency and increases the likelihood that epidural anesthesia will produce adequate surgical analgesia.

- An alternative recommendation places the patient with inadequate analgesia into the dependent position, and administers additional local anesthetic before withdrawing the epidural catheter.
- Evidence suggests this technique is less effective than first withdrawing the epidural catheter (91 % v. 74 % success rate); further, it wastes time and the patient remains uncomfortable but will eventually require catheter manipulation.

When patients develop adequate analgesia, administer a dilute solution of local anesthetic (most commonly bupivacaine 0.0625%–0.125%) plus opioid (usually fentanyl 2 mcg/ml) for maintenance. Although ultra-dilute solutions of bupivacaine (< 0.0625% concentration), fentanyl and epinephrine have been recommended in the literature, evidence suggests that approximately 50% of patients experience inadequate analgesia during labor. Therefore, the more concentrated solutions noted above, which produce better analgesia and reduce the need for further interventions, are recommended.

Maintenance Techniques

Labor analgesia can be maintained by intermittent bolus, continuous infusion, and patient-controlled epidural analgesia (PCEA) techniques.

Table 3.5 Recommended Solutions for Epidural Analgesia Maintenance

Technique	Concentration and Dosing Schedule
Intermittent bolus	0.125%–0.25% Bupivacaine + Fentanyl 3–5 mcg/ml + Epi 1:200,000 10 ml (5 + 5 ml) boluses, repeat as needed
Continuous infusion	0.0625%–0.125% Bupivacaine + Fentanyl 2 mcg/ml at 8–16 ml/h

PCEA with basal infusion	0.0625%–0.125% Bupivacaine + Fentanyl 2 mcg/ml at the following settings:
	  Basal rate: 6–12 ml/h
	  Bolus dose: 5–6 ml
	  Lockout: 8–12 min
	  Hourly limit: 20–30 ml

PCEA without a basal infusion	0.0625%–0.125% Bupivacaine + Fentanyl 2 mcg/ml at the following settings:
	  Bolus dose: 6–8 ml
	  Lockout: 8–12 min
	  Hourly limit: 30–40ml

In general, intermittent bolus techniques require the most anesthetic interventions and PCEA techniques the least. A recommended technique for each method is described Table 3.5. Patient-controlled epidural analgesia with a background infusion is recommended, since the basal infusion significantly reduces workload and improves efficiency by limiting the number of anesthesia provider interventions (re-boluses) required during labor.

Regardless of the maintenance technique used, analgesic requirements vary throughout labor and delivery and, occasionally, patients experience breakthrough pain or perineal pressure as labor progresses. The administration of additional boluses of bupivacaine or lidocaine 5–10 ml is recommended. If discomfort persists, epidural catheters can be manipulated as previously described.

Complications

Epidural analgesia is associated with side effects and rare complications (Table 3.6). Fortunately, the most common of these are easily treated. Back pain is usually self-limited and treated with oral analgesics and ambulation. Hypotension results from sympathetic blockade, which, if untreated, can lead to fetal bradycardia by reducing uterine artery blood flow and fetal oxygenation. Hypotension and/or fetal bradycardia after epidural placement should be treated promptly by

Table 3.6 Complications and Side Effects Associated with Epidural Analgesia*

Complication or Side Effect	Incidence
Backache at insertion site	75%–90%
Inadequate labor analgesia	15%–25%
Hypotension	Varies with dose
Motor block	Varies with dose
Urinary retention	Varies with dose
Require replacement	8%–10%
Fetal bradycardia	8%
Intravenous cannulation	1%–6%
Inadvertent dural puncture (Wet Tap)	1%–2%
Post dural puncture headache	1%
Inadvertent spinal catheter	<1%
Subdural catheter	Rare (1:1000)
High spinal block	Rare (1:10,000)
Permanent neurologic injury	Extremely rare (<1:10,000)
Epidural hematoma	Extremely rare (<1:100,000)
Epidural abscess	Extremely rare (<1:100,000)
Death	Extremely rare (<1:100,000)

* The listed incidence for each complication or side effect is an average value obtained from multiple sources within the literature.

ensuring left uterine displacement, giving intravenous fluid and either ephedrine 5–10 mg or phenylephrine 50–100 mcg intravenously as needed (see also Chapter 12).

Medications

Local anesthetics are the primary pharmacologic drugs used in obstetric anesthesia; they are used to provide regional analgesia for labor and delivery, as well as anesthesia for cesarean delivery. The most common local anesthetics used in obstetrics are listed in Table 3.7. At the author's institution, lidocaine is primarily used to test epidural catheters for location and establish labor analgesia, bupivacaine to maintain labor analgesia, and chloroprocaine to provide anesthesia for instrumental and operative deliveries. The bulleted sections that follow represent an overview of local anesthetic properties and toxicity.

Table 3.7 Commonly Administered Local Anesthetics in Obstetrics

Drug	Class	Concentration	Dose*	Onset	Duration of Labor Analgesia**	pka	Protein Bound
Chloroprocaine	Ester	2%–3%	10–30 ml	Rapid	30 min	8.7	0
Lidocaine	Amide	1%–2%	10–30 ml	Intermediate	45 min	7.9	70
Bupivacaine	Amide	0.04%–0.5%	10–30 ml	Slow	60 min	8.1	95
Levobupivacaine	Amide	0.04%–0.5%	10–30 ml	Slow	60 min	8.1	97
Ropivacaine	Amide	0.04%–0.5%	10–30 ml	Slow	60 min	8.1	94

* Local anesthetics should be administered incrementally rather than as a bolus (5 ml aliquots)
** Duration of labor analgesia from a single 15 ml epidural dose administered incrementally.

Local Anesthetics (see also Chapter 1)

Local anesthetics are classified as either esters or amides, according to the alkyl chain linking the lipophilic carbon ring and the tertiary amine.

Esters:

- Include cocaine, tetracaine, procaine, and chloroprocaine
- Are degraded in the plasma by pseudocholinesterase and nonspecific esterases
- Are hydrolyzed to produce para-aminobenzoic acid (PABA), which gives them greater allergic potential than the amides

Amides:

- Include lidocaine, etidocaine, mepivacaine, prilocaine, bupivacaine, ropivacaine, and levobupivacaine
- Are metabolized in the liver

All local anesthetics are weak bases with pKa values approximating 8.0. At physiologic pH, most of the local anesthetic molecules exist in the ionized form but only unionized molecules diffuse through tissues and cross cell membranes.

- Physiochemical properties such as pKa, lipid solubility, and protein binding determine the clinical properties of various local anesthetics, including variability in speed of onset, potency, and duration of action.
- Speed of onset is generally inversely related to pKa, since local anesthetics with lower pKa values have a higher fraction of unionized molecules.

Blood levels of local anesthetics are influenced by the total dose of drug administered, its physiochemical properties, the addition of vasoconstrictors, metabolism, and the vascularity of the site where administered. Using lidocaine as an example:

- Although 5 mg/kg administered within the epidural space is considered safe, 20 mg injected directly into the carotid artery will likely produce a seizure.
- A similar dose administered into the following compartments produces varying plasma levels that directly correlate with the vascularity of each site in the following order: intercostal > caudal > epidural > brachial plexus = femoral.
- The addition of epinephrine 1:200,000 lowers plasma concentrations and prolongs the duration of the block.

Local anesthetics have no adverse effects on uterine or umbilical artery blood flow at clinically relative doses.

- They can produce in uterine artery vasoconstriction and uterine hypertonus at higher concentrations.
- Unionized local anesthetic molecules freely cross the placenta.
- Since fetal pH is lower than the maternal pH, more local anesthetic becomes ionized and accumulates in the fetal circulation, in a phenomenon known as "ion trapping."
- This "ion trapping" effect may become clinically significant in a distressed, acidotic fetus.

Local Anesthetic Toxicity

All local anesthetics are toxic if administered in high enough doses. As blood levels increase, local anesthetics first cause excitatory neurologic symptoms, such as tinnitus, perioral numbness and seizures, followed by CNS depression, respiratory arrest, and eventual cardiac arrest (Table 3.8).

Cardiotoxicity is relative to the specific drug, total dose administered and the local anesthetic concentration in the blood. A small dose of local anesthetic administered directly into the carotid artery will produce a seizure but poses no risk of a cardiac arrest, while a large bolus (intended for the epidural space) inadvertently injected intravenously can cause cardiac arrest.

Table 3.8 Signs and Symptoms of Local Anesthetic Toxicity*

1. Tinnitus, perioral numbness
2. Inability to communicate appropriately (glassy-eyed look)
3. Loss of consciousness
4. Seizure
5. Respiratory arrest
6. Cardiac arrest

* All local anesthetics can produce these reactions. The signs and symptoms generally occur in the listed order as blood concentrations increase. A test dose containing local anesthetic should produce the first two symptoms but not loss of consciousness, seizures, or cardiopulmonary arrest. To prevent severe toxic reactions, local anesthetics should always be administered in fractionated doses (5 ml aliquots).

- Bupivacaine is the most cardiotoxic of clinically used local anesthetics. If the dose of bupivacaine required to produce cardiac toxicity is **1**, the equivalent dose of ropivacaine is **2**; for lidocaine it is **8–16** and for chloroprocaine >**16.**

- Chloroprocaine has the least potential for inducing cardiotoxicity, due to rapid metabolism.

Testing epidural catheters after placement, fractionated dosing, and vigilance are the keys to preventing local anesthetic toxicity.

- The *spinal test dose* will rule out an intrathecal catheter, and is intended to be large enough to produce pain relief and motor block but not high spinal block.
- The *intravenous test dose* will detect an intravenous catheter, and is intended to be large enough to produce early signs of CNS toxicity, but not so large as to produce seizures or cardiopulmonary arrest.

Fractionated dosing entails administering 5 ml aliquots at least 30–60 seconds apart, while observing the patient for signs and symptoms of intravascular or intrathecal injection.

- The relatively small doses and slow injection will lessen risk of a catastrophic toxic event.
- Large boluses of concentrated local anesthetic should never be injected as a single rapid bolus, even with a functioning epidural catheter, since catheters can migrate into epidural veins or intrathecally.
- Even in urgent situations, large volumes of local anesthetic (i.e., 30 ml) can be administered over 3–4 minutes in 5 ml increments.

Lipid Treatment of Local Anesthetic Toxicity

The term "lipid rescue" was first coined in 2003 and is a new treatment modality for local anesthetic toxicity that has shown promising results in animal models and in numerous case reports. Experimental models have shown that infusion of a lipid emulsion increases the dose of bupivacaine needed to cause asystole in rats. Infusion of a lipid emulsion has improved resuscitation success after bupivacaine-induced cardiac arrest in dogs, is superior to either vasopressin alone or vasopressin in combination with epinephrine for resuscitation of local anesthetic toxicity in rodents, and has been used successfully to treat many cases of local anesthetic toxicity in humans.

Recommendations for Use of Lipid Rescue:

- At present, no standard protocol exists
- Intralipid® (lipid emulsion) solution should be stocked on labor and delivery units for easy access in emergencies.
- If standard adult cardiac life support (ACLS) is not immediately successful after LA overdose, consider administration of Intralipid® (Table 3.9).

Specific Drugs Used in Obstetric Anesthesia

Bupivacaine

Bupivacaine is the most commonly used local anesthetic to maintain labor analgesia for a number of reasons:

- Dilute concentrations produce proportionally greater sensory block than motor block.
- Bupivacaine has limited placental transfer since it is highly protein-bound.
- Plain 0.25% bupivacaine or 0.125% bupoivacaine with opioid 10–15 ml produces analgesia in 10–15 min that lasts approximately 60 min before the patient requests additional analgesia.
- Continuous infusions of dilute bupivacaine 0.04%–0.125% at rates of 10–15 ml/h, with or without opioids, provide labor analgesia with minimal side effects.

Ropivacaine and Levobupivacaine

Bupivacaine is prepared as a 50/50% racemic mixture of D- and L-isomers. The D-isomer binds cardiac sodium channels more tightly than the L-isomer, and is consequently more cardiotoxic. Levobupivacaine and ropivacaine were developed as alternatives to bupivacaine, and are preparations of nearly pure L-isomers. Bupivacaine, levobupivacaine, and ropivacaine belong to the same pipecoloxylidide family and are structural analogs. Ropivacaine has a three-carbon side chain, while bupivacaine and levobupivacaine have four-carbon side chains.

Ropivacaine produces less motor block than either bupivacaine or levobupivacaine, at the same concentration; however, the three drugs produce clinically indistinguishable labor analgesia. Similar concentrations and dosing regimens of ropivacaine or levobupivacaine should be administered when used as alternatives to bupivacaine. While these newer agents result in slightly less motor block than bupivacaine at equal concentrations, several factors have slowed their clinical acceptance.

Table 3.9 Recommended Lipid Rescue Protocol for Local Anesthetic Induced Cardiac Arrest

- 20% Intralipid solution: 1.5 ml/kg as an initial bolus, followed by
- 0.25–0.5 ml/kg/min for 30–120 minutes
- Repeat bolus 1–2 times for persistent asystole
- Increase infusion rate by 0.25 ml/kg/min if the blood pressure declines

- Ropivacaine and levobupivacaine cost more than bupivacaine.
- The benefit of the reduced motor block in laboring parturients remains unproven.
- The incidence of local anesthetic induced cardiac arrest in obstetric anesthesia practice is exceedingly rare.

Lidocaine

Plain 1%–2% lidocaine 10–15 ml produces labor analgesia in 5–10 minutes that lasts approximately 45 minutes before the patient requests additional analgesia. Alkalinization with 8.4% sodium bicarbonate 1 meq/10 ml of local anesthetic decreases onset time to approximately 3–6 minutes. Lidocaine is commonly used to test epidural catheters, initiate labor analgesia, treat breakthrough pain, or produce anesthesia for instrumental or operative deliveries. It is not routinely used as a maintenance agent because it produces more motor block and has greater placental transfer than bupivacaine.

Chloroprocaine

Plain 2% chloroprocaine 10–15 ml produces labor analgesia in 3–6 minutes that lasts approximately 30 minutes before the patient requests additional analgesia. Chloroprocaine is not routinely used as a maintenance agent because its short duration of action makes management difficult.

3% chloroprocaine is well suited for producing surgical anesthesia for instrumental or operative deliveries.

- It has a very rapid onset of action.
- It produces dense sensory and motor block.
- It has a short duration of action.
- It has a very favorable safety profile; it is metabolized by plasma esterases, resulting in a plasma half-life of approximately 30 seconds, making it one of the least toxic local anesthetics.

Despite these benefits, chloroprocaine has several drawbacks. It has been associated with neurologic injury when administered intrathecally. In some patients, it may produce transient but uncomfortable back pain, and when administered together with epidural opioids, the opioid effect is inconsistent in both quality and duration. Although the exact mechanism is unknown, chloroprocaine reduces fentanyl and morphine analgesia, even after the block has receded. Although statistically significant, this effect does not appear to be clinically significant.

Chloroprocaine-induced neurotoxicity has been associated with both the pH of the solution and the use of the preservative sodium metabisulfite. Because of these concerns, a preservative-free preparation of chloroprocaine has been marketed. In addition, since the preparation's pH was increased from 3.0 to 7.0 several years ago, there have been no further reports of neurotoxicity. Nevertheless, in cases of unintentional dural puncture with the epidural needle avoiding chloroprocaine seems prudent.

Chloroprocaine induced back pain has been related to localized muscle hypocalcemia induced from the preservative EDTA (which binds calcium ions). Patients have developed severe muscle spasms of the upper back following large doses (> 50 ml) of chloroprocaine; usually after epidural analgesia has receded. Commercial preparations using EDTA are no longer available.

When considering a risk/benefit ratio for this drug, it is the author's opinion that the benefits of chloroprocaine clearly outweigh the risks of these rare complications.

Chloroprocaine should be avoided in patients with known abnormal psuedocholinesterase (1:3,000 patients).

Opioids (See also Chapter 5)

Opioids produce analgesia by binding to opioid receptors both in the spinal cord (spinal receptors) and within the brain (supraspinal receptors). Although opioids reliably produce analgesia in early labor, they are less effective during the later phases of labor and for delivery.

- Visceral pain fibers (early labor pain) are primarily located in the periphery of the spinal cord and have a larger population of opioid receptors, making them more amenable to opioid-induced modulation.
- Somatic pain fibers (late labor and delivery pain) are located more deeply within the spinal cord and have fewer associated opioid receptors.

Since opioids do not produce complete labor analgesia, they are most often co-administered with local anesthetics.

Lipid Soluble Opioids

Fentanyl (2–4 mcg/ml) and sufentanil (0.3–0.5 mcg/ml) are the most commonly used opioids in obstetrics (combined with local anesthetic to produce labor analgesia).

- Side effects produced by fentanyl and sufentanil are similar at equipotent doses.
- Pruritus is the most frequently encountered side effect (60%–100% incidence), but rarely requires treatment. If necessary,

pruritus is readily treated with an agonist-antagonist such as nalbuphine 5 mg.

- Less common side effects include nausea, urinary retention, dysphoria and respiratory depression.
- Lipid soluble opioids are associated with "early respiratory depression," which occurs within 30 min of administration. It is likely due to rapid systemic uptake or rapid cephalad distribution within the central nervous system and, may be more likely following repeat doses.
- All side effects, including respiratory depression, can be reversed with naloxone (40 mcg boluses titrated to effect are recommended).

Overview of Fentanyl Mechanism of Action in Obstetrics

The addition of fentanyl 2 mcg/ml to dilute concentrations of local anesthetic (typically bupivacaine 0.0625%–0.125%) for labor analgesia reduces local anesthetic use by 25%–30%.

- Epidural fentanyl at 20 mcg/h, a typical obstetric dose, and in contrast to intravenous fentanyl, reduces epidural bupivacaine use in laboring women, which indirectly indicates a spinal analgesic effect.

In contrast, epidural fentanyl alone offers little advantage over intravenous administration to treat postoperative pain.

- Fentanyl requirements, blood concentrations, analgesia and side effects are similar.
- Treatment of postoperative pain requires relatively large doses of fentanyl (>100 mcg/h).
- At these higher doses, epidural fentanyl is absorbed systemically and activates both spinal and supraspinal opioid receptors.

Hydrophilic Opioids

Morphine and meperidine (pethidine) have been used in obstetrics, but much less commonly than lipid soluble opioids. The onset of analgesia from neuraxial administration of morphine is slow (up to 1 hour). Epidural morphine is associated with biphasic "early and late respiratory depression."

- Early respiratory depression is probably due to rapid systemic uptake, and occurs within 1 hour of administration.
- Late respiratory depression occurs 6–18 hours after administration and is secondary to rostral spread within the CSF leading to brainstem depression of respiration.

In theory, parturients that deliver vaginally may be at increased risk of morphine-induced respiratory depression since they experience less postpartum pain than parturients requiring an operative delivery. Additionally, parturients are more sensitive to nearly all anesthetics, and are usually sent to unmonitored postpartum wards.

- For these reasons, epidural or intrathecal morphine is not recommended for vaginal delivery.

Neuraxial meperidine has local anesthetic-like as well as opioid properties, but clinical data are lacking, so recommendations about its use and safety for labor analgesia cannot be made at this time.

Adjuncts

The holy grail of analgesia in obstetrics is a medication or combination that produces long-lasting, complete pain relief without side effects. Since all current medications produce side effects, a variety of epidural and spinal adjuncts have been studied in an attempt to improve or prolong labor analgesia while minimizing side effects (Table 3.10). Unfortunately, each adjunct studied (e.g., epinephrine, neostigmine) produced undesirable side effects or, as is the case with clonidine, its routine use is precluded in the United States. The following is a summary of three adjuncts studied to date.

Epinephrine, an α-adrenergic receptor agonist, enhances analgesia, reduces blood levels of local anesthetics, increases onset times, and prolongs block duration.

- Epidural doses of 1:200,000–600,000 are often used for continuous epidural analgesia.
- Single-shot spinal doses of 200 mcg or less have been reported.
- Epinephrine increases the degree and duration of motor block, especially with continuous infusions.

Clonidine, an α_2 adrenergic receptor agonist, is the most promising epidural adjunct.

- At an epidural dose of 4 mcg/ml, clonidine significantly reduces PCEA bupivacaine/fentanyl use in laboring women without increasing side effects.
- Spinal doses of 15–50 mcg prolong labor analgesia from bupivacaine/sufentanil but produce sedation and hypotension.
- Clonidine is expensive in the United States, and has an FDA "Black Box Warning" against its use in obstetrics.

Neostigmine is an anticholinesterase that enhances analgesia by indirectly increasing spinal levels of acetylcholine.

- At a spinal dose of 10 mcg, neostigmine fails to enhance labor analgesia but produces severe nausea.
- At epidural doses up to 500 mcg, preliminary studies indicate that it enhances labor analgesia without producing nausea, but is still under investigation and cannot be recommended for routine use at this time.

Combined Spinal Epidural (CSE) Analgesia

A CSE anesthetic combines a single-shot spinal with continuous epidural analgesia, as one procedure that harnesses the advantages of each while minimizing risks. The development of small gauge pencil-tip spinal needles that minimize the risk of post-dural puncture headache and inadvertent spinal catheter placement have allowed CSE use to gain widespread acceptance in obstetrics.

Equipment
Specially designed CSE kits are commercially available. To increase the likelihood of successful dural puncture, the spinal needle tip should

When first introduced to clinical practice, CSE analgesia was believed to be particularly beneficial for patients in either early or late labor; it was viewed as a tool to reduce anesthetic interventions by speeding the progress of labor and by allowing more patients to deliver without requiring epidural analgesia. In practice, nearly all patients administered CSE analgesia in early labor, and 40% of multiparous women administered CSE with a cervical dilatation > 7 cm, require epidural analgesia prior to delivery.

Early CSE research often focused on prolonging the duration of the spinal analgesia. Although spinal analgesia can be prolonged to nearly 3.5 hours, the required combination of medications also produced side effects such as motor block, hypotension, sedation and nausea (Table 3.10). Consequently, CSE has evolved into a true combined spinal-epidural technique that increases efficiency, limits side effects, and increases patient satisfaction.

extend 11–15 mm past the tip of the epidural needle (Figure 3.2a and 3.2b; Figure 3.3c). Although epidural needles with separate spinal and epidural catheter lumens are available, to theoretically minimize the risk of unintentionally placing a spinal catheter, they are expensive. Further studies have failed to demonstrate an increased risk, especially when the CSE is technically easy. As a result, the "needle through needle" approach is recommended (Figure 3.2b).

- A standard epidural needle is used to identify the epidural space.
- A long spinal needle is inserted through the lumen of the epidural needle.
- Spinal medications are administered via the spinal needle into the intrathecal space, and the spinal needle is removed.
- The epidural catheter is inserted as usual.

Anesthetic Technique

The contraindications to regional analgesia and anesthesia and the guidelines for regional anesthesia previously described (Tables 3.1 and 3.2)

Table 3.10 Summary of Spinal Analgesia from Various CSE Solutions			
Drugs	Dose	Duration (min)	Side Effects*
Fentanyl	25 mcg	90	
Fentanyl	25 mcg	108	
Bupivacaine	2.5 mg		
Sufentanil	10 mcg	105	
Sufentanil	10 mcg	150	
Bupivacaine	2.5 mg		
Sufentanil	10 mcg	188	Motor block
Bupivacaine	2.5 mg		
Epinephrine	200 mcg		
Sufentanil	5 mcg	205	Sedation
Bupivacaine	2.5 mg		Hypotension
Clonidine	50 mcg		
Sufentanil	5 mcg	205	Sedation
Bupivacaine	2.5 mg		Hypotension
Clonidine	50 mcg		Nausea
Neostigmine	10 mcg		

* Nearly all patients administered spinal opioids experience pruritus although it rarely requires treatment.

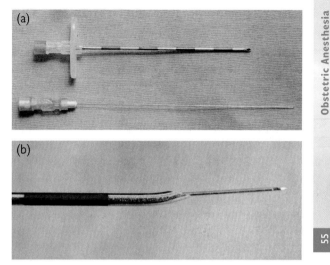

Figure 3.2 (a) An epidural needle and a spinal needle from a standard CSE kit are pictured. The epidural needle is a 17g winged needle with a 9 cm barrel. The hub is specially designed to receive this particular spinal needle, which is a 27g 4–11/16" Whitacre needle. (b) The tips of the epidural and spinal needle using the recommended "needle through needle" technique are pictured. Once the epidural space has been located with the epidural needle, the spinal needle is inserted through the lumen of the epidural needle. It is recommended that the spinal needle tip extend 11–15 mm past the tip of the epidural needle to facilitate dural puncture. The tip of the spinal needle pictured extends 11 mm past the tip of the epidural needle.

also apply to CSE techniques. Procedurally, CSE and epidural techniques are similar, with only a few exceptions (also see recommended technique described in Table 3.11).

The sitting position, rather than the lateral decubitus position, is recommended for CSE placement. The sitting position offers several advantages.

- Identification of the midline is easier, which is essential for successful dural puncture.
- The position increases lumbar intrathecal pressure, making the dura more taut and increasing the likelihood of a successful dural puncture.

Table 3.11 Recommended Technique for CSE Labor Analgesia

- Sitting position
- Sterile prep and drape, any interspace between L_2 and S_1
- LOR with air or saline
- CSE kit (spinal needle tip should extend 11–15mm past epidural needle tip)
- Small gauge pencil tip spinal needle (25–27 g)
- Firmly secure spinal and epidural needle hubs with index finger and thumb
- Spinal injectate:
  - Bupivacaine (0.25%) 1.75–2.5 mg (0.7–1 ml) + Fentanyl 15–20 mcg (0.3–0.4 ml)
- If possible, aspirate CSF to total 2 ml prior to injection
- Remove spinal needle, insert multiport epidural catheter 5–6 cm, remove epidural needle
- Have patient assume lateral position
- Secure catheter
- Test dose (if desired):
  - 2 ml 2% lidocaine (40 mg), or
  - 3 ml 1.5% lidocaine (45 mg) + epi 15 mcg
- Begin epidural maintenance infusion as described in Table 3.5

Either air or saline can be used for loss of resistance. After placing the spinal needle, secure the spinal needle by pinching both the spinal and epidural needle hubs between the thumb and index finger during aspiration and injection, to reduce needle movement and the failure rate.

- The dura does not hold the spinal needle firmly in place as does the ligamentum flavum during a one-shot spinal technique.

Since CSE solutions are hypobaric, aspiration of spinal fluid 1 ml makes the injectate more isobaric, and theoretically limits cephalad spread.

- Once the epidural catheter is inserted and the epidural needle removed, have the patient assume the lateral decubitus position and secure the catheter.

A spinal test dose may be administered to rule out an intrathecal catheter. Some clinicians prefer to avoid the use of this test dose, feeling it may result in an unnecessarily dense block. The epidural infusion can be initiated immediately.

- If using PCEA, ask the patient to press the demand button approximately 45 min after spinal injection; this augments the epidural dose and increases the likelihood of the patient remaining pain free when the spinal analgesia recedes.

Initiation of CSE with the spinal injection noted in Table 3.11 (bupivacaine/fentanyl) will produce about 90–120 minutes of analgesia. The onset of analgesia is approximately 5–7 minutes faster than epidural analgesia.

- The rapid onset of profound analgesia improves patient satisfaction compared to epidural techniques.
- The low drug doses minimize side effects such as motor block and hypotension.
- Initiating the epidural infusion soon after the spinal injection eliminates the need for independent dosing of the epidural catheter.
- Less than 20% of patients should require interventions for inadequate analgesia.

The primary drawback of the CSE technique is that the correct epidural catheter placement remains unproven for some time after the spinal injection. As a result, the routine use of CSE anesthetics in parturients at high risk for operative delivery is not recommended. Inducing traditional epidural analgesia in high-risk patients is recommended, since a well-functioning epidural catheter reduces the need for general anesthesia should urgent cesarean section be required.

When to Consider Avoiding CSE

- Morbid obesity
- Severe preeclampsia
- History of previa or abruption
- Abnormal presentation
- Multiple gestation
- Fetal macrosomia
- Abnormal fetal heart rate tracing
- Anticipated difficult airway

Reasons for CSE Failure

Assuming the use of appropriately sized spinal and epidural needles, the most likely reason for failure to obtain CSF is deviation from the midline (Figures 3.3).

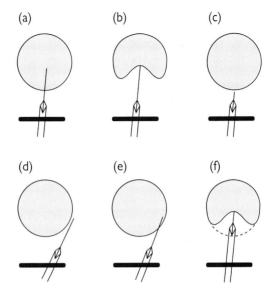

Figure 3.3 The figure illustrates a successful dural puncture, and a number of possible scenarios that lead to CSE failure or the inability to aspirate spinal fluid. (a) A successful dural puncture, (b) The dura is "tented" rather than punctured. (c) A short spinal needle fails to reach the dura. (d) Lateral deviation of the epidural needle causing the spinal needle to miss the dural sac. (e) Similar to (d) except that the dura is punctured laterally, which may result in the inability to aspirate CSF. (f) "Tenting" of the dura with a "too short" spinal needle. Further advancement of the epidural needle may result in the dura rebounding over both the spinal and epidural needle tips, causing an accidental "wet tap" with the epidural needle.

Should CSF fail to return when the spinal needle is passed, the following steps can be performed:

- Remove the spinal needle.
- Withdraw the epidural needle 1–2 cm.
- Reassess the angle of epidural needle placement and redirect either right or left, using LOR to re-enter the epidural space in a slightly different position.
- If still unsuccessful following the second attempt, abandon the CSE technique and proceed with an epidural technique.

If CSF is observed but cannot be aspirated, this is most likely due to lateral penetration of the dura.

- Attempt to aspirate while rotating the spinal needle.
- If still unsuccessful but there is no persistent paresthesia, it is recommended to inject the spinal solution and proceed with epidural catheter placement.
- If the patient fails to develop spinal analgesia (which should be rapidly apparent), dose the epidural catheter.

Complications

In general, the risks associated with CSE and epidural analgesia are similar. Although concerns of meningitis, high spinal block, abscess, permanent neurologic injury, hematoma, and metallic fragments introduced into the spinal space have been suggested as possible complications of the technique, the incidence of these complications has not increased since the advent of CSE. The incidence of post-dural puncture headache should not be significantly different from standard epidural techniques with the use of very small gauge spinal needles.

- Some series have indicated that use of the CSE technique actually avoids inadvertent dural punctures with the epidural needle by using the spinal needle as a "finder needle" to confirm correct epidural needle placement.

Initial reports of fetal bradycardia associated with CSE led to speculation that fetal heart rate changes were related to uterine hypertonicity, induced by a precipitous decrease in circulating maternal epinephrine as a consequence of rapid onset analgesia.

- Clinical studies, however, suggest that the incidence of fetal bradycardia is similar with both CSE and epidural anesthetics, and approximates 10%.
- Fetal bradycardia following either technique is usually self-limiting and generally persists only a few minutes. Ensuring left uterine displacement, administering oxygen and supporting maternal blood pressure, if necessary, are recommended.

It is imperative that interspaces below the L_2 spinous process be used during CSE placement, to minimize the risks of permanent neurologic injury; spinal cord damage can occur if interspaces above L_2–L_3 are used (see also Positioning and Choice of Interspace above).

- A "**walking epidural**" is simply any epidural or spinal technique that produces analgesia without inhibiting the ability to ambulate. Although the concept is based on the theory that ambulation during active labor shortens labor and reduces the incidence of instrumental or operative deliveries, prospective studies have failed to support this hypothesis.

- In many respects, having patients ambulate tends to increase the workload, since many walking epidural protocols require multiple anesthetic interventions. Time is required to not only place and initially dose with local anesthetic, but also to perform subsequent re-dosing. Further, allowing patients to ambulate after inducing any regional anesthetic incurs medicolegal risk. Even if the patient can perform a deep knee bend prior to ambulating, the anesthetic would most likely be implicated should she sustain an injury during an accidental fall.

- For these reasons, allowing patients to ambulate following CSE placement is not recommended. On the other hand, allowing parturients who are able to do so to sit in a chair at the bedside, with only minimal nursing assistance, may enhance patient satisfaction.

Continuous Spinal Analgesia

The advantages of continuous spinal analgesia over either one-shot spinal or the continuous epidural techniques include rapid-onset, reliable analgesia that can be titrated to varying labor conditions over a prolonged duration. Despite these benefits, a continuous spinal anesthetic poses technical challenges.

To reduce the incidence of post-dural puncture headache, small gauge spinal catheters (< 24 g) were introduced in the late 1980s; however, these catheters were withdrawn form the market in the United States following reports of permanent neurologic injuries. These injuries are believed to result from maldistribution of local anesthetic within the CSF. Safe use of a 24 g spinal catheter was investigated in a recent series, but the catheter is not commercially available in the United States. As a consequence, relatively large gauge epidural catheters must be used for continuous spinal techniques and these catheters increase the likelihood of a post-dural puncture headache.

Recommended Clinical Scenarios for Spinal Analgesia

Most often, the use of a continuous spinal technique for labor analgesia is a consequence of difficulty placing an epidural catheter, and the decision to use the catheter via the spinal route. Such scenarios might include:

- Unintentional dural puncture in parturients that are nearing delivery (multiparous women presenting in late phase labor).
- Unintentional dural puncture during difficult placement (multiple attempts in a morbidly obese patient or a patient with previous scoliosis surgery).
- Unintentional dural puncture in a patient with an anticipated difficult airway.

Planned use of a continuous spinal technique can be useful in several clinical scenarios:

- The patient with prior back surgery who desires regional analgesia for labor, or anesthesia for surgical delivery. Even if an epidural catheter can be placed in such patients, the spread of local anesthetic may be inadequate, resulting in an unacceptable block.
- The patient considered likely to be extremely difficult or impossible to intubate, secondary to deformity or airway anomaly. A planned continuous spinal anesthetic in these patients is a means of minimizing the risk of losing the airway should emergent operative delivery be required.

Continuous spinal anesthesia can reduce the likelihood of a high spinal block from a one-shot spinal technique, by allowing for the careful titration of the anesthetic to a desired sensory dermatomal level.

In all cases the "spinal catheter" should be boldly marked to clearly stand out from a regular epidural catheter, properly documented on the anesthesia record, and all anesthesia providers in the labor suite should be personally notified.

- The potential for accidental administration of epidural doses into the CSF or inaccurate dosing into the spinal catheter increases the likelihood of a high spinal block. A high spinal block in the uncontrolled setting of a labor room potentially increases the risks of catastrophic loss of airway.

Recommended dosing regimens are outlined in Table 3.12. Caution must be used when administering opioids, as repeat doses may increase the risk of respiratory depression. With the intermittent bolus technique, the catheter should be flushed after each injection with a 2 ml bolus, since the epidural catheter and filter may contain up to 1 ml of dead space.

Anesthesia for Vaginal Delivery

Vaginal Delivery

Pain during early labor is primarily visceral in nature, and nociceptive input enters the spinal cord at the T_{10}–L_1 levels. As labor progresses, pain arises due to stimulation of spinal cord at S_2–S_4 (the pudendal nerve). These dual pain pathways result in varying analgesic requirements over the course of labor and during delivery. It is not uncommon for patients to experience increasing rectal pressure or perineal pain (sacral sparing) as labor progresses. The S_2–S_4 nerve roots are relatively large, and may require higher concentrations of local anesthetic to anesthetize than thoracic or lumbar nerve roots.

Table 3.12 **Recommended Solutions for Maintenance of Spinal Catheter Analgesia**	
Technique	*Solution**
Labor Analgesia:	
Intermittent Bolus:	0.25% Bupivacaine 1.75–2.5 mg + Fentanyl 15–20 mcg as needed (CSE doses every 1–2 hours)
Continuous Infusion:	0.05%–0.125% Bupivacaine + Fentanyl 2–5 mcg/ml @ 0.5–3.0 ml/hr and titrated to a T_{10} block
Surgical Anesthesia:	Preservative free 0.5% Bupivacaine 5.0 mg (1 ml) + Fentanyl 15 mcg for the initial dose followed by 0.5 ml boluses of 0.5% bupivacaine (2.5 mg) every 5 min until the desired block height is obtained. Repeat the 0.5 ml bupivacaine dose as needed to maintain the desired block height

* The epidural catheter and filter has >1 ml of dead space; therefore, a continuous spinal catheter should be flushed with 2 ml of saline after each bolus dose.

Treatment for Breakthrough Pain during Labor

- Administer 5–10 ml of epidural 0.125%–0.25% bupivacaine with fentanyl 25 mcg.
- If ineffective, administer 5–10 ml of 2% lidocaine with fentanyl 25 mcg.
- If discomfort persists, withdraw the epidural catheter so that 3–4 cm remains within the epidural space and administer additional local anesthetic.
- For vaginal delivery, perineal analgesia can usually be produced with 5–15 ml of either 2% lidocaine or 2% chloroprocaine (Table 3.13).

Forceps or Vacuum Assisted Delivery

Indications for assisted vaginal delivery include maternal exhaustion, cardiovascular or neurologic disorders that preclude maternal pushing, fetal distress, arrested rotation and abnormal fetal position.

- Forceps deliveries are classified as either outlet, low, mid, or high depending on the relation of the fetal head to the introitus and ischial spines, although high forceps deliveries are almost never indicated.

Anesthetic requirements vary with the type of forceps delivery attempted. In general, higher fetal stations and rotation of the fetal head require more force by the obstetrician for delivery, which in turn increases the risk of fetal and maternal complications, as well as anesthetic requirements.

Anesthesia Requirements for Forceps or Vacuum Delivery

The dilute local anesthetic solutions used to provide labor analgesia are usually insufficient for forceps delivery. For outlet or low forceps, a dense T_{10} sensory block will usually suffice.

Table 3.13 Recommended Epidural Local Anesthetics for Vaginal or Assisted Vaginal Delivery

	Perineal (Sitting) Solution	Outlet Forceps	Mid Forceps	Initial Volume*
Agent	%	%	%	(ml)
Lidocaine	2	2	2	10–15
Chloroprocaine	2	2	3	10–15
Bupivacaine	0.25	0.25–0.5	0.5	10–15

*Volume should be varied to individual patient requirements. A dense T_{10} sensory block is desirable for vaginal deliveries or low-risk assisted vaginal deliveries, while a dense T_6 sensory and motor block is desirable for a mid-forceps trial.

- Mid-forceps delivery with head rotation (mid-forceps trial) typically requires a dense T_6 sensory block.
- Mid-forceps trials can result in prolonged fetal bradycardia, requiring cesarean section.
- Consider attempting a mid-forceps trial in the operating room prepared for an operative delivery (double set-up) rather than in the labor room.
- 3% chloroprocaine 15–20 ml should produce sufficient anesthesia for the forceps trial, and for a lower abdominal incision should an emergent cesarean section be required.

Vacuum deliveries generally require anesthetic levels similar to those of low and outlet forceps.

- Each patient should be evaluated individually, and the dose of local anesthetic titrated to effect.

Alternative Regional Anesthetic Techniques

Although alternative regional anesthetic techniques can be used in obstetrics, they do not afford the flexibility of epidural or CSE analgesia. In general, alternative techniques are technically more difficult to perform, and produce more frequent complications, than epidural or CSE techniques. Nevertheless, they can be used in patients who are not candidates for epidural or CSE analgesia and who do not have contraindications to regional anesthesia.

Lumbar Sympathetic Block

This technique produces analgesia for early labor by blocking pain originating in the lower uterine segments and cervix. Local anesthetic is administered near the lumbar sympathetic chain to provide 2–3 hours of analgesia.

- The technique is ineffective for later phases of labor or delivery. Although a lumbar sympathetic block has minimal effects on the fetus, it is technically difficult to perform, requires multiple needle sticks, and occasionally produces significant complications, such as accidental intravascular, subarachnoid or epidural injection, retroperitoneal hematomas, Horner's Syndrome, and post-dural puncture headache.
- Approximately 20% of patients develop hypotension that requires treatment. Because of these risks, and the fact that this technique is

ineffective for delivery, lumbar sympathetic blocks are rarely used in obstetrics.

Technique

- The patient is placed in the sitting position
- Identify the transverse process of the L_2 vertebra using a 10 cm, 22 g needle
- Redirect the needle medially below the transverse process
- Advance approximately 5 cm into the anterolateral surface of the vertebral column (tip of the needle lies just anterior to the medial attachment of the psoas muscle)
- Use a loss of resistance technique to identify when the needle has passed beyond the psoas fascia and near the sympathetic trunk
- Following a negative aspiration, administer 10 ml 0.5% bupivacaine or ropivacaine/1:200,000 epinephrine solution
- Repeat the procedure on the opposite side
- A continuous catheter method has also been described

Paracervical Block

This technique produces analgesia of the lower uterine segment, cervix, and upper vaginal canal by anesthetizing the paracervical (Frankenhauser's) ganglion. Similar to a lumbar sympathetic block, a paracervical block provides analgesia only for early labor. Analgesia typically occurs within 5 minutes and lasts 45–120 minutes. However, this technique produces a high incidence of maternal and fetal side effects. Maternal toxicity results from systemic absorption or direct intravascular injection, while fetal bradycardia results from direct absorption, vasoconstriction of uterine arteries or from accidental injection of local anesthetic into the fetal presenting part. In addition, hematomas of the broad ligament and retropsoal or subgluteal abscesses have been reported. Because of these risks, paracervical blocks are rarely used in obstetrics.

Technique

- The patient is placed into the lithotomy position
- A special 12–14 cm 22 g needle with a depth guard is introduced 2–3 cm under the mucosa of the vaginal fornix adjacent to the cervix
- Approximately 10 ml of local anesthetic is injected at both the 3 and 9 o'clock positions

- Dilute concentrations reduce the risk of intravascular absorption and fetal bradycardia

Pudendal Nerve Block

This technique blocks the S_2–S_4 nerve roots and the pain originating from the perineum, lower vaginal wall, and vulva. It is most effective for late-phase labor and delivery. Disadvantages include risk of systemic toxicity from intravascular injection, potential trauma to the pudendal artery or to the fetal presenting part, formation of vaginal wall hematomas, and retropsoas or subgluteal abscesses. In addition, unless the block is timed correctly, many patents do not develop effective analgesia until after delivery, since it takes 6–15 minutes to produce analgesia. This block is also rarely used now.

Technique

- The patient is placed in the lithotomy position
- A special needle with depth guard is inserted into the vaginal mucosa slightly medial and posterior to the ischial spine
- The needle is advanced through the sacrospinous ligament by using a loss of resistance technique
- Dilute local anesthetic 10 ml is administered
- The procedure is repeated on the opposite side
- Aspiration prior to injection is critical because of the proximity of the pudendal artery

Perineal Infiltration

Perineal infiltration is the most commonly used regional anesthetic technique in patients that deliver without preexisting epidural analgesia. It provides anesthesia for repair of lacerations or an episiotomy, and may also be used to supplement poorly functioning epidural analgesia. Since the perineum lacks major nerves, local anesthetic must be injected subcutaneously and submucosally to provide anesthesia. Anesthetic requirements vary with the amount of injury sustained during delivery.

Improving Anesthetic Efficiency in Obstetrics

Maximizing efficiency without compromising patient safety is a reasonable goal for any labor epidural service. This discussion focuses on four factors that accomplish this goal: CSE analgesia, multiport epidural catheters, fentanyl, and PCEA.

CSE

CSE techniques produce analgesia faster than epidural techniques. Although minimal time is saved in any individual patient, efficiency can be considerably improved in a busy labor service (estimated savings of 600 man hours/year at 5,000 vaginal deliveries per year).

- Use CSE for all patients at low risk of urgent cesarean section.
- Initiate epidural infusion immediately following the spinal injection.
- If CSF is not obtained after 2 attempts at spinal needle placement following epidural space location by loss of resistance (time required usually 6–7 minutes), convert to epidural analgesia.

Epidural Catheters

Multiport epidural catheters reduce the incidence of inadequate analgesia and the number of catheters that require manipulation compared to uniport epidural catheters.

- Flexible wire-reinforced epidural catheters also reduce the incidence of venous cannulation.
- Insert multiport catheters 5–6 cm into the epidural space to reduce the risk of intravenous cannulation and subsequent catheter dislodgement.
- If analgesia is inadequate 15 min after initial dosing:
  - Withdraw the catheter so that 3–4 cm remains within the epidural space
  - Administer additional local anesthetic
  - Remove the catheter and replace it (consider using CSE) if the patient is not comfortable within 5 minutes.

Fentanyl

- Fentanyl 2 mcg/ml added to dilute local anesthetic for labor analgesia reduces local anesthetic use by approximately 25%–30%.
- This may translate into fewer side effects, thus reducing workload.

PCEA

PCEA reduces analgesic requirements and motor block compared to intermittent bolus and continuous infusion techniques.

- Use of a basal infusion significantly reduces anesthesia provider interventions (breakthrough pain).
- The patient self-administers most of the required supplementary doses.
- Recommended PCEA settings are 6–12 ml/h basal rate, 5–6 ml bolus, 8–12 min lockout, 20–30 ml hourly limit.

Epidural Analgesia and the Progress of Labor

For several decades, epidural analgesia suffered from the perception that it prolongs labor and increases the incidence of instrumental and operative deliveries. Numerous independent maternal, fetal, obstetric and anesthetic factors influence obstetric outcome, however. The majority of studies over 10 years old addressing this issue are complicated by retrospective analysis, selection bias, a lack of randomization, the inability to blind participants, crossover, and ethical issues related to withholding treatment. In addition, women requesting epidural analgesia may be inherently different from those who do not (Table 3.14). Intense pain may actually be a marker for abnormal or dysfunctional labor, which in itself results in longer labors and increases not only the likelihood of instrumental or operative delivery, but also the probability the parturient will request epidural analgesia.

Despite limitations with any study design, the vast majority of sentinel event or "catastrophe" model (sudden offering of an epidural service, for example) studies suggest that epidural analgesia has no clinically significant effect on the progress of labor or the incidence of cesarean section. A recent series of 750 parturients randomized to either CSE labor analgesia or systemic IV opioid analgesia in early labor (<4 cm cervical dilatation) found that patients in the CSE group had *shorter* first and second stages of labor. There was no difference between groups in cesarean delivery rate and, of course, the CSE patients had much lower pain scores than the systemic analgesia group.

Table 3.14 **Characteristics of Parturients Requesting Epidural Analgesia**
1. Frequently nulliparous
2. Earlier stages of labor and with higher fetal station
3. Slower cervical dilatation prior to requesting analgesia
4. More likely to be receiving oxytocin
5. Deliver larger babies
6. Have smaller pelvic outlets
7. Greater pain of labor (dysfunctional labor)
8. Higher risk of operative delivery (poor fetal status or maternal disease)

Systemic and Alternative Analgesia for Labor

General Considerations and Alternatives

Attitudes toward analgesia for labor and analgesic methods are diverse. Despite the justifiable enthusiasm of obstetric anesthesiologists for epidural analgesia, pain during labor and delivery is contextually unique and individual-specific.

- Globally, the vast majority of pregnant women have no access to epidural analgesia (or any form of pharmacological pain relief).
- In developed countries, many parturients manage very well without epidural analgesia but most request some method of pain relief.
- If ready access to epidural analgesia is available, 50%–90% of women will use it.

The popularity of non-epidural methods varies with cultural, regional and local influences (Table 3.15). For example, transcutaneous electrical nerve stimulation (TENS; Figure 3.4) and "water blocks" (Figure 3.5) appear more widely used in Scandinavia; ketamine in India; nitrous oxide inhalation in the UK and Australia; and intramuscular opioids in much of Europe.

Nitrous Oxide

Nitrous oxide was described as an analgesic for labor pain in 1880, and became popular after the manufacture of the Minnitt apparatus for self-inhalation of mixtures with air. This was followed by Entonox, a 50:50 mix with oxygen (Figure 3.6).

Nitrous oxide has very rapid onset and offset due to low blood-gas solubility. The parturient inhales in conjunction with each contraction via a mouthpiece or face mask.

- Concentrations of 30%–70% provide modest analgesia for 10%–40% of parturients.
- Side effects include drowsiness, reduced awareness, and occasionally nausea.
- Risks include oversedation, dizziness, hyperventilation-induced hypocarbia and tetany, and compensatory hypoventilation between contractions that leads to maternal and fetal hypoxemia. This is more likely after opioid analgesia or in the obese parturient.
- Atmospheric pollution in the delivery unit to 300 ppm has been measured, and is beyond the recommended limits of 25–100 ppm. This raises concerns about abortion and bone marrow effects among staff working in the unit.

Table 3.15 Features of Nonpharmacological Methods of Labor Analgesia

In general

Aid relaxation and ability to cope with pain
- no or minimal pain reduction

High levels of maternal satisfaction
- especially if patient-controlled

Popular and widely available
- useful alone or as adjuncts to other methods

Excellent safety record
- avoid hyperventilation during breathing exercises if the fetus is compromised

Specific techniques

Water baths/massage
- readily available; no antenatal preparation required

Learned relaxation techniques/biofeedback/hypnosis
- motivation or investment of time or money essential

Transcutaneous electrical nerve stimulation (TENS)/acupuncture
- mainly a placebo analgesic effect
- safe, but may limit mobility

Water block
- painful injection may need repetition
- modest efficacy and short duration

Other inhalational agents can also be used.

- Inhalational of subhypnotic concentrations of various inhalational anesthetic drugs (e.g., 0.25% isoflurane or 1%–4.5% desflurane with 50 % nitrous oxide and oxygen) has shown modest efficacy.
- Such techniques are not popular because of practical problems with drug delivery.

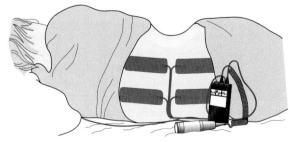

Figure 3.4 Position of TENS electrodes for labor.

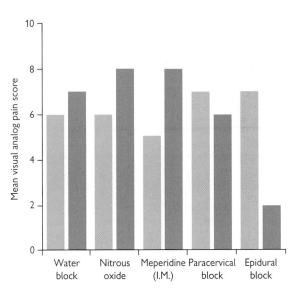

Figure 3.5 Visual pain scores (0–10) before and after pain management in the first stage of labor in the various pain relief groups. Minimum, lower (25th) quartile, median, upper (75th) quartile, maximum. Reprinted with permission from Ranta P, Jouppila P, et al. Parturient's assessment of water blocks, pethidine, nitrous oxide, paracervical and epidural blocks in labour. *Int. J Obstet Anesth.* 1994;3(4):196.

Opioid Analgesia

Morphine and scopolamine injection were introduced for labor pain in 1902, but little systematic evaluation of neonatal effects was attempted until Virginia Apgar developed her simple scoring system in 1953. Meperidine (pethidine) was introduced in the 1940s and was promoted as having minimal respiratory depressant effects.

- Morphine has more favorable kinetics, the neonatal half-life is shorter, and plasma levels remain low or undetectable.
- In Europe and the United States, partial μ- or κ-opioid receptor agonists (e.g., meptazinol, pentazocine, nalbuphine, butorphanol) and tramadol (a mixed μ-opioid, serotonergic and α_2-adrenergic agonist) are also available. Administration of some opioids by midwives is permitted in some countries, including the UK and Australia.

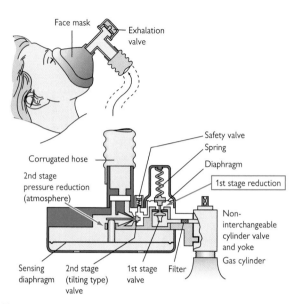

Figure 3.6 The Entonox nitrous oxide/oxygen analgesic apparatus (British oxygen). Reprinted with permission from Crawford JS, *Principles and Practice of Obstetric Anaesthesia 5th ed.* 1984, Wiley-Blackwell.

- κ-opioid agonists are particularly effective at polymodal visceral nociceptors sensitized by chemical or thermal stimuli, and females are more sensitive to their effect, so these drugs show some experimental promise.

Conventional Systemic Opioid Administration

Over the course of a labor, intramuscular [IM] or intravenous [IV] opioids (morphine or meperidine) are usually restricted to one or two injections.

- Opioids delay gastric emptying.
- Normeperidine, a metabolite of meperidine, is proconvulsant.
- Both meperidine and morphine cross the placenta rapidly due to their low molecular weights and lipid solubility. This may diminish fetal heart rate variability.

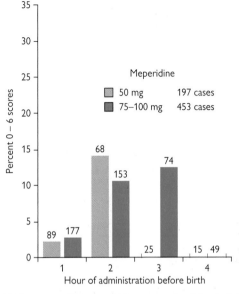

Figure 3.7 Percentage of low neonatal Apgar scores in relation to timing of intramuscular meperidine administration before delivery. This article was published in the American Journal of Obstetrics and Gynecology, Vol. 89, Shnider SM and Moya F, Effects of meperidine on the newborn infant, pg. 1011, Copyright Elsevier (1964).

- Although dose-related, even a single dose of opioid can cause neonatal respiratory depression (Figure 3.7); this is maximal 2–3 hours after IM administration.
- The long elimination half-lives in newborns (compared with adults) of both meperidine (13–23 hours) and its active metabolite, normeperidine (60 hours) depress newborn sucking behavior for up to 4 days.

Opioids generally result in poor pain relief, with only 25%–40% of women reporting benefit. Most women report no reduction, or only a small reduction, of pain scores, but benefit from euphoria and relaxation. Opioids also commonly cause confusion, reduced awareness and nausea, and are associated with low maternal satisfaction.

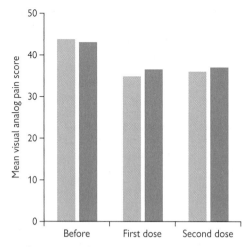

Figure 3.8 Pain intensity before and following intravenous morphine (dose 0.05 mg/kg body weight) or meperidine (dose 0.5 mg/kg body weight). Values are presented in box plot (median with interquartile range). No significant effect was found after each dose. ▨ morphine; ▨ meperidine (pethidine). Reprinted with permission from Olofsson C, et al. Lack of analgesic effect of systemically administered morphine or pethidine on labour pain. Br J Obstet Gyenaecol. 1996;103:969.

Non-opioid systemic analgesia with ketamine is employed in some countries because the drug is cheap and readily available.

- Intravenous or subcutaneous ketamine infusion (250 mcg/kg/h), after a bolus of 0.25 mg/kg, reduces labor pain scores.
- Small intravenous doses result in 3–5 minutes of analgesia in late labor or at delivery.
- Maternal amnesia and aspiration are recognized hazards.

Patient-Controlled Intravenous Analgesia (PCIA)

Contraction pain scores diminish very little after systemic opioids (Figure 3.8), with the exception of the potent μ-opioid receptor agonist remifentanil. Patient-controlled intravenous analgesia (PCIA) with fentanyl results in modest analgesia but total doses > 600 mcg are likely to cause neonatal depression and require reversal at birth with naloxone.

Although usually reserved for specific indications (such as a contrain-dication to requested epidural analgesia), the potent ultra-short acting opioid remifentanil is being used for PCIA in many countries, despite use during labor being "off-label."

Remifentanil—

- Reaches peak effect site concentration within 2–3 minutes of IV administration.
- Has a very short, 3-minute, context-sensitive half-life (i.e., the time for plasma concentration to fall by 50% from a steady-state level during drug infusion), independent of the duration of infusion, due to tissue and blood esterase metabolism.
- Shows very rapid placental transfer, but is rapidly metabolized by the fetus; neonates rarely appear affected after remifentanil in labor.

Remifentail often causes maternal drowsiness and hypoxemia, requir-ing oxygen therapy in approximately 15% of parturients. It can cause profound respiratory depression, muscle rigidity and severe hypox-emia after a rapid bolus or accidental injection of very small volumes of drug, so protocol-based monitoring and application of safety guide-lines are essential (Table 3.16).

Remifentanil PCIA is not as effective as epidural analgesia, but is a valid option when epidural techniques cannot be employed (Table 3.17 for a potential regimen).

- The optimum dosing regimen is unclear, but titration of bolus doses (0.1–0.5 mcg/kg) over 1 minute, or adjustment of infusion, is fre-quently required to optimize outcomes.
- Short lockout intervals (1–3 minutes) are used to allow frequent repeated dosing, despite peak effect site concentrations usually occurring after the contraction.
- Alternative regimens provide fixed bolus doses but a titrated con-tinuous infusion or an infusion alone. In one study, an infusion of 0.025–0.15 mcg/kg/min (mean infusion rate 0.075–0.1 mcg/kg/min) resulted in analgesia that was not as good as neuraxial analgesia for labor, but lower pain scores than those reported in most series of remifentanil PCIA. Mild sedation occurred in 4% but no respiratory depression or fetal heart rate effects were reported.

Alternative Techniques

When using "alternative techniques" for labor analgesia, several points should be considered.

- For some patients, use of a holistic approach to preparation for labor is important. Patient education is very helpful, and anesthesiologists as well as midwives can play an important role.
- Women accompanied by a duola (support person) or using relaxation, breathing exercises, psychological support and physical therapies such as water baths or counter-irritation by back rubbing, experience modest reductions in pain and are more likely to express that labor was a positive experience.
- Patient-controlled techniques, whether non-pharmacological, intravenous, inhaled or epidural, should be encouraged. Maternal satisfaction with the experience of childbirth is largely determined by perception

Table 3.16 Safety Guidelines when Using Remifentanil for Labor Analgesia

- Dosing regimen must be protocol-based
- Use dedicated equipment, clearly labeled
- Use a dedicated administration line and avoid dead space within tubing or intravenous cannula
- Provide continuous observation for sedation and respiratory depression
- Use continuous or regular, frequent intermittent pulse oximetry monitoring of arterial oxyhemoglobin saturation (SpO_2)
- Encourage the woman to breathe if SpO_2 < 95% but > 90% on air
- Give supplemental oxygen if SpO_2 remains < 95% on air & modify the patient-controlled analgesia variables
- Give naloxone 200 mcg IV and stop remifentanil administration if SpO_2 remains < 90%

Table 3.17 Potential Dosing Regimen for Remifentanil PCIA during Labor

- Choose a fixed concentration of remifentanil for the protocol (e.g., 20 mcg/ml)
- Administer remifentanil using a dedicated pump via a dedicated intravenous infusion line or limb with an anti-reflux valve and minimal dead space
- Demand bolus 0.4 mcg/kg (maximum dose 40 mcg)
  - titrate down to 0.1 mcg/kg if side effects excessive
- Continuous infusion (either routine or as an extra if maximum bolus doses prove inadequate)
  - 0.05 mcg/kg/min, titrated to maximum 0.15 mcg/kg/min
- Lockout interval 1 minute (1–3 min depending on pump used)

of personal control, rapport with support staff, and participation in decision making.

Non-pharmacologic alternatives include acupuncture and transcutaneous electrical nerve stimulation (TENS). These methods are rarely used in developed countries, and are not of proven efficacy.

A technique known as "water block" is sometimes employed, especially in Scandinavian countries.

- Sterile water 0.1 mL is injected intra- or subcutaneously at 4 points corresponding to the sacral borders.
- This is transiently painful but reduces back pain during labor for up to 60 minutes.

Further Reading

1. Bloom SL, McIntire DD, Kelly MA, et al. Lack of effect of walking on labor and delivery. N Engl J Med. 1998;339:76-79.

2. Bricker L, Lavender T. Parenteral opioids for labor pain relief: A systematic review. Am J Obstet Gynecol. 2002;186:S94-109.

3. Bucklin BA, Hawkins JL, Anderson JR, et al. Obstetric anesthesia workforce survey: twenty-year update. Anesthesiology. 2005;103:645-653.

4. D'Angelo R. New Techniques for labor analgesia: PCEA and CSE. Clin Obstet Gynecol. 2003;46:623-632.

5. D'Onofrio P, Novelli AM, Mecacci F, et al. The efficacy and safety of continuous intravenous administration of remifentanil for birth pain relief: An open study of 205 parturients. Anesth. Analg. 2009;109:1922-1924.

6. Halpern SH, Carvalho B. Patient-controlled epidural analgesia for labor. Anesth Analg. 2009;108:921-929.

7. Halpern SH, Leighton BL, Ohlsson A, et al. Effect of epidural vs parenteral opioid analgesia on the progress of labor: a meta-analysis. JAMA. 1998;280:2105-2110.

8. Hawkins JL. American Society of Anesthesiologists' practice guidelines for obstetric anesthesia: update 2006. Int J Obstet Anesth. 2007;16:103-105.

9. Hill D, Van de Velde M. Remifentanil patient-controlled analgesia should be routinely available for use in labour. Int J Obstet Anesth. 2008;17:336-342.

10. Palmer CM. Continuous spinal anesthesia and analgesia in obstetrics. Anesth Analg. 2010;111:1476-1479.

11. Rosen M. Nitrous oxide for relief of labor pain: A systematic review. Am J Obstet Gynecol. 2002;186:S110-126.

12. Rowlington JC. Lipid rescue: a step forward in patient safety? Likely so! Anesth Analg. 2008;106:1,333-336.

13. Wong CA, Scavone BM, Peaceman AM, *et al.* The risk of cesarean delivery with neuraxial analgesia given early versus late in labor. *N Engl J Med.* 2005;352:655-665.

14. Wong CA. Epidural and Spinal Analgesia/Anesthesia for Labor and Vaginal Delivery. Chapter 23: 429-92. In: Chestnut DH, Polley LS, Tsen LC, Wong CA, eds. *Chestnut's Obstetric Anesthesia Principles and Practice (4th Ed.)* Philadelphia, PA: Mosby Elsevier; 2009.

Chapter 4

Anesthesia for Cesarean Delivery

Michael J. Paech, FANZCA

What to Tell the Woman

Cesarean delivery is probably the most frequently performed surgical operation in developed countries today, and shows no sign of diminishing. For most women the procedure is not urgent and for many, if not most, it is also the first time they will have surgery. Given the concern many women have about anesthetic effects on the baby, and their anxiety about having a major operation while wide awake, these circumstances often result in women (and their spouses) having numerous questions about their impending anesthesia. Whenever possible, the anesthesiologist should take the time and effort necessary to explain the procedure thoroughly, and work with the patient to develop a mutually agreeable plan for the anesthetic.

Reasons for Recommending Regional Anesthesia

The 1982–1984 report of the Confidential Enquiries into Maternal Deaths in the United Kingdom recommended greater use of regional anesthesia, which is now used in the vast majority of elective and nonelective cesarean deliveries (80%–95%) in developed countries. Consequently the public has come to expect a regional anesthetic. There are three main reasons for this emphasis on regional techniques.

- Greater maternal safety compared with general anesthesia
  - Epidemiological data from the United States during the period 1997–2002 indicate case fatality rates for general anesthesia twice those of regional anesthesia, although rates for all types of anesthesia, especially general anesthesia, have fallen.
  - The maternal mortality data from the Confidential Enquiries into Maternal Deaths in the United Kingdom, and the Confidential Enquiries into Maternal and Child Health (CEMACH), also indicate far fewer deaths from regional anesthesia.
- Enhanced parental satisfaction (Table 4.1).
- Less neonatal depression at birth.

Obtaining Consent for Anesthesia

The key elements defining adequate consent (also see Chapter 13) are:
- explanation of the procedure
- explanation of risks, benefits and alternative options
- answering any questions the patient may have

Cesarean delivery represents an occasion of great significance to the parents, but sometimes generates considerable psychological stress. Elements unique to cesarean delivery include having major surgery while fully alert and potentially consenting to major surgery while in severe pain or under great stress, with little time to reflect on options. In urgent cases, consent is often given in a busy, noisy environment, when surrounded by a large number of unfamiliar staff, and while facing the possible loss of a child or serious personal risks.

General principles to note are:
- Spending time obtaining informed consent establishes rapport and may contribute to avoiding litigation should complications arise.
- Most women want to maximize the information they receive about anesthesia (and analgesia) and are not made more anxious by full disclosure of complications.

Table 4.1 Advantages and Disadvantages of Regional Anesthesia for Cesarean Delivery

Advantages

Maternal safety
- No airway management difficulties with consequent risks of aspiration of gastric content or hypoxic organ injury
- Less blood loss

Neonatal outcome
- Immediate resuscitation at birth less likely to be required than after general anesthesia

Desirable postoperative outcomes
- Less risk of nausea and vomiting
- Delayed recovery of consciousness and drowsiness avoided
- Early interaction with the newborn
- Early resumption of oral intake
- High quality analgesia achievable by several means

Consumer satisfaction
- Presence of mother and father/support person at birth enhances birth experience for parents
- Early skin-to-skin contact improves maternal-infant bonding
- Early attachment of infant to the breast

Disadvantages

Potential for hypotension, leading to maternal syncope, nausea or vomiting symptoms, and fetal compromise

Potential for post-dural puncture headache

Anesthesia cannot be established as quickly as general anesthesia

- The provision of information through pamphlets or other patient education resources in the antenatal period, at anesthetic or preadmission clinics, improves opportunities for frank discussion at the time of surgery.
- Providing an opportunity for the woman to ask questions is important.
- The details of the discussion should be documented (consent forms can be used as a checklist or aid).

Some of the difficulties facing the obstetric anesthesiologist in particular include:

- The anesthesiologist is often expected to provide effective and safe anesthesia within minutes of meeting the patient for the first time. However, in very few (only 20%) of unplanned cesarean deliveries was there *no* prior indication of the potential need for operative intervention.
- The amount of time for informed discussion may be significantly constrained. Nevertheless, even in emergent situations, it is

important to explain as much as possible about what is happening, while obtaining a brief history and performing a basic physical examination of vital signs and the airway.

- Always visit the woman postoperatively, to answer any questions or concerns which may remain.

Consent for Regional Anesthesia

When obtaining consent for a regional anesthetic, the anesthesiologist has a valuable opportunity to establish rapport, assuage anxieties, and order drug therapy, if necessary.

- The effects of regional anesthesia should be explained, and a treatment plan agreed upon (Table 4.2).
- The fear of pain during needle insertion or during surgery can be minimized by empathetic reassurance. In rare instances, the application of topical local anesthetic cream, if time allows, may be helpful.
  - Although rarely necessary, the use of light sedation (intravenous midazolam 1–2 mg, fentanyl 0.5–1 mcg/kg or remifentanil 0.1–0.25 mcg/kg) may be considered. These drugs are unlikely to affect neonatal outcomes, but should be timed to avoid maternal amnesic effects that detract from the birth experience.

Closed claims and similar studies indicate that litigation often results from maternal dissatisfaction with the management of pain during cesarean delivery, so it is critically important to explain common sensations. The patient should be aware that.

- Pressure and stretching are normal parts of the experience.
- Mild intraoperative pain is not uncommon (5%–20% depending on the situation).
- More severe pain will not be ignored.

If pain leads to a complaint, the anesthesiologist should be able to demonstrate that they had taken reasonable steps to warn about it, and about conversion to general anesthesia. In addition,

- The regional technique used must have been reasonable.
- The block should have been tested and noted to be adequate prior to surgery.
- Pain should have been treated when it was reported.
- The anesthesiologist should have provided follow-up and support.

Dealing with a Patient Refusing Regional Anesthesia

Many contraindications to regional anesthesia (Table 4.3) are relative. In most instances, regional anesthesia will remain the anesthetic of choice. Despite this, some women will initially refuse regional

Table 4.2 Discussion Points at Consent for Regional Anesthesia
Advantages compared with general anesthesia
Enjoyment of the birth experience (including the father)
Fewer life-threatening complications (high-block, local anesthetic toxicity)
Possibly lower mortality rate (extremely rare)
More alert neonate at birth
Procedural events
Positioning and needle insertion
Onset and testing of block
Intraoperative positioning
Postoperative analgesic options (pros and cons, side effects)
Post-block effects
Shaking
Nausea and vomiting
Syncope
Itch
Insertion site tenderness
Intraoperative events
Abdominal stretching and pressure
Pain (incidence/location/timing/severity/treatment plan including conversion to general anesthesia)
Infrequent complications
Post-dural puncture headache
Rare complications
Neuraxial infection
High block requiring intubation
Neurological injury
Extremely rare complications
Death

anesthesia due to fear of pain either during block placement or during the surgery, or because of cultural unfamiliarity. In this situation -

- Attempt to allay the patient's concerns with compassionate but realistic discussion, pointing out the advantages.
- Respect the patient's final decision. Some women may have had a distressing experience previously (for example, multiple failed attempts at insertion or severe pain during surgery) and will refuse any reasoned argument.

Regional Anesthesia for Nonelective Cesarean Delivery

Cesarean deliveries can be classified by their degree of urgency, and this classification can be useful in determining an appropriate anesthetic

Table 4.3 **Potential Contraindications to Regional Anesthesia**
Infection risk   • bacteremia and sepsis
Infection   • septic shock   • local skin infection at insertion site
Severe immunocompromise in the presence of other risk factors
Exacerbation of preexisting disease states   • raised intracranial pressure   • severe aortic stenosis   • severe pulmonary hypertension
Maternal hypovolemia with cardiovascular instability   • obstetric or non-obstetric major hemorrhage
Vertebral canal hematoma risk   • severe thrombocytopenia   • coagulopathy   • anticoagulation   • vertebral canal vascular pathology

(Table 4.3). For emergency or urgent cesarean delivery (Categories 1, 2 and 3), if a functioning epidural catheter is in place, it can be used to rapidly achieve a surgical anesthetic block (within 10–20 minutes), or spinal anesthesia can be established (within 10–20 minutes). General anesthesia is occasionally preferable, and may be mandated by failure of regional anesthesia or as the quickest means of anesthetizing the parturient (5–15 minutes) when there is life-threatening fetal compromise (Table 4.4).

In addition to the advantages of regional anesthesia noted above, a number of other factors have led to decreased use of general anesthesia. These include:

• liberalization of the limits traditionally applied to define when regional anesthesia is safe

• greater use of epidural analgesia during labor

• better interdisciplinary communication, leading to earlier maternal anesthetic assessment and preparation for operative delivery

• greater expertise in rapidly establishing safe regional anesthesia.

The American College of Obstetricians and Gynecologists (ACOG) suggests that when risk factors are identified, "the obstetrician obtain antepartum consultation from an anesthesiologist" and that strategies such as early intravenous access and placement of an epidural or spinal

Table 4.4 Categorization of Cesarean Delivery*

Category 1: Non-elective cesarean delivery because there is an immediate threat to the life of the mother or fetus

Category 2: Non-elective cesarean where delivery is indicated because of maternal or fetal compromise that is not immediately life-threatening

Category 3: Non-elective cesarean where early delivery is needed but there is no maternal or fetal compromise

Category 4: Elective cesarean delivery scheduled at a time to suit the mother and the medical team

* Adopted by many hospitals based on Lucas DN, et al. J Royal Soc Med. 2000;93:346–350.

catheter be developed "to minimize the need for emergency induction of general anesthesia in women in whom this would be especially hazardous".

Consent for General Anesthesia

When obtaining consent for general anesthesia for cesarean delivery, a number of topics need to be discussed (Table 4.6). Place emphasis on:

- Benefits and risks
- Common events and symptoms
- Preparation, and postoperative sequele

If the patient's request for general anesthesia appears inadvisable, document in detail how her decision was reached.

Table 4.5 When to Consider General, Rather than Regional, Anesthesia

Category 1 cesarean delivery (immediate threat to the life of the fetus or mother)

After two attempts to establish regional anesthesia have failed

Following eclampsia or other seizure or maternal collapse, when the mother is not fully alert, medically stable, or has focal neurological signs

When intraoperative pain under regional anesthesia is severe or uncontrolled by other means

Cardiac disease when reduction in systemic or pulmonary vascular resistance may lead to a critical event

Cardiac or respiratory disease when the patient cannot tolerate the supine or semi-supine position

Respiratory disease when postoperative ventilation will be required

An uncooperative patient

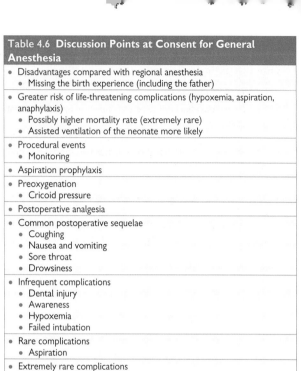

Table 4.6 Discussion Points at Consent for General Anesthesia
• Disadvantages compared with regional anesthesia   • Missing the birth experience (including the father)

• Greater risk of life-threatening complications (hypoxemia, aspiration, anaphylaxis)
  • Possibly higher mortality rate (extremely rare)
  • Assisted ventilation of the neonate more likely

• Procedural events   • Monitoring
• Aspiration prophylaxis
• Preoxygenation   • Cricoid pressure
• Postoperative analgesia

• Common postoperative sequelae
  • Coughing
  • Nausea and vomiting
  • Sore throat
  • Drowsiness

• Infrequent complications
  • Dental injury
  • Awareness
  • Hypoxemia
  • Failed intubation

• Rare complications   • Aspiration

• Extremely rare complications
  • Neurological injury
  • Death

Explaining the Effects of Anesthesia on the Baby

Factors Affecting Neonatal Outcome

Much of the evidence about neonatal outcome and its relation to the method of anesthesia is of poor quality and pertains only to elective delivery of healthy women and fetuses. At emergency cesarean delivery, neonatal acid base balance can be improved irrespective of the method of anesthesia.

Meta-analysis comparing regional and general anesthesia suggests that neonatal umbilical cord blood pH and base deficit is:

- worse with spinal anesthesia compared with general anesthesia (although the magnitude of difference is small)
- affected by the severity and duration of maternal hypotension and the duration of the uterine incision to delivery interval

- possibly made worse by the arterial occlusion associated with inadequate pelvic tilt (indicating the lateral position may be preferable when establishing regional anesthesia).

Effects of Regional Anesthesia

- Fetal and neonatal effects of local anesthetic or opioid are usually undetectable.
- Only a Venturi type face mask delivering at least 60% inspired oxygen will improve fetal oxygenation, but this should be considered if the fetus is thought to be hypoxemic.
- The biochemical and metabolic condition of the healthy fetus is unaffected by regional anesthesia, provided ephedrine and sustained or profound hypotension are avoided (Table 4.7).
- Control of hypotension with ephedrine results in lower umbilical artery pH and higher base deficit than control with phenylephrine or metaraminol.

Table 4.7 Anesthesia and Neonatal Acid-Base Status at Elective Cesarean Delivery 1kPa = 7.5mmHg

	General (n = 30)	Epidural (n = 30)	Spinal (n = 30)
Maternal			
pH	7.36 (0.04)[a]	7.44 (0.06)	7.42 (0.03)
pO$_2$ (kPa)	30.80 (1.37)	31.73 (1.56)	32.10 (1.50)
Base deficit (mmol/l)	5.10 (1.82)	2.43 (2.13)	3.21 (1.79)
Umbilical vein			
pH	7.33 (0.05)	7.34 (0.04)	7.34 (0.05)
PO$_2$	5.80 (0.33)	5.67 (0.36)	5.92 (0.51)
Base deficit	4.00 (2.10)	4.80 (1.81)	4.78 (2.23)
Umbilical artery			
pH	7.28 (0.04)	7.29 (0.07)	7.28 (0.02)
PO$_2$	2.90 (0.19)	2.91 (0.23)	2.87 (0.23)
Base deficit	4.31 (1.79)	4.58 (1.99)	4.53 (2.01)

Values are mean (SD). [a]$P < 0.01$ compared with other groups. Reprinted from the *International Journal of Obstetric Anesthesia*, Vol. 2. Mahajan J, *et al*. Anaesthetic technique for elective caesarean section and neurobehavioural status of newborns, 89–93, Copyright (1996), with permission from Elsevier.

- Uncorrected hypotension may cause subtle neurobehavioral changes in infant responsiveness and sucking.

Effects of General Anesthesia

- Fetal drug exposure is limited by factors regulating placental transfer.
- Fetal oxygenation is improved by giving the woman 100% inspired oxygen, but no improvement in neonatal clinical outcome has been shown.
- The sedative effects of the inhalational anesthetics and the respiratory depressant effects of opioid may be evident at birth, especially after a prolonged induction to delivery interval (> 15 minutes).
  - A person experienced in neonatal resuscitation should be available, because active resuscitation is more likely to be necessary (although usually confined to assistance in establishing first breaths).
  - In cesarean delivery for fetal compromise, lower Apgar scores and neonatal intubation may be more likely than after regional anesthesia (Figure 4.1).

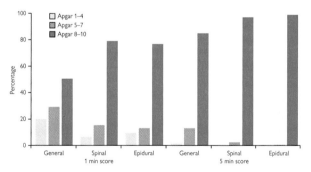

Figure 4.1 Influence of anesthetic technique on neonatal condition after urgent cesarean section for fetal distress. Data derived from Marx, G.F., *et al.* (1984) Fetal-neonatal status following cesarean section for fetal distress. *Br J Anaesth.* 56:1011. Reprinted with permission from Reisner LS and Lin D, Anesthesia for cesarean section. In: Chestnut DH, *Obstetric Anesthesia 2nd ed.* 1999, Elsevier.

Patient Preparation

Preoperative Assessment

Ideally, a thorough pre-anesthesia assessment should be completed, including:

- Patient characteristics (age, weight, fasting status).
- Past medical and surgical history.
- Systems review, medications and allergies.
- Physical examination focusing on the cardiovascular and respiratory systems, and the relevant airway investigations and imaging.
- Additional elements related to pregnancy and cesarean delivery. (Table 4.8)

Fasting

The American Society of Anesthesiologist's (ASA) practice guidelines recommend a fasting interval of at least 6 hours for solids prior to elective cesarean delivery.

- In laboring women, oral intake should be limited to clear fluids alone, due to difficulty predicting which women are at risk of surgical delivery.
- In many cases, the urgency of delivery will take precedence over fasting status. In parturients who have not been "nil per oris" (NPO),

Table 4.8 Pre-Anesthesia Assessment Related to Pregnancy and Cesarean Delivery
Past obstetric history

Current obstetric history
  Indication for cesarean delivery
  Gestational age
  Pregnancy-related diseases and disorders and their management
  Presence of ruptured membranes or labor
  Fetal status during pregnancy and current fetal status

Relevant surface landmarks, especially vertebral column

Relevant investigations and laboratory tests
  Hemoglobin concentration / hematocrit
  Platelet count
  Blood group and hold or blood crossmatch

Relevant imaging
  Placental location
  Spinal anatomy

regional anesthesia is preferable in terms of avoiding the risk of aspiration.

Preoperative Optimization

Preoperative optimization is an important goal, irrespective of the urgency of delivery. Recent data from the CEMACH database noted the failure of staff to recognize the severity of maternal illness. Undiagnosed or inadequately treated sepsis and cardiac failure are examples of conditions in which induction of anesthesia may precipitate a fatal event.

The timing of delivery in critically ill pregnant women requires careful consideration, preferably decided by a multidisciplinary team including obstetricians, obstetric physicians, neonatologists and anesthesiologists. Even if delivery appears mandated by an immediate threat to the life of the fetus, intrauterine resuscitation (see Chapter 15) may improve the fetal condition significantly and gain preparation time. The life of the mother must always take priority over that of the fetus.

Airway Assessment

Difficult intubation (incidence 1 in 30–60) or failed intubation (incidence 1 in 250–1500) leading to hypoxemia, aspiration, and cardiac arrest, represents the most common fatal complication of obstetric anesthesia in developed countries (fatal complications of regional block are very rare except in developing countries).

Although difficulties may arise unexpectedly, in many cases good airway assessment will be predictive and critical to management planning. A high false positive rate (low specificity) is not an issue, and a difficult airway cart should be available in all units, preferably housed beside the operating table when general anesthesia is induced.

Airway assessment should be routine and performed at patient admission or as early as possible in labor. Ideally there are hospital-based systems of referral to the anesthesiology department of women of known or suspected high risk of airway difficulty.

Risk Factors for a Difficult Airway

Risk factors must be sought and a comprehensive evaluation performed (Table 4.9 and Figure 4.2). Review of documentation of previous airway management is valuable, but unless reasonably contemporaneous it may not reflect the patient's current condition.

Table 4.9 Indicators of Potential Difficulty with the Airway

History
- Previous anesthesia and airway management details (known difficulty)
- Breath sounds (stridor associated with airway infection or severe preeclampsia)

Examination and Tests
- Morbid obesity (associated with difficult ventilation and intubation)
- Limited cervical spine or atlanto-occipital joint extension (including due to large hair knots or buns)
- Short neck (thyromental distance < 6 cm)
- Reduced laryngoscope access (e.g., anterior neck mass or large breasts)
- Small oral cavity or large tongue (Grade 3 or 4 Mallampati view)
- Temporomandibular joint dysfunction or reduced mouth opening (inter-incisor distance < 3 cm)
- Prominent upper incisors (inability to protrude lower teeth past upper teeth or to bite upper lip)
- Receding mandible
- Height to thyromental distance ratio > 21
- Poor dentition (missing, loose, or prosthetic teeth)
- Oral pathology

Most individual tests show poor specificity and positive predictive value. Combinations (e.g., Mallampati test and upper-lip bite test) are more accurate, and multiple factors multiply the relative risk of difficult airway management.

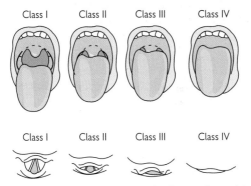

Class I   Class II   Class III   Class IV

Class I   Class II   Class III   Class IV

Figure 4.2 Airway assessment. Upper panel: classification of view of the pharyngeal structures during airway assessment. Lower panel: Classification of direct laryngoscopic view. Upper panel modified from Mallampati SR, *et al.* A clinical sign to predict difficult intubation: a prospective study. Can Anaesth Soc J. 1985; 32: 429-434. Lower panel modified from Comarck RS and Lehane J. Difficult intubation in obstetrics. Anaesthesia 1994; 39: 1105-1111. Reprinted with permission from Samsoon GLT and Yount JRB. Difficult tracheal intubation: a retrospective study. Anaesthesia 1987; 42: 488.

Airway management plans are best based on established algorithms, such as those endorsed by the ASA, with appropriate modifications for the obstetric population. Such plans include:

- Avoiding nasal instrumentation if possible because of the risk of epistaxis (due to increased vascularity and edema of the nasal mucosa).
- Early placement of an epidural catheter during labor in women at increased risk of difficult airway management (e.g., morbidly obese, known or suspected difficult intubation). This allows for rapid induction of surgical anesthesia if necessary.
- Repeat airway assessment in laboring women to exclude changes within the airway (e.g., mucosal or tongue swelling or laryngeal edema due to deteriorating preeclampsia).
- Use of awake fiberoptic intubation when general anesthesia appears necessary in a woman at high risk of difficult airway management.

If difficulty is anticipated the anesthesiologist should be familiar with and have prepared a range of equipment for intubation, aids to intubation, and both supraglottic and transtracheal airway devices. The patient should be warned about possible dental and soft tissue injury. Experienced assistants are essential.

Minimization of Aortocaval Compression

Physiology

Once the gravid uterus rises from within the pelvis (at approximately 20 weeks gestation) it may obstruct the inferior vena cava and/or the aorta (usually just below the bifurcation of the iliac arteries) when the woman lies supine.

- At term, imaging shows that 90% of women lying supine have partial or complete inferior vena caval obstruction (with diversion of venous flow via the azygous system) and 10%–15% become symptomatic (syncope, nausea) due to reduced cerebral perfusion.
- Aortic obstruction and impaired placental flow may be silent but cause fetal hypoxemia and acidosis.
- These effects are exaggerated by anesthesia, due to venous pooling, reduction in blood pressure, impaired compensatory vasoconstriction, and reduced cardiac output.

In combination with other events, the hemodynamic disturbance of aortocaval compression has contributed to case fatalities.

Prevention

Although impossible to prevent entirely during the period of surgery (even more so in women with polyhydramnios or multiple pregnancy), steps should be taken to minimize aortocaval compression.

- Place the woman in the left lateral position (preferable to right lateral, tilted, semi-erect or sitting) whenever possible, including during transfer to the operating room or prior to surgery.
- Maximize left pelvic tilt if the full left lateral position is not feasible (e.g., during establishment of anesthesia and during surgery).
- If initial steps are unsuccessful in increasing uterine displacement (preferably to the left), increase tilt, or use manual uterine displacement.

In practice, purpose-designed pelvic or lumbar wedges or inflatable devices can be used, or the operating table can be inclined laterally. The degree of tilt will be limited by surgical considerations and patient safety, but up to and at least 15-degree tilt is recommended (although aortic compression may persist at up to 30-degree tilt).

Prophylaxis against Pulmonary Aspiration of Gastric Content

Aspiration Risk

Hall in 1940, and Mendelson in 1946, drew attention to the potentially fatal complication of aspiration in pregnant women.

- Aspiration appears to be more common in pregnancy as a result of the physiological changes (see Chapter 2) that predispose to regurgitation. These changes occur in early pregnancy and increase in incidence until term gestation.
- Regurgitation occurs in 1 in 100–200 general anesthetics for cesarean delivery.
- Aspiration pneumonitis is rare (estimated 1 in 1,000 general anesthetics in pregnancy) but occurs twice as frequently in nonelective cesarean delivery.
  - Aspiration is more frequently encountered outside the immediate perioperative period (e.g., in sedated or unconscious women in the intensive care unit, or in women who have collapsed or had a seizure).
- Improvements in critical care have led to a reduction in mortality rate (estimated as < 5%).

Aspiration Prophylaxis

The current low incidence of aspiration in obstetrics has been attributed to several factors. These include:

- the predominant use of regional anesthesia for operative delivery
- the teaching that rapid sequence induction should always be part of general anesthesia
- pharmacological prophylaxis against aspiration.

The role of drug prophylaxis is controversial; it has not been proven to improve clinical outcome, but the physiological benefits of reducing and alkalinizing gastric secretions (to achieve small volumes < 30 ml of pH > 3.5) appear of high benefit versus risk. Options are:

- Nonparticulate antacids (e.g., 0.3 molar sodium citrate 30 ml). These cause mild nausea in some women, but have a long history of safe use.
- H_2-receptor antagonists (e.g., ranitidine 150–300 mg PO or 50 mg IV). These have a benign side effect profile and are as effective as more expensive proton-pump inhibitors.
- Metoclopramide (20 mg IV). Metoclopromide is prokinetic but has limited efficacy. It increases lower esophageal sphincter tone and is antiemetic.

Eating during labor has no benefits. The pain of labor and its treatment with opioids results in profound delay in gastric emptying, with solids retained for many additional hours. Most anesthesiologists argue that women in labor should confine oral intake to energy-containing clear fluids; but, given lack of evidence of harm, some units take a more pragmatic approach of allowing women to eat if they wish. An example policy for aspiration prophylaxis is shown in Table 4.10.

Assessment of Regional Block

Early and regular assessment and documentation of the regional anesthetic sensory and motor block (Table 4.11) serves several purposes.

- It provides confirmation of a successful block that is likely to be associated with a low risk of intraoperative pain.
- It reassures the patient that the anesthetic will be effective.
- It serves as a safety check for impending high block.
- It provides protection against a charge of negligence if sued because of intraoperative pain.

Table 4.10 **Suggested Aspiration Prophylaxis Regimen for Cesarean Delivery**
Avoid intake of solids by women in labor at increased risk of operative delivery
Give an H2-receptor antagonist • Oral ranitidine 300 mg 1–2 h prior to elective surgery • Oral ranitidine 150 mg 6 hourly regularly to women in labor who are at high risk
Give oral 0.3 molar sodium citrate 30 ml within 45 minutes of surgery to all women having non-elective surgery *or* Give IV ranitidine 50 mg (or similar) at the time of decision to deliver a woman in labor by cesarean delivery and add oral sodium citrate as above if general anesthesia planned
Consider passing an orogastric tube to aspirate the stomach during general anesthesia at non-elective cesarean delivery

Block Management

An effective sensory block is required if a patient is to remain awake and comfortable during cesarean delivery.

- The block should reduce nociceptive input from not only the wound (T_{12}–L_1 for Pfannenstiel and T_{10}–T_{12} for lower abdominal

Table 4.11 **Assessment of Regional Block**
Initially confirm immediate paresthesia sensations or warmth in buttocks and feet
Check for loss of cold or touch on outer border of the foot (S_1)
Test in a cephalad direction using loss of temperature to cold and/or light touch or pin-prick
Prior to surgery confirm: • satisfactory bilateral cephalad sensory block (e.g., loss of cold to T3–T4 and/or loss of light touch to T5–T6) • presence of motor block in the legs
Consider having the obstetrician test loss of pain at the level of incision (e.g., T_{12})
If the woman complains of tingling in the arms or dyspnea: • test sensation in the upper limbs • test grip strength • reassure, monitor respiration and maternal symptoms, observe for further progression of block • intervene if clinically indicated (hypoxemia, respiratory distress, impaired conscious state, severe hypotension)

midline incision) but also relevant visceral structures and the peritoneal cavity, which is supplied by splanchnic nerves from an upper to mid thoracic spinal level.

- Symmetric and complete bilateral loss of light touch from the fifth to sixth thoracic (T_5–T_6) to the fifth sacral (S_5) dermatome or loss of temperature sensation from T_3–T_4 to S_5 is usually adequate. (Figure 4.3)
- Partial block above these levels is common.
- The inter-patient variability in assessment of light touch appears greater and some anesthesiologists use loss of pin-prick because some patients find light touch discrimination difficult.
- A two-dermatome differential between complete loss of temperature and light touch is typical.
- If neuraxial opioid is included, pain-free conditions may be present with slightly lower cephalad distributions of block.

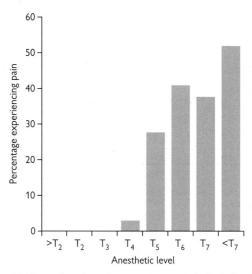

Figure 4.3 The number of parturients attaining a particular level of analgesia or anesthesia after spinal or epidural anesthesia, and the number of women subsequently experiencing pain within that subgroup. Reprinted from the *International Journal of Obstetric Anesthesia, Vol. 4*, Russell IF, Levels of Anaesthesia and intraoperative pain at caesarean section under regional block, p. 74, Copyright (1995), with permission from Elsevier.

- Sensory changes may reach upper thoracic and occasionally lower cervical nerve root dermatomes, but rarely cause clinical concern.

The woman may need reassurance, given that motor block is usually of slower onset, may be incomplete (especially with epidural anesthesia), and is of more caudad distribution. These factors help protect against significant impairment of ventilation (the function of the diaphragm and the lower intercostal muscles is adequately preserved). Because vital capacity and peak expiratory flow are reduced, some women experience mild dyspnea or note a less powerful cough.

- Check for normal grip strength, which indicates a functioning median nerve (C_5–C_8, T_1) and thus also intact phrenic innervation (C_3–C_5) and a functioning diaphragm.
- Reassure the patient that ventilation at rest is likely to remain satisfactory and oxygenation adequate, and give supplemental oxygen if required.

Monitoring

Respiratory Monitoring (Ventilation and Oxygenation)
Under regional anesthesia, clinical observation of respiratory rate and depth and pulse oximetry for oxyhemoglobin saturation are sufficient in routine circumstances.

Under general anesthesia, a number of routine monitoring techniques are mandatory and informative.

- **End-tidal oxygen.** Prior to induction, end-tidal (ET)-oxygen should be elevated to 90% or more, if possible, by "preoxygenation" with 100% oxygen. This confirms satisfactory denitrogenation of the lung and maximizes the period before hypoxemia commences once apnea is induced.
- **Capnography.** A normal trace after intubation confirms tracheal intubation.
  - Target an ET-carbon dioxide of 30–32 mmHg. In patients in whom the arterial-alveolar difference may be increased (e.g., morbid obesity, heavy smoking, other lung disease) consider assessing ventilation with arterial blood gas analysis.
  - Inspiratory dips indicate spontaneous ventilatory efforts and may influence use of neuromuscular blocking drugs.
  - Falling or low end-tidal carbon dioxide may indicate an inadequate cardiac output.

- **Pulse oximetry.** Oxygen saturation > 95% confirms adequate oxygenation.
- **Spirometry and/or arterial blood gas analysis** is useful in the presence of significant respiratory disease.
- **Airway pressure** should be kept below 40 cm water (due to the risk of barotrauma, although this may be difficult in the morbidly obese patient).

Cardiovascular Monitoring

Blood pressure (BP) monitoring should commence before anesthesia and be continued frequently during the case. Immediately post-spinal and after general anesthesia induction, it should be measured each minute until stable.

- BP should be measured at least every five minutes throughout surgery and after the fetus is delivered.
- Continuous BP measurement via an arterial cannula may be necessary in patients at high risk (e.g., severe preeclampsia, intrapartum hemorrhage, major cardiac and respiratory disease) or when noninvasive monitoring is unreliable (e.g., morbid obesity).

Automated devices (noninvasive oscillotonometry) are usually employed, but have limitations such as:

- Failure to read due to movement or shaking
- Under-reading of diastolic pressure in particular, and reduced accuracy in the presence of hypertensive disease or severe hypotension.

Electrocardiography (ECG)

An ECG should be used routinely during general anesthesia. Changes are common (25%–60%), although rarely clinically significant.

- If chest pain is experienced, ST-segment changes (> 1–2 mmHg) should be sought and a postoperative troponin assay considered.

Other Parameters

In specific situations, other monitoring may be valuable.

- **Central venous pressure** or pulmonary wedge pressure measurement is usually reserved for selected critically ill patients, especially those having inotrope infusions.
- **Pulse pressure and stroke volume variation** measurement (e.g., Doppler esophageal cardiac output monitors) may be more reliable guides to adequate fluid administration or fluid responsiveness.

- **Transthoracic or transesophageal echocardiography** may guide therapy in critically ill patients in relation to ventricular filling, systolic and diastolic cardiac function, pulmonary artery pressure, and response to fluid challenges.
- **Cardiac output monitoring** (including noninvasive methods such as arterial pulse waveform analysis or transesophageal Doppler measurement of stroke volume) is usually reserved for patients with specific indications. Cardiac output changes are as relevant as blood pressure changes, but currently most monitoring systems are not sufficiently reliable to follow acute physiological changes such as those occurring at the time of cesarean delivery.

Brain Monitoring

Depth of anesthesia (hypnosis) monitors are potentially useful during general anesthesia for cesarean delivery. For example, the bispectral index (BIS) monitor has been validated in a large randomized trial as a means of reducing the risk of awareness in high-risk groups such as pregnant women.

- BIS monitoring displays an index from 0 to 100, with 60 or less associated with a very low risk of recall and 40–55 a target for adequate depth of anesthesia.
- BIS is quick and easy to apply immediately prior to induction of anesthesia.
- In combination with ET-anesthetic drug monitoring, BIS monitoring can guide depth of anesthesia assessment and help avoid overdosing that leads to myometrial relaxation and neonatal drowsiness.

Fetal Monitoring

Cardiotocographic fetal heart rate monitoring is difficult to interpret in severe prematurity infants (< 26–28 weeks), but thereafter, the fetal heart rate should be checked:

- While regional block is developing
- Near the time of induction of general anesthesia
- Regularly or continuously in the presence of fetal compromise.

Some nonreassuring patterns (e.g., severe fetal bradycardia, Chapter 12) require urgent attention, including intrauterine resuscitation (Chapter 14) and expeditious delivery (which may involve a change in anesthetic plan).

Spinal Anesthesia

Advantages and Disadvantages (Table 4.12)

In most developed countries, spinal anesthesia is the most commonly used anesthetic technique for both elective (scheduled) and nonelective cesarean section if an epidural catheter has not been placed.

- Dose requirements in pregnant patients fall by approximately 30% from early in pregnancy, suggesting a hormone-induced change in neural sensitivity. A reduction in the size of the lumbar intrathecal sac, and a higher cephalad location of the lowest point of the thoracic spine when supine, also contribute in later pregnancy.
- Maternal satisfaction with spinal anesthesia is high, providing hypotension is well managed and post-dural puncture headache (PDPH) is minimized by use of non-cutting bevel needles (see Chapter 13).

Table 4.12 Advantages and Disadvantages of Spinal Anesthesia

Advantages

Establishes *de novo* regional anesthesia more rapidly than epidural anesthesia

Rapid onset of dense sensory and motor block
- reassuring for the patient
- valuable for Category 1 and 2 non-elective cesarean deliveries
- good surgical conditions

Low failure rate (0.5%–4%)

Low incidence of paresthesia during insertion (~ 10%)

Low incidence of intraoperative pain (~ 5%)

Low incidence of post-dural puncture headache with 26–27 gauge pencil point or similar needles (~ 0.5%–1%)

No risk of local anesthetic toxicity

Effective postoperative analgesia achievable with "single-shot" injection including intrathecal morphine

Disadvantages

Reduction in cardiac output greater than with epidural anesthesia and higher incidence of hypotension (~ 60%–80%, especially first 4–8 minutes)

Single-shot technique requires choice of a fixed dose of subarachnoid local anesthetic, with little ability to influence low or high block

Finite duration of surgical anesthesia (~ 90–150 minutes)
- making a single-shot approach unsuitable for complex or difficult cases when surgical time is likely to be prolonged

Incidence of high block requiring intubation approximately 1 in 2,000–5,000

The rapid onset of block, within 5–15 minutes, makes spinal anesthesia feasible for all but the most emergent of cesarean deliveries. However, sensory block regression begins after 60–180 minutes (with subarachnoid bupivacaine, dependent on dose) or 45–90 minutes (with subarachnoid ropivacaine), so if surgery is delayed or unduly prolonged, block failure may occur.

Techniques and Equipment

Patient Positioning

The block may be placed with the woman positioned in either the lateral decubitus or sitting position. The sitting position:

- Makes insertion easier in obese women, because it helps visualization of the midline and increases the rate of efflux of cerebrospinal fluid (CSF) from a small gauge spinal needle.
- Improves ventilation
- Should be avoided if the umbilical cord is presenting, if the woman is hypovolemic or has syncope.

In the lateral patient position, the onset of sensory block to T_{10} (but not to T_3–T_5) is more rapid and there may be a slightly lower incidence of hypotension.

After the subarachnoid injection of drugs, apply a left lateral or left pelvic tilt position while surgical anesthesia establishes.

- Once the woman is lying down, accentuate her upper thoracic curve (e.g., by placing pillows under the shoulders, neck and head, or elevating the bed head) to restrict cephalad spread of local anesthetic to mid-thoracic dermatomes, especially if spinal anesthesia was used to rescue failed epidural anesthesia.
- In the lateral decubitus position, the vertebral canal is not horizontal but slopes slightly head down.
- Tipping the bed head-down should be done cautiously and the sensory block monitored frequently when attempting to improve cephalad spread of local anesthetic.

Safe Insertion Technique

In most patients the spinal cord terminates at the L_1 level (range T_{12} to L_3). To minimize the risk of spinal cord injury, select a low lumbar vertebral interspace. L_3–L_4 is frequently used, being the largest and most superficial interspace.

- Use surface landmarks to help identify the interspace. The imaginary supracristal line across the top of the iliac crests ("Tuffier's line") crosses the L_4 spinous process in most patients, but shows variability and is difficult to visualize in obese patients.

- Anesthesiologists only correctly identify the vertebral interspace in 25%–35% of cases.
- A higher level than appreciated is often mistakenly selected for needle placement.
- The use of ultrasound imaging improves the accuracy of identifying vertebral interspaces, and assists in visualizing spinal canal anatomy.

A suggested approach to needle insertion is shown in Table 4.13. If experiencing difficulty, try to identify the epidural space first using loss-of-resistance, then insert the spinal needle.

Spinal Needles

Every attempt should be made to use only a non-cutting-edge spinal needle (e.g., 24–27 gauge pencil-point Whitacre or Sprotte style spinal needle, Figure 4.4) to reduce the rate of PDPH (see Chapter 13). In general, these small gauge needles are easy to use in the pregnant

Table 4.13 Suggested Approach to Spinal Needle Insertion
Infiltrate intradermal, subcutaneous ± ligamentous tissue with local anesthetic; e.g., 0.5%–1% lidocaine with epinephrine 1:200,000–400,000
Insert an introducer needle 1–2 cm into the interspinous ligament (to prevent lateral deflection of a fine gauge spinal needle away from the midline)
Use a pencil-point spinal needle • Whitacre style 26–27 gauge • Sprotte style 24–26 gauge
Feel for "dural pop" as needle penetrates the dura-arachnoid after tenting • Incidence approximately 70–80% with 26–27 gauge spinal needles
If paresthesia occurs (approximately 10% of cases) this should be very transient. • If the paresthesia is not transient, contact with neural tissue is implied and the needle should be withdrawn. Drug or solution must not be injected because of the risk of intraneural injection and disruption, leading to injury.
Withdraw the stylet, confirm free efflux of cerebrospinal fluid (CSF) and attach drug syringe carefully with slight twisting motion (to avoid loss of drug at connection when injecting) but without moving the needle tip
Aspirate CSF easily, then inject spinal drugs
If using a Quincke cutting edge spinal needle, replace the stylet prior to withdrawal (weak evidence for reduced post-dural puncture headache rate)

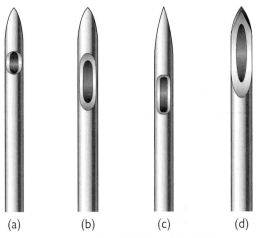

(a)   (b)   (c)   (d)

Figure 4.4 Spinal needle tip design for (a) Gertie Marx, (b) Sprotte, (c) Whitacre, (d) Atraucan needle. These needles result in a lower incidence of post-dural puncture headache than sharp-bevel (Quincke) needles of equivalent size. Modified from Holdcroft A and Thomas TA. Regional Anaesthetic techniques. In: Principles and Practice of Obstetric Anaesthesia and Analgesia, p. 248. 2000 Wiley-Blackwell.

population, provide tactile indication of entry into the subarachnoid space in most patients (the "dural pop"), and have an acceptable rate of PDPH (1 in 100–200).

Oxygen Therapy

During regional anesthesia, the administration of oxygen in a concentration above 21% via an air-entraining face mask is not justified routinely in healthy women having elective cesarean delivery; because 35%–40% inspired oxygen does not increase fetal oxygenation of a healthy fetus.

- For nonelective cesarean due to fetal compromise consider providing 60%–100% inspired oxygen to modestly increase fetal umbilical venous oxygen content. In the preterm or nonlaboring parturient this concentration of oxygen should probably be limited to less than 10 minutes because of an associated increase in lipid peroxidation and oxygen free radicals that are injurious to lipid cell membranes.
- An inspired concentration of 100% can be achieved, if needed, using an anesthetic circuit and tight-fitting face mask.

Subarachnoid Drug Selection

In choosing drugs and drug doses for spinal anesthesia, aims are:

- A mid to upper thoracic sensory block, but a low incidence of clinically relevant "high block."
- Minimization of the incidence of intraoperative pain.
- A low incidence of hypotension, nausea and vomiting, and shivering.
- An adequate block duration to meet the anticipated duration of surgery.
- Motor block of the shortest possible postoperative duration.
- Postoperative analgesia.

Drug Distribution

An adequate sensory block distribution can be achieved with a wide range of doses of local anesthetic, but the incidence of intraoperative pain, the degree of motor block, and duration of effective surgical anesthesia are all partly dose-related (Figure 4.5). Individual variability in spread of local anesthetic is also significant, such that altering the dose administered based on patient factors such as weight, height or vertebral column length or on administration factors such as the lumbar interspace or direction of needle bevel is not recommended except in exceptional cases (e.g., achondoplastic dwarfism).

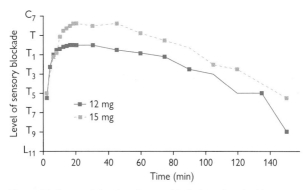

Figure 4.5 Onset and duration of sensory block after subarachnoid hyperbaric bupivacaine, 12 mg or 15 mg, showing more spinal segments blocked for a significantly longer time with the higher dose. Reprinted with permission from De Simone, C., et al. Spinal anesthesia for cesarean delivery: A comparison of two doses of hyperbaric bupivacaine. *Reg. Anesth.* 1995;20(2):91.

Choice of Drug

Local Anesthetics

Suitable intrathecal local anesthetics are:

- Hyperbaric bupivacaine (in dextrose 8%–8.25%)
  - This is readily available and widely used.
  - Inject at least 10 mg if used alone (range 10–15 mg).
  - Inject at least 8 mg (range 8–12.5 mg) if opioid is added.
  - Hyperbaric solutions are favored over plain 0.5% bupivacaine (slightly hypobaric in CSF) because they result in shorter duration of motor block, spread more consistently in patients who are sitting and cause fewer high blocks (both formulations in combination have also been used safely).

- Tetracaine or Lidocaine
  - These are less satisfactory, have other problems and are not recommended.

- Ropivacaine
  - Has few advantages over bupivacaine.
  - Requires larger doses (15–25 mg, depending on whether combined with opioid).
  - Has shorter duration than bupivacaine (regression begins after approximately 45–60 minutes, which may prove to be a problem).
  - Produces less intense motor block (movement intraoperatively can be a problem, although normal function returns more rapidly).

Higher doses of local anesthetic give a better quality and longer duration of block, with a lower incidence of intraoperative pain but also make hypotension or high block more likely.

Adjuncts

A number of analgesic adjuncts are safe to add, the most valuable being opioids. Opioids:

- Lower the effective dose of local anesthetic.
- Reduce intraoperative pain (number-needed-to-treat [NNT] of 4).
- Reduce intraoperative nausea.

  Examples are:

- Fentanyl (6.25–15 mcg)
- Sufentanil (2.5–5 mcg)
- Diamorphine (300–400 mcg)
- Morphine (50–150 mcg)

Intrathecal morphine analgesia is of slow onset (30–60 minutes), which limits its effectiveness during surgery. Like diamorphine (which is metabolized in neural tissue to morphine and 6-mono acetylmorphine) or hydromorphone, morphine produces clinically useful postoperative analgesia (duration 4–24 hours, median 12 hours, so supplementary analgesia must usually be provided). The risk of clinically relevant opioid-induced respiratory depression is very low (1 in 250–500 for mild depression), being greatest and most delayed in timing (6–18 hours) after morphine, but its safety record with respect to serious morbidity is excellent (see also Chapter 5).

Other Adjuvants

- Epinephrine (adrenaline) 200 mcg does not enhance the efficacy of local anesthetic with opioid.
- Clonidine 60–150 mcg prolongs the duration of block and has a moderate postoperative analgesic effect (up to 6 hours), but causes intra- and postoperative sedation.
- Ketamine, midazolam and magnesium enhance local anesthetic efficacy but are experimental and should not be used routinely.

An example of an effective and safe regimen for "single-shot" spinal anesthesia for cesarean delivery is:

- Hyperbaric bupivacaine 12.5 mg
- Fentanyl 15 mcg
- Morphine 100 mcg

Epidural Anesthesia

Advantages and Disadvantages

A comparison of epidural and spinal anesthesia is shown in Table 4.14. Even in resource-rich countries where the equipment is readily available, epidural anesthesia is now rarely used for elective (scheduled) cesarean delivery. Spinal anesthesia has advantages and combined spinal-epidural anesthesia is preferable when prolonged anesthesia and/or postoperative analgesia are desired (for example a multiple repeat cesarean or when cesarean hysterectomy is planned).

Epidural anesthesia should be considered when:

- A slowly titrated technique (over 45–90 minutes) is appropriate to prevent hemodynamic changes associated with sympathetic block (e.g., certain stenotic valvular diseases, cardiac failure, pulmonary hypertension; see also Chapter 10).

Table 4.14 Epidural Anesthesia: Differences from Spinal Anesthesia

Mechanisms

Primarily conduction block of spinal nerve roots and ganglia, as well as subarachnoid effects after drug transfer into cerebrospinal fluid

Anatomical distribution through epidural and paravertebral tissues less consistent than intrathecal distribution

Distribution affected by multiple factors including level of injection, dose, and volume, but less influenced by patient position

Onset and Efficacy

Slower onset 10–30 minutes

Higher failure rate (3%–10%)

Less effective block
- incidence of intraoperative pain 5%–20%
- incidence of conversion to general anesthesia 1%–3% (versus < 1%)

Other Effects and Complications

Cardiac output better maintained and lower incidence and severity of hypotension

Risk of shivering possibly greater

Risk of local anesthetic toxicity

Headache only if inadvertent dural puncture (incidence 0.5%–4%)

- Sudden changes in subarachnoid space pressure or dural puncture are best avoided (e.g., raised intracranial pressure; see also Chapter 10).

The principal indication for epidural anesthesia is nonelective cesarean delivery when an epidural catheter has already been placed, usually for labor analgesia.

- Ideally the epidural catheter should have been functioning satisfactorily already; otherwise, attempting conversion to epidural anesthesia may fail and delay surgery. This is particularly important when an emergency (Category 1) cesarean delivery is a significant risk (e.g., women with fetal compromise during labor) or where general anesthesia is a major issue (e.g., the morbidly obese woman or a patient with a difficult airway).
- If the epidural catheter is functioning well, epidural anesthesia can be established within 10–15 minutes (making it suitable for all categories of nonelective cesarean delivery with the exception of the most urgent Category 1 cases, for which general anesthesia is potentially faster).
- The incidence of intraoperative pain is higher (5%–20%) than under spinal anesthesia, but changing to a spinal technique is

usually unnecessary. It also results in a greater risk of a high and less predictable block, due to the reduced volume of the lumbar intrathecal CSF compartment as a result of compression by recently injected epidural solution.

Techniques and Equipment

There are many approaches to epidural catheter insertion (see Chapter 3). With the patient lying in the lateral position, aortocaval compression is minimized and the risk of epidural vein puncture is reduced. With the patient sitting, it may be easier to identify the midline.

- It is usually easier if the epidural needle is first inserted in the lower half of the lumbar interspace.

In difficult cases and obese women, the use of **ultrasound imaging** assessment is increasing in popularity, serving to locate the midline, identify specific interspaces and scolioisis, and calculate the skin to epidural space depth. Real-time ultrasound-guided paramedian epidural insertion using a spring-loaded loss-of-resistance syringe (Episure™, Indigo Orb, U.S.A) has been described.

- If the epidural catheter needs to be replaced, it will usually be necessary to remove the original catheter, both to ensure an aseptic technique and to avoid the potential risk of damaging the original catheter during reinsertion.
- Rarely, if a low bilateral block will not extend cephalad, it is appropriate to move several interspaces cephalad to a low thoracic interspace and to insert a second epidural catheter, limiting catheter insertion to < 5 cm.

Management of Epidural Anesthesia

The spread of epidural solution is minimally influenced by gravity, so when converting ("topping up") labor epidural analgesia to epidural anesthesia for surgical delivery, keep the woman in the left lateral position throughout. This minimizes aortocaval compression without compromising successful bilateral block.

- Use an incremental dosing approach to extend the block (5–10 ml, 2–5 minutes apart depending on urgency). Test for intravenous placement between each injection by repeated catheter aspiration through a liquid containing filter and connector, or (under strict aseptic conditions) via the connector only.

- Consider a test-dose for intrathecal placement if the catheter is newly inserted (see Chapter 3).

Epidural Drug Selection

Local Anesthetic

A number of local anesthetics are suitable for either extending epidural analgesia or instituting a block to establish surgical anesthesia for cesarean delivery. Mixtures have been used, but do not offer any real advantages. The preferred drugs for "topping-up" are:

- 3% 2-chloroprocaine.
  - Onset is very rapid (5–15 minutes) but this drug is not available in some countries.
- 2% lidocaine (lignocaine) with epinephrine (adrenaline) 1:200,000 plus sodium bicarbonate 8.4% 0.1 ml/ml
  - Adding bicarbonate to alkalinize the pH of the solution to approximately 6.5 results in a more rapid onset (7–10 minutes) and decreases the incidence of intraoperative pain.

Other epidural local anesthetics of slower onset are:

- 0.5% bupivacaine.
- 0.5% levobupivacaine or 0.75% ropivacaine
  - Onset is similar or slightly faster than bupivacaine (10–30 minutes) and cardiotoxicity potential is less.

Table 4.15 Suggested Approach when Converting Epidural Analgesia to Anesthesia

- Position the patient on the left side throughout
- Check the epidural catheter site to exclude dislodgement
- Check the location of the epidural catheter by aspiration to exclude intravascular placement
- Check the location of the epidural catheter by aspiration to exclude presence of cerebrospinal fluid (subarachnoid placement)
- Consider an intrathecal test-dose (see Chapter 3)
- Administer 5–10 ml 2% lidocaine (lignocaine) with epinephrine (adrenaline) 1:200,000 plus sodium bicarbonate 8.4% 0.1 ml per ml of lidocaine, or use 3% 2-chloroprocaine
  - repeat again 2–5 minutely until block adequate (usually 10–20 ml total)
  - use the larger dose and shorter interval for Category 1 or 2 non-elective cesarean delivery
  - consider adding fentanyl 50 mcg and/or clonidine 75 mcg if no recent epidural opioid, or bilateral symmetric block not present

Adjuncts

The addition of epinephrine (concentration 1 in 200,000–400,000 or 2.5–5 mcg/ml) to lidocaine is recommended to reduce peak plasma concentrations and permit safe administration of larger doses, but is not of benefit with other local anesthetics.

Addition of a lipophilic opioid decreases intraoperative surgical pain, but can increase the incidence of pruritus and sedation. Nevertheless it is strongly recommended if there has been no previous exposure to opioid (see Table 4.15). Choices include:

- Fentanyl 50 mcg
- Sufentanil 15–20 mcg
- Diamorphine 3 mg
- Clonidine (dose 75–300 mcg) is an α_2-adrenergic agonist that prolongs the duration of block and provides postoperative analgesia for 4–6 hours, but causes significant dose-dependent sedation. It is not used in the United States.

Combined Spinal-Epidural Anesthesia (CSEA)

Advantages and Disadvantages

This dual technique delivers the advantages of both spinal and epidural techniques (Table 4.16), making it very useful logistically and in a number of high-risk patients. The combination of a conventional spinal anesthetic technique with placement of an epidural catheter as back-up and for postoperative analgesia is recommended when:

- A risk exists that surgery may be delayed.
- Prolonged surgery is likely because of known difficult surgical conditions (e.g., morbid obesity), the presence of intra-abdominal pathologies, or the likelihood of obstetric hemorrhage and complex additional surgery.
- Postoperative analgesia is likely to be challenging (e.g., major abdominal surgery in addition to cesarean delivery, or an opioid-tolerant patient).
- "Topping up" an epidural catheter has failed to produce epidural anesthesia, and consent has been obtained to repeat a regional block.

The disadvantages of CSEA are relatively minor, although for routine elective cesarean delivery there is no evidence for outcome benefits compared with single-shot spinal anesthesia and additional equipment and time costs are incurred.

Table 4.16 Advantages and Disadvantages of Combined Spinal-Epidural Anesthesia

Advantages

Lowest failure and conversion to general anesthesia rate (both ~ 1% or less)
High quality spinal block of rapid onset
Regional anesthesia of prolonged duration
Good hemodynamic stability • low doses of intrathecal bupivacaine (5–10 mg) with lipophilic opioid • aid cephalad distribution using epidural volume extension (5–10 ml normal saline or local anesthetic) or use a sequential technique with epidural augmentation of low spinal anesthesia (T_{12}–S_5)
High quality postoperative epidural analgesia
Possibly lower rate of post-dural puncture headache

Disadvantages

Possibly higher incidence of paresthesia during insertion (versus spinal anesthesia alone)
Marginally slower insertion time
May require conversion to • epidural anesthesia alone (if the subarachnoid space cannot be located) • spinal anesthesia alone (if the epidural catheter cannot be inserted)

Techniques and Equipment

Insertion

There are two alternative insertion techniques:

- A single vertebral interspace, needle-through-needle technique.
  - This is by far the most popular approach because it is quicker to perform and is preferred by most patients (Figure 4.6).
- Separate vertebral interspace technique, with low thoracic or upper lumbar epidural insertion, then low lumbar spinal anesthesia.
  - This allows better titration and lower drug doses when establishing the block and has a potential safety advantage in the morbidly obese woman or when hemodynamic stability is vital.

Kits

Although CSEA can be performed using separate needle components, there are also a number of purpose-designed "kits" available for a single interspace approach. This equipment:

- Ensures an adequate protrusion of the spinal needle through the tip of the epidural needle (> 11 mm).
- May incorporate a means of guiding the spinal needle (through a separate hollow passage or epidural needle back-eye).

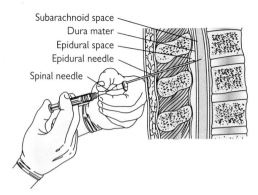

Figure 4.6 Combined spinal-epidural insertion using the single intervertebral space needle-through-needle approach. Reprinted with permission from Rawal N. *et al.* The combined spinalepidural technique, p. 166. In: Birnbach DJ, Gatt SP, Datta S., *Textbook of Obstetric Anesthesia.* 2000, Elsevier.

- May secure the spinal needle so that its tip remains immobile after penetrating the dura and arachnoid, reducing needle movement and possible failure to inject some or all the spinal drug solution.

If the entry of the epidural needle into the epidural space is not in the midline, the spinal needle may not enter or remain within the subarachnoid space (Figure 4.7). For this reason, especially in obese women in whom the distance to the epidural space is increased, the sitting rather than lateral patient position is preferred by many anesthesiologists.

There are three methods of establishing CSEA.

- Conventional spinal anesthesia (using bupivacaine 10–12.5 mg with or without opioid)
  - In this case use of the epidural catheter is reserved to supplement the block if necessary and for postoperative analgesia.
- Sequential CSEA, using a low dose of intrathecal drug (bupivacaine 3.5–8 mg with fentanyl or sufentanil)
  - This limits the spinal block (e.g., T_{10}–S_5) which is later extended (to T_3–T_5) using epidural local anesthetic.
- CSEA by "epidural volume extension" (EVE) using a low dose of intrathecal drug (bupivacaine 3.5–8 mg with fentanyl or sufentanil) followed immediately (at most within 5–10 minutes) by injection of epidural local anesthetic or saline 5–10 ml

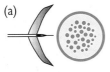

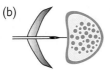

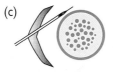

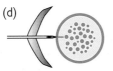

Figure 4.7 Position and direction of the spinal needle during combined spinal-epidural anesthesia. (a)–(c) result in technical failure. Similar mechanisms may apply for failure of spinal anesthesia. Reprinted with permission from Rawal N., *et al.* The combined spinalepidural technique, p. 176. In: Birnbach DJ, Gatt SP, Datta S., *Textbook of Obstetric Anesthesia.* 2000, Elsevier.

- The epidural injection extends spread of the intrathecal drug in a cephalad direction.
- This method is suitable for routine use only when the time from establishing block to completion of surgery can be guaranteed to be rapid (maximum 60–90 min).
- If the woman is sitting this method is associated with a higher risk of inadequate cephalad spread of subarachnoid drug.

Choice of Method

Situations when the sequential or EVE CSEA methods are clinically useful are when:

- A low incidence of maternal hypotension and hemodynamic disturbance is particularly important (e.g., maternal cardiac disease)

- Control of cephalad sensory block height is likely to be more difficult or titration of spread is important (e.g., after failed epidural anesthesia, or in a patient who has previously experienced a high block)
- A shorter duration of motor block and earlier postoperative mobilization (for greater patient satisfaction) are desired.

The main disadvantages of conventional CSEA are that it is slower and more costly. Sequential CSEA and especially EVE may be associated with a higher risk of intraoperative pain if the cesarean is not commenced and completed rapidly, and additional epidural local anesthetic injection after 45–60 min is advisable if surgery is ongoing.

Drug Selection for CSEA

The usual spinal and epidural anesthetic drugs and concentrations apply (see above). Because low doses of bupivacaine are most appropriate for sequential approaches, it is essential to include adjuncts, most commonly a lipophilic opioid.

Continuous Spinal Anesthesia

This technique, first used in obstetrics in the 1940s, is used only in select circumstances. Interest in it reemerged in the late 1980s when small gauge intrathecal microcatheters were introduced, but neural injuries resulted in their withdrawal from the market in some countries. Currently, both purpose-designed microcatheters (available in some countries) and standard epidural "macrocatheters" are used. The latter approach is popular in tertiary units as an alternative to reinsertion of the catheter into the epidural space when the epidural needle has punctured the dura and arachnoid mater (a "wet tap").

Advantages, Disadvantages and Applications

The advantages of continuous spinal anesthesia (CSA) are:

- Successful block can be established in patients with abnormal or altered neuraxial anatomy, in whom epidural or single-shot spinal anesthesia has a substantial risk of failure (e.g., severe scoliosis or previous vertebral canal surgery).
- A safe, reliable anesthetic can be performed when attempts to achieve epidural or spinal anesthesia have previously failed (e.g., in a morbidly obese woman).
- The ability to titrate drug in women at high risk for morbidity from high block, or from general anesthesia (e.g., severe asthma or impossible intubation).

- Stable hemodynamics in those likely to tolerate sympathetic-induced cardiovascular changes poorly (e.g., certain cardiac diseases, pulmonary hypertension, aortic stenosis, cardiomyopathy, adult congenital heart disease).
- Effective anesthesia for operative delivery after an epidural catheter has been placed intrathecally for labor analgesia.

The disadvantages include:

- Difficulty with microspinal catheter placement, contributing to a high overall failure rate (as high as 20% in some reports, though with frequent use the failure rate falls).
- The possibility of catheter misuse, in particular, unintentional injection of epidural drug doses resulting in high or "total spinal" block.
- A high incidence of PDPH, though the incidence is lower among the morbidly obese.
- The risk of microcatheter breakage during insertion or withdrawal, possibly necessitating surgical removal.

Equipment and Technique

Equipment

There are two main types of catheter and kits:

- An epidural catheter (20 or 22 gauge) inserted through an epidural needle (unintentionally or deliberately) placed into the subarachnoid space (designated a "macrocatheter"). Pediatric epidural catheters, 24 gauge, which pass through a 20 gauge Tuohy needle, can also be used.
- Catheter-over-needle kits available with 22 or 24 gauge catheters mounted over an internal needle or stylet, which can be withdrawn after placement. The catheter is introduced with a Crawford style needle placed in the epidural space.

Insertion Technique

Technical issues with placement are common, irrespective of the proceduralist's experience. Successful and safe insertion depends on:

- Accurate needle placement
- Insertion of only 3–4 cm of catheter (the direction and final tip location cannot be predicted)
- Rapid injection of drugs (local anesthetic maldistribution is more likely with slow injection)
- Titration of bolus doses (e.g., bupivacaine 1.25–2.5 mg in volumes of 0.25–0.5 ml)

- Dose requirements vary widely (range for surgical anesthesia with bupivacaine may be 5–17.5 mg).
- For safety, pay attention to detail with respect to use of small syringes, filling of the dead space within the catheter (and filter, if used) and frequent block assessment.

Drug Selection

Plain 0.5% bupivacaine is usually titrated to the desired level or effect. Hyperbaric solutions can be used but may contribute to maldistribution of local anesthetic in the CSF. Opioid adjuncts as used for single-shot spinal anesthesia are often a good idea.

Local Infiltration or Field Block

In developing countries in particular, some obstetricians gain experience in performing cesarean delivery under progressive local anesthetic infiltration of the abdominal wall (Figure 4.8), with or without instillation of local anesthetic into the peritoneal cavity and wound, or field block of the lower abdomen (bilateral iliohypogastric and ilioinguinal nerve blocks). As large volumes of local anesthetic are required, solutions of low to medium concentration are used, and total dose must be considered. Maximum recommended doses of bupivacaine (up to 150 mg) or ropivacaine (300 mg) are very unlikely to result in plasma concentrations reaching the toxic range. Sedation, including subanesthetic doses of ketamine, may be added.

The transversus abdominis plane (TAP) block also appears to be a suitable technique, but has not yet been evaluated as a component of anesthesia.

Dealing with Failed Regional Anesthesia

Management of Failed Block before Surgery

Failed Spinal Anesthesia

Technical failures (failed or abandoned insertion, or inadequate block) are infrequent. Inability to obtain a satisfactory spinal block (incidence approximately 0.5%–4% for spinal anesthesia and 0.5%–2% for CSEA) may be due to several factors:

- Delivery of an inadequate dose of local anesthetic (dose selection errors, loss from the syringe-needle connection or deposition outside the dura).
- Maldistribution of local anesthetic due to anatomical factors (high CSF volume, subarachnoid and extradural cysts, arachnoid adhesions

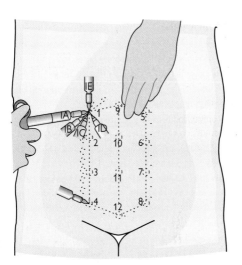

Figure 4.8 Method of local field block of the lower abdominal wall.
Reprinted with permission from Ranney B. and Stanage WF.
Advantages of local anesthesia for cesarean section. *Obstet Gynecol.*
1975;45(2):165.

and trabecula, previous surgery or severe scoliosis), poor patient
positioning, or low injection level

- Mistaking infiltrated local anesthetic for CSF, leading to injection in
  the wrong anatomic compartment or space

- Other rare causes.

A good assistant who helps position the patient optimally is very helpful. Manipulation of patient position post-injection (e.g., changing sides
for unilateral or asymmetric spread or head-down posture) can also
be an important factor in obtaining a good block.

Strategies to "rescue" a bilateral but low spinal block include:

- Repositioning the patient head-down with her hips fully flexed
  (although caution is required with these maneuvers, and sensory
  distribution should be checked very frequently to avoid a high
  block).

- Insertion of an upper lumbar or low thoracic epidural catheter,
  after which often only a small volume of local anesthetic (3–5 ml)
  will be sufficient to establish surgical anesthesia.

- Dosing the epidural catheter if a CSEA was performed.

Failed Epidural Anesthesia

This is more common than failed spinal anesthesia (incidence 5%–15%) and is predicted by factors such as:

- Unsatisfactory analgesia previously, during labor
- A large number of supplementary bolus doses during labor
- Failure to add opioid to the local anesthetic
- Morbid obesity.

If time allows a "top-up," up to 85% of these cases will ultimately develop satisfactory epidural anesthesia. Strategies to improve the quality or height of the block include:

- Withdraw the catheter slightly (about 1 cm) before re-dosing (provided at least 4 cm of catheter remains in the epidural space).
- Re-dose with a high concentration of local anesthetic.
- Add adjuncts such as lipophilic opioid (e.g., fentanyl 50 mcg) and/or clonidine 75–150 mcg.

The decision to abandon use of the epidural catheter and perform a repeat regional anesthetic technique, or to change to general anesthesia, must be based on personal experience, individual risk-benefit assessment, the urgency of delivery and the woman's wishes. An essential part of the consent process is to warn women that regional analgesia and anesthesia may fail or prove to be unsatisfactory intraoperatively, despite having established an apparently satisfactory surgical anesthetic.

Management of Intraoperative Pain

Despite good somatic (abdominal wall) block, visceral pain, particularly from pelvic organs such as the ovary, fallopian tubes, or the peritoneum, is not uncommon during cesarean delivery, even in the presence of apparently adequate sensory anesthesia to light touch, pinprick or cold at mid-thoracic dermatomes. The incidence of pain is lower with spinal compared with epidural anesthesia, but with either can reach 20%–50% (typically 5%–20% if neuraxial opioid has been used), especially when surgery takes more than 45–60 minutes. The anesthesiologist must be prepared to deal with pain in an unsedated and anxious patient, and with their support person.

Assessment of the patient is imperative.

- The patient should already have been aware that the experience will involve sensation, and the block distribution must be re-checked and documented.

- The timing of pain in relation to surgery is important.
  - Pain during initial incision is highly indicative that general anesthesia will be required.
  - Pain arising during pelvic organ inspection and peritoneal closure is not uncommon and can normally be managed satisfactorily.
- The severity of pain (e.g., on a verbal numerical 0–10 rating score) and the location of the pain should be noted.
  - Surgical exteriorization of the uterus increases the likelihood of intraoperative pain.
  - Up to 5% of women experience upper chest or shoulder pain in the skin distribution of the cervical nerve roots of the phrenic nerve (C_3–C_5). This is thought to result from irritation of the subdiaphagmatic peritoneum by blood and amniotic fluid. Shoulder tip pain can be reduced by head-up table tilt and sometimes counter-irritation, with vigorous rubbing of the painful shoulder.
- Psychological support and reassurance can be crucial.
  - Reassure the woman that the pain will be dealt with, that mild pain is often short-lived and resolves fully, and let the patient know how you intend to treat it.
  - Ascertain her feelings about the proposed treatment, maintain rapport, and if pain is severe, immediately raise the possibility of conversion to general anesthesia.
  - Use distraction techniques, especially by encouraging maternal–infant contact and interaction.
  - Inform the obstetrician of the situation and the plan. Unless at the time of delivery, consider asking them to stop surgical manipulation briefly in order to gain control.
- Consider a small dose of an analgesic drug and also an anxiolytic drug if the patient is obviously fearful. Anxiolysis with 50%–70% nitrous oxide in oxygen via the anesthetic circuit, or intravenous midazolam 1–2 mg, can be helpful.
  - Document the events and management.
  - Follow up with the patient, and counsel the woman postoperatively.

There are a number of analgesic options, which can be used if necessary.

- Start with IV opioid (e.g., fentanyl 25–100 mcg or remifentanil 0.01–0.02 mcg/kg/min).

- Inject epidural local anesthetic (especially if near the end of surgery or at a time of possible block regression).
- Give epidural adjuncts (fentanyl or sufentanil, clonidine), recognizing that these and local anesthetic will take 5–15 minutes to take effect.
- Ask the obstetrician to inject local anesthetic (e.g., 20–30 ml 0.5% ropivacaine) either into the peritoneum (for adnexial or generalized abdominal or pelvic pain) or beneath the rectus sheath (for somatic abdominal wound pain during closure).
- As a last resort, consider IV ketamine (e.g., 5 mg repeated as required until sedated). Care must be taken not to give so much that general anesthesia is induced and airway reflexes are lost. Specific consent from the patient should be obtained before administration because of potential oversedation and the undesirable psychomimetic effects.

Management of Failed Regional Anesthesia due to Complications

The anesthesiologist must be prepared for complications of regional anesthesia that require intervention (see the following and Chapter 13). This includes induction of general anesthesia during the operation. Some like to keep drugs for induction and intubation of the patient (e.g., sodium thiopental and succinylcholine) at hand. If propofol is prepared, it should be used within 4 hours because it supports bacterial growth.

Management of Early Complications of Regional Anesthesia

Maternal Hypotension

Regional anesthesia for cesarean delivery is associated with significant and potentially life-threatening cardiovascular changes.

- Modest blood pressure reduction is anticipated due to sympathetic block and decreased peripheral vascular resistance.
- Venodilation may, in some circumstances, also cause reduction of venous return.
- Caval compression may reduce venous return.
- A reduction in heart rate via various mechanisms may occur.
- A combination of effects can reduce blood pressure, left ventricular preload, stroke volume, and heart rate (thus cardiac output), leading to underperfusion of maternal vital organs and the placenta.

Organ perfusion depends on adequate cardiac output and blood pressure. Given the inability to readily measure cardiac output under typical clinical conditions, changes in maternal blood pressure and heart rate and maternal symptoms have been used to infer the state of organ perfusion, including that of the uteroplacental unit. The importance of maintaining cardiac output as well as blood pressure is well recognized, because a significant decrease in cardiac output correlates with increased umbilical artery pulsatility indices and neonatal arterial academia, both of which reflect inadequate uteroplacental blood flow. New technologies, such as analysis of arterial pulse waveforms and noninvasive Doppler flow assessments, are potential means of estimating acute changes in cardiac output during pregnancy.

Attention to maternal blood pressure and heart rate is fundamental during anesthesia for cesarean delivery. The clinical impact of similar degrees of hypotension differs between individuals, and the degree and duration of reduced uteroplacental flow that leads to significant fetal compromise is undetermined. Different studies variably define hypotension, but typically use a fall in systolic arterial blood pressure from baseline of 10%–30%, or an absolute value of 80–100 mmHg. Hypotension occurs in 80%–90% of women having cesarean delivery under regional block, depending on the definition.

- Blood pressure falls within 5–10 minutes of induction of spinal anesthesia, but bedside methods to predict women at higher risk of significant hypotension currently do not show clinical utility.
- Blood pressure changes appear less severe in women who are in active labor or who have severe preeclampsia.
- Maternal nausea almost always reflects moderate to severe hypotension, while maternal syncope or a fall in fetal oxygenation typically occur with severe hypotension or fall in cardiac output (Figure 4.9).

Treatment of falling blood pressure is warranted if the woman becomes symptomatic (nausea, vomiting, syncope, collapse and potential aspiration or cardiac arrest) or if the fetus appears compromised (nonreassuring fetal heart rate patterns appear).

- Neonatal acid-base status is best maintained by keeping maternal blood pressure as close as possible to pre-anesthetic baseline values.

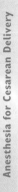

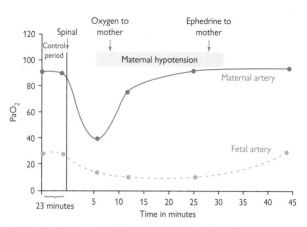

Figure 4.9 Changes in arterial oxygen tension in the fetus after spinal anesthesia-induced hypotension, hypoxia, oxygen and ephedrine administration to the mother. This article was published in the *American Journal of Obstetrics and Gynecology, Vol. 102*, Shnider SM, *et al.* Vasopressors in obstetrics. I. Correction of fetal acidosis with ephedrine during spinal hypotension, p. 917, Copyright Elsevier (1968).

Prevention of Maternal Hypotension

Intravenous crystalloid administration is of no or limited efficacy in preventing or treating maternal hypotension. Crystalloid administration induces atrial natriuretic hormone-related vasodilation, and fluid rapidly redistributes to the extravascular fluid compartment. Preventative measures that are helpful include:

- Lower limb compression stockings combined with leg elevation.
- Preloading or coloading (concurrent with the onset of block) with colloid 500–1,000 ml. This is associated with a low risk of colloid-related allergic reactions, however.
- Slow establishment of epidural anesthesia, or use of sequential CSEA, starting with low doses of spinal local anesthetic (4–8 mg with opioid).
- Titrated infusion of a vasopressor drug (e.g., starting with IV phenylephrine 25–50 mcg/min, metaraminol 250 mcg/min).
- Vasopressor boluses (e.g., phenylephrine 50–100 mcg, metaraminol 0.25–0.5 mg, ephedrine 5–10 mg).

Vasopressor Therapy

The efficacy of vasopressor therapy is dose-dependent, with generally better control from higher doses. This also produces more iatrogenic hypertension and α_1-adrenergic agonists such as phenylephrine may reduce cardiac output (due to a reflex fall in heart rate). Routine use of ephedrine is now controversial-it has been shown to have a direct metabolic effect on the fetus, which reduces fetal pH in a dose-dependent fashion. The magnitude of effect is small and of unknown clinical significance. While it is almost certainly detrimental to the acidotic neonate, it arguably may benefit the healthy neonate.

• Prophylactic vasopressor infusion is more effective than treatment.
• A combination of strategies, including α_1-adrenergic agonists, will prevent maternal hypotension and nausea in 90% of women.

The choice of vasopressor is influenced by factors such as availability, ease of use, direct and indirect fetal effects, and other pharmacodynamic properties (Table 4.17).

Ephedrine was considered the vasopressor of choice for over 30 years, based on animal research of effects on uteroplacental blood flow. Although still widely used, many anesthesiologists now routinely use α_1-adrenergic agonists such as phenylephrine (Figure 4.10). Phenylephrine has been better evaluated than other α_1-adrenergic agonists, and compared with ephedrine:

• Is more effective in preventing maternal symptoms when titrated by infusion.
• Is associated with better maternal and neonatal acid-base outcomes.

A prophylactic infusion of phenylephrine (e.g., 10 mg in 100 ml saline or 100 mcg/ml) run at 25–75 mcg/min from the time of subarachnoid drug injection, or treatment with 100–150 mcg boluses:

• Minimizes maternal symptoms related to hypotension (incidence 10% versus > 50% without vasopressor).
• May reduce maternal cardiac output due to reflex bradycardia (avoid < 50 bpm). Bradycardia can be corrected by decreasing the dose rate, stopping the infusion changing to a β_1-agonist such as ephedrine, or treating with glycopyrrolate (0.2–0.4 mg) or atropine (0.2–0.6 mg).

Once a full autonomic and sensory block has been achieved and oxytocin administered, vasopressors are seldom required.

Systemic Local Anesthetic Toxicity

Background

This potentially lethal complication of epidural techniques was a significant cause of maternal death 20 years ago, but is now a very rare

Table 4.17 Features of Three Vasopressor Drugs for Blood Pressure Control at Regional Anesthesia for Cesarean Delivery

Ephedrine
- Considered the vasopressor of choice for many years but many authorities now disagree, partly due to limited efficacy
- Direct and predominantly indirect β-plus weak α1-adrenergic agonist
  - increases heart and cardiac output with mild peripheral vasoconstriction
  - tachyphylaxis may be a problem
- Typical intravenous doses 5–15 mg (bolus) or 1–5 mg/min (infusion)
- Onset slightly delayed (1–2 minutes)
- Results in a small reduction in umbilical artery pH and increase in base deficit
- Rarely induces ventricular tachyarrhythmias

Phenylephrine
- The most thoroughly evaluated alternative to ephedrine and 80 times more potent
- Potent direct α1-adrenergic agonist
  - marked peripheral vasoconstriction with reflex reduction in heart rate
  - cardiac output increases slightly initially but may fall with bradycardia
- Rapid onset and short duration (5–10 min post-bolus) facilitates titration
- Typical intravenous doses 100–150 mcg (bolus) or 25–75 mcg/min (infusion)
- No effect on fetal acid-base status

Metaraminol
- Potent direct and indirect α1-adrenergic agonist with some β-activity
  - increases peripheral vascular resistance
  - cardiac output stable or falls
- Rapid onset and easily titrated
- Typical doses 0.2–0.5 mg (bolus) or 0.25–0.5 mg/min (infusion)
- No effect on fetal acid-base status

event (estimated incidence 1 in 10,000). Possible factors contributing to this improvement in safety are shown in Table 4.18.

The pregnant woman appears more susceptible to systemic toxicity from bupivacaine and ropivacaine because of reduced plasma protein binding, reduced clearance of local anesthetics, and progesterone-induced changes in the myocardium. Yet, despite the frequency of epidural analgesia during labor and "topping up" for cesarean delivery, when careful attention is paid to maximum recommended doses, a rise in local anesthetic blood concentrations leading to clinical toxicity is exceptionally rare.

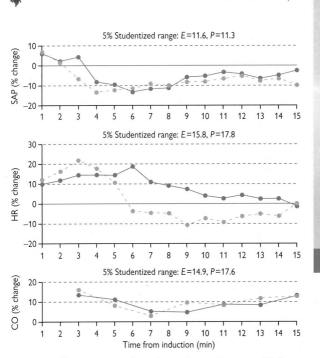

Figure 4.10 Mean percentage changes in systolic arterial pressure (SAP), heart rate (HR) and cardiac output (CO) from baseline values after induction of spinal anesthesia in the ephedrine bolus (▇) and phenylephrine bolus (▇) groups. Reprinted with permission from Thomas DG et al. Randomized trial of bolus phenylephrine or ephedrine for maintenance of arterial pressure during spinal anaesthesia for caesarean section. *Br J Anaesth.* 1996;76(1):63.

Intravenous Injection

Intravenous local anesthetic injection is the most likely cause of serious toxicity. Epidural vein cannulation occurs more frequently during pregnancy (incidence 5%–10%) as a result of the dilated azygous venous system and prominent veins in the lateral and, particularly, anterior epidural space. Intravenous catheter placement is reduced by:

- Use of a flexible, soft-tip epidural catheter.
- Epidural insertion with the woman in the lateral position.
- Epidural saline (5–10 ml or more) injected prior to catheterization.

Table 4.18 Factors Possibly Contributing to the Decline in Deaths from Local Anesthetic Toxicity

- Publicity and education
- The decline in use of caudal blocks (much higher risk of intravenous injection than lumbar epidural)
- The increased use of spinal anesthesia for elective cesarean delivery
- The reduction in local anesthetic doses for epidural analgesia for labor and delivery
- Better prevention and detection of intravascular catheter placement (catheter aspiration, test-dosing, use of multi-holed catheters)
- Incremental epidural dosing, observing for signs and symptoms of toxicity
- Newer drugs with higher therapeutic indices (e.g., ropivacaine and levo-bupivacaine)
- Management of toxicity with intravenous Intralipid "lipid rescue"

After accidental intravenous injection of local anesthetic, the blood concentration and toxicity depend on the drug, the dose injected, and the rate of rise of arterial concentration in vital organs. The individual's response may be modified somewhat by other drugs (e.g., benzodiazepines). A number of strategies should be applied to increase the safety of epidural local anesthetic injection:

- Always aspirate the catheter looking for blood. A fluid-filled filter and catheter system are highly sensitive for detection of intravascular placement of multi-holed epidural catheters.

Test-Dosing

Intravenous but not epidural epinephrine (adrenaline) 15 mcg will increase systolic blood pressure by 15 mmHg and heart rate by 10 bpm (after 30–90 seconds) in the absence of β-blockade or a concurrent painful uterine contraction. The response is transient, however, so continuous monitoring of heart rate and blood pressure are necessary to reliably detect the changes.

- Epinephrine test-doses have limitations, especially during labor when false-positive responses occur, and should be avoided in women with hypertension, cardiac disease, or arrhythmias.
- Lidocaine or chloroprocaine 100 mg, bupivacaine 25 mg, ropivacaine 30 mg, or fentanyl 100 mcg, may produce clinical symptoms but not serious complications.
- Incremental injection of local anesthetic, in 5 ml aliquots, waiting 30–50 seconds between doses (to reduce peak plasma concentration and allow detection of subjective symptoms before seizures or

cardiac arrest) is recommended. Failure of an epidural block to develop may indicate intravascular injection.

Systemic Toxicity

When lidocaine is accidently injected intravascularly, in addition to seizures, myocardial depression and peripheral vasodilation may be evident—but, in contrast to bupivacaine and other long-acting amide local anesthetics, cardiac arrest is unlikely because it has anti-arrhythmic properties. After accidental intravenous injection, probably no more than 1 in 10 patients experience typical symptoms:

- Central nervous system excitation (tinnitus, circumoral tingling, visual disturbance, altered mentation, restlessness, slurred speech, twitching, seizures) then depression.
- Cardiotoxicity (myocardial depression, bradycardia, hypotension, sudden onset re-entrant ventricular arrhythmias, ventricular fibrillation and cardiac arrest).

The management of systemic toxicity (Table 4.19) is based on:

- Airway management, avoiding hypoxia and hypercarbia.
- Suppression of seizures.
- Circulatory support.
- Intravenous lipid infusion. This improves the success of resuscitation in animal models and also, it appears, in humans. The mechanism appears related to binding of local anesthetic in plasma and improvement in myocardial mitochondrial function (see Chapter 3).

High Block and Respiratory Depression

Regional block to a level that meets the clinical requirements for surgical anesthesia has an impact on respiratory function, reducing peak expiratory flow and vital capacity. The parturient should be monitored and reassured while awaiting block regression. In cases where sensory block to ice and pinprick extends well above T_2, even though motor weakness is usually at least two dermatomal levels lower, a more complete motor block of abdominal and thoracic intercostal muscles can be expected and even greater vigilance is required.

If hypoventilation leads to a change in mental state or hypoxemia, oxygen must be given and immediate preparation made for intubation and ventilation.

In women for whom high block has particularly undesirable physiological consequences, a titrated technique such as sequential CSEA or epidural anesthesia is recommended. This includes women with

Table 4.19 **Management Plan for Local Anesthetic Toxicity**
Get help
Airway and Breathing <ul><li>Maintain a clear airway, give oxygen and ventilate</li><li>Avoid hyperventilation as well as hypoventilation</li><li>Watch for post-ictal airway obstruction</li></ul>
Seizures: Avoid patient injury <ul><li>Give an anticonvulsant as required (usually self-terminating)<ul><li>IV midazolam 2–5 mg</li><li>IV diazepam 5–10 mg</li><li>IV thiopental 50–100 mg or propofol 25–50 mg</li></ul></li></ul>
Circulation <ul><li>Check heart rate, blood pressure and apply ECG monitoring</li><li>Avoid aortocaval compression</li><li>Treat hypotension and bradycardia aggressively<ul><li>IV phenylephrine 100–200 mcg then 50–100 mcg/min</li><li>IV norepinephrine 0.05–0.5 mcg/kg/min</li><li>IV epinephrine 10–100 mcg boluses</li><li>IV atropine 0.6–1.2 mg</li></ul></li><li>Treat arrhythmias<ul><li>IV amiodarone 300 mg and avoid phenytoin, calcium channel blockers</li></ul></li></ul>
Give lipid infusion <ul><li>20% Intralipid 1.5 ml/kg bolus (repeat up to twice at 3–5 minute intervals) and infuse 0.25 ml/kg/min</li></ul>
Use Advanced Life Support algorithms for cardiac arrest during pregnancy

IV – intravenous

severe respiratory or cardiac disease; those for whom judging the correct dose may be difficult (e.g., achondroplasia); or those who have had a high block in the past. In approximately 1 in 3,000–5,000 women, a high block leads to impaired phonation or swallowing, hypoventilation or apnea, or loss of consciousness. Such an event will mandate intubation (preferably with cricoid pressure) and ventilation, and usually also cardiovascular support.

Causes of High Block

The exact mechanism of high regional block is often unclear.

- Exaggerated spread within the planned area of distribution may occur (epidural or subarachnoid), involving cervical nerve roots, cranial nerves and autonomic nerves (e.g., Horner's syndrome).
- Drugs may be unintentionally injected into the incorrect space (for example subarachnoid injection of epidural solution through a catheter thought to be entirely located in the epidural space). Immediate withdrawal of 20–30 ml of local anesthetic contaminated CSF and

replacement with saline has been suggested, but is of unproven benefit.

- Epidural drug may transfer through a breach in the dura and arachnoid after replacement of an epidural catheter following dural puncture (thus, all bolus doses must be given cautiously, preferably only by an anesthesiologist, and the effects monitored).
- Subdural or intradural block may occur, with drug spread by iatrogenic dissection of a cellular layer between the dura and arachnoid mater, leading to high cephalad and intracranial extension.

Subdural Block

During an apparently uneventful epidural needle insertion, the bevel can become subdural or intradural. A multi-holed epidural catheter may also occupy or traverse this tissue plane. No CSF is seen because the arachnoid mater remains intact. The incidence of subdural block is undetermined, but it is not rare.

- Presentation is varied, but usually extensive cephalad and asymmetric spread is seen, even after small volumes of injected solution.
- Approximately 5% of cases result in a restricted low block.
- Onset is usually more than 20 minutes, with relative sparing of anterior nerve roots, and thus motor and autonomic nerves (motor paralysis and severe hypotension are rare).
- Respiratory failure may occur, but is uncommon.
- In theory, large fluid volumes may rupture the arachnoid mater, allowing the drug to enter the subarachnoid space and result in a high spinal block.

The diagnosis of subdural block is clinical, so once suspected the catheter should be removed (although confirmation by radiological imaging may be worthwhile to enable counseling of the patient). The typical appearance of subdural contrast on X-ray is "railroad tracks" on the lateral view, with smooth central distribution of contrast medium across the spinal canal, but no extension outlining lateral spinal nerve roots, as is seen with epidural spread. (Figure 4.11).

Total Spinal Block

The clinical characteristics of extensive subarachnoid spread of local anesthetic include:

- Rising sensory and motor block leading to dyspnea or apnea (at any time within 30 minutes of spinal injection, sometimes in association with a change in the patient's posture).

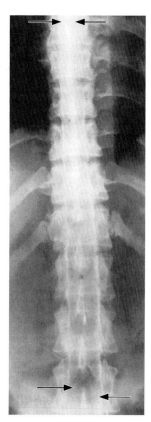

Figure 4.11 Typical appearance of subdural spread on anteroposterior epidurogram after injection of radiographic contrast through the epidural catheter. Arrows indicate "railroad track" bilateral distribution of subdural contrast from the mid-lumbar to the mid-thoracic region. Reprinted with permission from Collier CB, Epidural blocks investigated. In: *An Atlas of Epidurograms*. 1998, Taylor and Francis.

- Confusion, restlessness, severe drowsiness or unconsciousness.
- Moderate to severe hypotension (and possible cardiac arrest).

The most common cause is undetected intrathecal placement of an epidural catheter, although rarely spinal block occurs after previously normal epidural drug responses. Some case series note that high spinal block is more likely when spinal anesthesia is repeated, or initiated after recent "topping up" of an epidural catheter had proved unsuccessful. Attention to patient positioning immediately after injection is important, with elevation of the shoulders and upper thoracic spine to accentuate the thoracic curve and limit spread to the mid-thoracic segments.

No method of detection of catheter location is completely sensitive.

- Before each injection, an epidural catheter should be aspirated, looking for CSF.
- A test-dose looking for rapid onset of sacral block (by injecting a "safe" dose of local anesthetic, such as 3 ml of 1.5% lidocaine or 0.5% ropivacaine or 2 ml of 0.5% bupivacaine) should be considered, in particular after initial insertion.
- Bedside tests for CSF (as opposed to saline, epidural solutions, or tissue fluid) are unreliable. However, glucose content of fluid is highly suggestive for CSF, and the warmth of CSF or failure of the aspirated solution to precipitate in sodium pentothal are also indicative.

Management

The management of very high block is supportive (Table 4.20). Some patients remain conscious and clinically stable enough to observe and monitor. In most cases, treatment will require intubation and ventilation, along with naloxone, oxygen, cardiovascular support and sedation, until block regression is sufficient for the return of consciousness and adequate ventilation. A full recovery is expected, although substandard care still leads to maternal deaths.

Opioid-Induced Respiratory Depression

The incidence of severe respiratory depression due to neuraxial opioids given prior to cesarean delivery has not been quantified, but appears exceptionally rare.

- Rarely, intrathecal lipophilic opioids such as fentanyl or sufentanil cause sensory changes in a cervical or cranial nerve distribution, with or without respiratory depression, within 5–30 minutes of injection.
- Epidural fentanyl 100 mcg or sufentanil 10–50 mcg have the potential to cause hypoventilation but worrisome case reports are very rare.
- Intrathecal morphine is widely used, but doses <250 mcg (evidence supports an optimum dose of 100–150 mcg) do not affect minute ventilation or ventilatory responses to carbon dioxide.

Table 4.20 **Management Plan for High Block**
Get help
• Airway, oxygenation and ventilation: give high inspired oxygen
• Give naloxone if opioid may be contributing to respiratory depression
• Determine if intubation and ventilation is required (unconscious, apneic)
Intubate (with or without sedation and paralysis as required) using cricoid pressure and ventilate using continued intravenous sedation
Extubate once ventilation adequate and patient is conscious (usually within 2–4 hours)
Monitoring and circulatory support
• Monitor maternal hemodynamics (including noninvasive or continuous arterial blood pressure)
• Correct hypotension and bradycardia
• IV phenylephrine 100–200 mcg then 50–100 mcg/min
• IV norepinephrine 0.05–0.5 mcg/kg/min
• IV vasopressin 20 units then 0.2–0.4 units/min
• IV atropine 0.6–1.2 mg
• IV crystalloid infusion
• Avoid aortocaval compression if undelivered
Monitor the fetus if undelivered (urgent cesarean delivery is not likely to be required if well managed)
Make a diagnosis and counsel the patient later

IV – intravenous

Nevertheless, after neuraxial morphine, clinically detectable respiratory depression occurs in approximately 1 in 500 cases.

- Presentation is typically delayed 3–12 hours, and thus postoperative.
- Depression is usually mild, and naloxone is infrequently required.
- Administration of epidural or intrathecal morphine mandates at least observational monitoring, such as sedation, respiratory rate and depth, based on practice guidelines such as those of the ASA Task Force on Neuraxial Opioids (see also Chapter 5).

General Anesthesia

Indications

General anesthesia is infrequently the preferred option for cesarean delivery and even women who initially request it usually consent to regional anesthesia after adequate discussion. Nevertheless there are a number of circumstances and patients for whom general anesthesia may be a safer or more sensible option (Tables 4.4 and 4.21).

Table 4.21 Indications for General Anesthesia

- Emergency (category 1) cesarean delivery because there is the threat of immediate fetal death
- Maternal refusal of regional anesthesia
- Previous traumatic experience with regional anesthesia or cesarean delivery under regional anesthesia
- Anatomical abnormalities where regional techniques are unlikely to be successful
  - severe scoliosis
  - extensive lumbar surgery
  - certain spinal muscular disorders
- Uncooperative patient
- Recent eclamptic seizure with signs of possible further seizures or a suspected neurological complication
- Mental state disturbance
  - psychiatric illness
  - drug-induced state
  - severe needle phobia
- Potential contraindication to regional anesthesia
  - infection concerns (systemic sepsis, lumbar skin infection, acute viral disease)
  - neuraxial canal hematoma concerns (severe thrombocytopenia, e.g., platelet count < 50 x 109/dl; coagulopathy, e.g., international normalized ratio > 1.5; therapeutic anticoagulation; certain hereditary or acquired bleeding disorders)
  - circulatory collapse concerns (e.g., hemodynamically unstable due to hypovolemia, severe sepsis)
  - concern re consequences of dural puncture in the presence of raised intracranial pressure (e.g., cerebral tumor)
  - cardiac diseases where excessive reduction in afterload or reduction of venous return may be disastrous (e.g., severe aortic stenosis or pulmonary hypertension)
  - raised intracranial pressure or central nervous system pathology where change in cerebrospinal fluid pressure may be detrimental (e.g., large intracranial tumor)
- Severe respiratory impairment when supine
- Respiratory failure requiring ventilation (e.g., severe pneumonia or uncorrected pulmonary edema)

The use of general anesthesia for women at risk of major intraoperative and postpartum hemorrhage (e.g., anterior placenta previa, morbidly adherent placenta) is controversial. Regional anesthesia may reduce blood loss, and in many cases clinical experience supports beginning with a regional technique but maintaining a low threshold to convert to general anesthesia in the event of massive hemorrhage. Prerequisites are informed consent, full preparation and planning to manage hemorrhage, and a maternity setting with resources and familiarity with such an approach.

Technique and Drugs

The recommended approach for nearly all cases of general anesthesia for cesarean delivery is an intravenous rapid sequence induction, followed by tracheal intubation while maintaining cricoid pressure. Maintenance of anesthesia is with inhalational anesthesia prior to delivery; postdelivery, intravenous opioid is used for analgesia and to allow lower concentrations of inhalational anesthetic. Alternative techniques are reserved for special circumstances.

- Awake intubation followed by intravenous induction may be used in patients with a compromised or expected difficult airway.
- An inhalational induction with sevoflurane may rarely be indicated in a predicted difficult airway or severely needle-phobic patient.
- Total intravenous anesthesia can be used when malignant hyperthermia is a risk.
- Airway control with a supraglottic airway (i.e., laryngeal mask airway) has been used in fasted women of low body weight, with no risk factors for aspiration and having elective cesarean delivery. This remains controversial practice.

Principles of Induction and Maintenance

Pregnant women, being considered to have a "full stomach" (see Chapter 2), are at risk for regurgitation and aspiration. Although cricoid pressure (Figure 4.12) has not been proven to reduce the incidence of aspiration, and causes problems when applied incorrectly, it will reduce regurgitation into the hypopharynx and is recommended for general anesthesia for cesarean delivery. Supraglottic airways do not offer the same protection against aspiration as a correctly sited tracheal tube, so until we have more safety data, rapid sequence induction and intubation is recommended for pulmonary protection. The endotracheal tube remains in place until the return of consciousness and return of protective airway reflexes at the end of surgery.

Prior to or at induction, anxiolytic drugs such as midazolam and opioids are not usually used, to minimize fetal exposure. Intravenous opioid is also usually omitted.

- Administration of opioid (or other drugs, Table 4.22) is warranted in selected patients to obtund the "stress response" (sympathetic nervous system, adrenal catecholamine and neuroendocrine activation) to laryngoscopy and intubation. This response causes

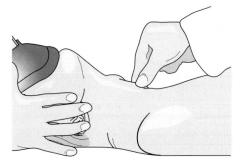

Figure 4.12 Application of cricoid pressure to prevent regurgitation of gastric content into the pharynx.

hypertension, tachycardia and increases the risk of a cerebrovascular event in hypertensive women.

- Opioids are considered for women with severe preeclampsia, poorly controlled hypertension, ischemic heart and severe cardiac disease.
- Inform the staff member responsible for neonatal resuscitation if maternal opioids have been given.

Intravenous remifentanil is the most effective opioid to obtund the intubation response, but may cause post-intubation hypotension and occasionally neonatal respiratory depression. A number of other options, which may be used in combination, are suitable to obtund intubation responses (Table 4.22).

Inhalational (volatile) anesthetic drugs can be used. They are easily titrated, can be monitored and do not achieve fetal concentrations sufficient to cause significant neonatal drowsiness, provided there is only a few minutes' exposure before birth.

Patient Preparation and Positioning

Details of patient assessment and preparation have been described previously. Prior to general anesthesia, a checklist of requirements and equipment is useful. This should include:

- Aspiration prophylaxis (with at least an oral antacid shortly before induction)
- Ready access to a "difficult airway" cart and equipment
- Free-flowing intravenous access

Table 4.22 Intravenous Drugs that Reduce Hypertension and Tachycardia in Response to Intubation

Opioids
- fentanyl 5–10 mcg/kg (bolus)
- alfentanil 7.5–10 mcg/kg (bolus)
- remifentanil 1 mcg/kg (slow bolus over 60 seconds, with risk of post-intubation hypotension and occasionally transient neonatal respiratory depression)

Beta-blockers
- esmolol 0.5–1 mg/kg
- labetolol 25–50 mg

Magnesium 30–60 mg/kg (after intravenous anesthetic induction, to avoid maternal side effects of severe burning, flushing and headache)

Vasodilators
- nitroglycerin (glyceryl trinitrate) 250–500 mcg
- hydralazine 10–15 mg

Local anesthetics
- lidocaine (lignocaine) 1 mg/kg slowly

- Full preparation for tracheal intubation
- Attention to patient positioning (pelvic tilt and airway)
- Thorough preoxygenation (denitrogenation)

To minimize the duration of fetal exposure to maternal drugs, induction usually takes place after positioning the patient on the operating table (not in an induction room) and with the patient already, or ready to be, prepped and draped. The surgical team should likewise be gowned and gloved, and ready to start as soon as the airway is secured.

- Patient positioning must include lateral pelvic tilt (preferably to the left) by means of a pelvic or lumbar wedge or table tilt. (15 degrees table tilt may make the woman feel insecure about falling.)
- Access to the airway, especially in the morbidly obese woman, is improved by elevating the thorax and then the head on pillows, creating space at the anterior neck for easier access to the mouth and aligning the view to the larynx (Figure 4.13).
- Consider placing the woman head up 30 degrees during preoxygenation, especially if she is obese, before laying her down (this results in more rapid and effective denitrogenation and arguably less risk with regurgitation).
- Consider placing a bolster to the left side of the head, using a support or pillow, to prevent the head falling to the left after induction.

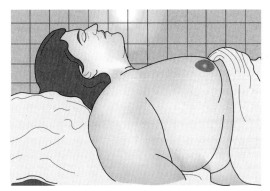

Figure 4.13 Positioning of the obese parturient to improve access to the neck and mouth and the view at direct laryngoscopy at induction of anesthesia. Note elevation of the upper torso and head and neck.

Preoxygenation

Pregnant women have higher oxygen consumption and lower oxygen stores (i.e., a reduced functional residual capacity) compared with nonpregnant individuals.

- Maternal oxygen tension falls at twice the rate of the nonpregnant woman at the onset of apnea, leading to cyanosis before intubation can be attempted if preoxygenation is not performed.
- A healthy pregnant woman given 100% inspired oxygen for two minutes achieves an arterial oxygen tension of 350–550 mmHg, such that oxygen saturation is > 90% for approximately 3–5 minutes after apnea.
- This safe period in which to control the airway and start ventilation is reduced by factors such as obesity, labor, sepsis, smoking and respiratory disease (leading to higher oxygen consumption and/or small airway closure in the supine position).

Thus, it is mandatory that all women having cesarean delivery are pre-oxygenated prior to general anesthesia.

- 100% oxygen (FiO_2 1.0) should be delivered through a circuit and tight-fitting face mask at 10 L/min (a normal capnography trace confirming no large leak).
- If the patient talks and the mask is removed briefly, the time to adequate denitrogenation is increased.

- The 25–30 degree semi-erect position may improve respiratory mechanics and speed the process, especially in the morbidly obese woman.
- End-tidal oxygen concentrations should be monitored, aiming for > 90% prior to induction (this usually requires 3 minutes at tidal ventilation but in emergency cases where time is at a premium, 6–10 repeated vital capacity breaths is sufficient).
- For obese parturients having nonelective cesarean delivery, nasopharyngeal insufflation of oxygen at 5 L/min will help maintain saturation after induction.

Intravenous Anesthetic Drugs

Sodium thiopental (thiopentone or Pentothal) has a long history of safe and effective use. It must be mixed with diluent, and high alkalinity can cause tissue necrosis if extravascular spread occurs.

- Pentothal is a barbiturate that causes more myocardial depression and less mood-enhancement during the recovery phase, compared with propofol.
- With succinylcholine, it may increase masseter tone, and airway reflexes show more activity than after propofol.

Propofol (2–2.5 mg/kg) is a phenol that controls hypertension more effectively (due to peripheral vasodilation), and shows a flatter dose-response curve (thus requiring some titration during rapid sequence induction and arguably a greater chance of "light" anesthesia post-induction) compared with pentothal.

- Propofol has good recovery characteristics, and although not endorsed for use in pregnancy, it is now widely used, especially because the availability of pentothal is diminishing in some places.
- Some anesthesiologists prefer to use propofol because of familiarity, while others reserve it for specific indications. These include severe asthma (less active airway reflexes versus pentothal) or malignant hyperthermia risk (total intravenous anesthesia).
- If continued as a maintenance infusion, propofol results in more neonatal sedation than an inhalational anesthetic.

Ketamine (1.5 mg/kg initially) is widely used in developing countries for induction and then infused for maintenance and analgesia. It is rarely used in developed countries because of its postoperative psychomimetic effects, in particular hallucinations and nightmares, although these appear less common than in nonpregnant patients.

- Ketamine increases maternal blood pressure (so is best avoided in hypertensive patients).

- It is associated with good neonatal outcomes.

- It provides more stable hemodynamics in patients who are hypovolemic (e.g., from prepartum hemorrhage), and may be combined (in reduced dose) with propofol or pentothal.

Etomidate (0.3 mg/kg) has not been adequately evaluated in obstetrics. It causes myoclonic movement and pain on injection; it may cause nausea. It provides good hemodynamic stability in the hypovolemic patient.

Rapid Sequence Induction, Cricoid Pressure and Muscle Relaxants

A typical induction sequence after preoxygenation is:

- Intravenous sodium pentothal 4–5 mg/kg or propofol 2–2.5 mg/kg.

- Application of cricoid pressure by an assistant as consciousness is lost (Figure 4.12). Cricoid pressure physically prevents regurgitated gastric content reaching the laryngeal inlet and bronchial tree by occluding the hypopharynx against the paravertebral tissues and cervical vertebrae. A trained assistant applies sufficient pressure (2–3 kg or 20–30 Newtons of force toward C_6) under instruction from the anesthesiologist. If applied too forcefully or too high near the thyroid cartilage, it may distort the laryngeal view and require remanipulation or removal, to allow intubation. Ideally, cricoid pressure should not be released until tracheal tube placement and isolation of the lungs has been confirmed.

- Intravenous succinylcholine (succinylcholine) 1.5 mg/kg (to a maximum of 150 mg).

- After fasciculations have ceased (or after 45 seconds if they are not seen) laryngoscopy and intubation are performed, and correct tube location (in trachea, above carina) confirmed clinically and by capnography.

- When neuromuscular function returns (typically 5–15 minutes after succinylcholine, the longer duration resulting from lower plasma pseudocholinesterase concentrations during pregnancy), a nondepolarizing neuromuscular blocking drug may be given (based on clinical need, such as abdominal muscle laxity and tolerance of ventilation).

- Small doses of short-acting drugs are preferable (e.g., mivacurium 0.15 mg/kg or atracurium 0.1 mg/kg) because surgery may be fast (sometimes only the initial dose of succinylcholine is required).
- Neuromuscular block should be monitored by nerve stimulation (e.g., ulnar nerve and adductor pollicis response).
- Residual paralysis should always be reversed.

Succinylcholine has some disadvantages—it is contraindicated in malignant hyperthermia and some other muscle diseases, and the risk of a serious reaction is 1 in 4,000. Myalgia however, is less frequent than in the nonpregnant population. Bradycardia may follow repeat administration. It has the fastest onset, creating good intubating conditions within 45–60 seconds.

Rocuronium has its proponents for intubation because of a good side effect profile (other than rare allergic reactions). It provides suitable intubating conditions in 60–90 seconds after a dose of 0.6–1.0 mg/kg, but until recently the resulting duration of paralysis (30–60 minutes before reversal could be attempted) was often excessive and considered dangerous in a "can't intubate, can't ventilate" scenario. **Sugammadex** (16 mg/kg) will fully reverse an intubating dose within 3 minutes, and this new drug may influence future practice.

Inhalational Anesthetics

The minimum alveolar concentration, or MAC (which reflects anesthetic drug potency for inhibition of spinal cord responses to noxious stimuli), is reduced by approximately 25% during pregnancy. Labor reduces the response to nociceptive surgical stimuli and increases the response to pentothal and sevoflurane.

To minimize periods of "light" anesthesia, aim to reach an ET-anesthetic concentration equivalent to 0.75–1 MAC (e.g., ET-sevoflurane 1.5%) as rapidly as possible after intravenous induction. The myometrium will maintain normal contractility despite the tocolytic effect of 0.5 MAC volatile anesthetic. Blood loss only increases at > 1 MAC, and the uterus responds to oxytocin at up to 1.5 MAC.

Isoflurane (ET-0.6%–0.8%), sevoflurane (ET-1.5%) and desflurane (ET-3%) are all suitable inhalational anesthetics, with slightly differing pharmacologic properties. The latter two are popular because of their rapid onset and offset. Post-induction this allows up-titration as the intravenous anesthetic effect site concentration falls rapidly. At completion of surgery, rapid arousal for awake extubation is achieved. Nitrous oxide is a useful adjunct, reducing inhalational anesthetic and analgesic requirements, and has no disadvantages after short periods of administration.

The Delivery Phase, including Fetal and Neonatal Considerations

Despite rapid placental transfer, the rapid decline in maternal intravenous anesthetic concentration after bolus injection produces a rapidly falling concentration gradient across the placenta to the fetus, which tends to minimize fetal exposure. In addition, fetal central nervous system drug exposure is limited by dilution and hepatic metabolism, such that neonatal sedation is minimal at birth irrespective of the induction to delivery interval.

- Polar drugs such as the neuromuscular blocking drugs are highly ionized, so show minimal placental transfer.
- Opioids produce dose-dependent respiratory depression in the neonate, but this is seldom severe.
- To minimize fetal exposure to inhaled anesthetics, delivery should preferably occur with 15 minutes of induction. Nitrous oxide equilibrates in maternal blood within 20–30 minutes, but umbilical venous concentrations lag well behind. Other inhalational anesthetics are even slower to equilibrate.

The impact of maternal physiological derangements, such as hypotension, hypoxemia, hypocarbia (< 25 mmHg) or hypercarbia (> 34 mmHg) on placental blood flow and gas exchange are likely to be more important than drug effects in influencing neonatal acid-base status and clinical condition at birth. The uterine incision to delivery interval is especially important, because placental blood flow declines significantly during this period.

Physiological aims during anesthesia are to:

- Ventilate to normocarbia (30–32 mmHg or 4–4.3 kPa).
- Maintain blood pressure at pre-anesthetic levels.
- Keep oxygenation saturation satisfactory (> 95%).

Although fetal oxygen tension in the umbilical vein and artery increase with higher maternal inspired oxygen and oxygenation (Figure 4.14), this confers no apparent benefit to the healthy neonate

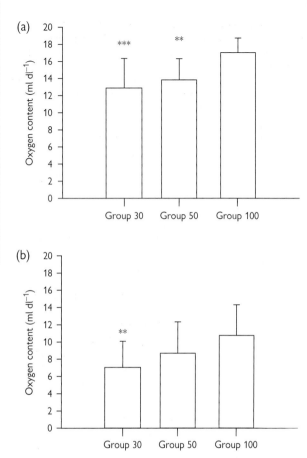

Figure 4.14 Effect of maternal oxygenation on neonatal oxygenation during general anesthesia for cesarean delivery. Umbilical venous (a) and arterial (b) cord blood oxygen content after administration of maternal inspired oxygen of 30%, 50% or 100% from induction of general anesthesia at cesarean delivery. ** P < 0.01 compared with group 100. *** P < 0.001 compared with group 100. Reprinted with permission from Ngan Kee WD, et al. Randomized double-blind comparison of different inspired oxygen fractions during general anaesthesia for Caesarean section. *Br J Anaesthesia.* 2009;103:559 Figure 1.

at birth. The hypoxemic fetus may achieve higher oxygen tensions when 100% inspired maternal oxygen is supplied, but toxic oxygen free radical formation increases, so it is unclear whether high maternal inspired oxygen is of outcome benefit.

Intravenous synthetic oxytocin is given immediately after delivery to reduce postpartum bleeding and increase uterine tone, usually by IV bolus (1–5 iu) and by infusion (5–30 iu/h).

- Oxytocin has a rapid onset (within 1–2 minutes) but a short half-life and brief duration of clinical effect (5–15 minutes).
- The optimal uterotonic dose is uncertain. The "Product Information" dose of 5 iu is commonly used but at elective cesarean delivery the 95% effective dose is < 1 iu (with down-regulation of receptors increasing this to 3 iu after oxytocin exposure during labor). A dose of 2 iu appears as effective as 5 iu at scheduled cesarean delivery.
- Oxytocin causes vasodilation (mild blood pressure reduction), tachycardia, and increased cardiac output after rapid administration.
- Side effects such as palpations, nausea, headache and flushing occur. Bolus administration should be omitted for women in whom the increase in cardiac work might precipitate cardiac failure, ischemia or even cardiac arrest (e.g., severe valvular or subvalvular stenosis; ischemic heart disease, uncompensated hypovolemia).

Postdelivery, an intravenous opioid such as fentanyl 3–5 mcg/kg or morphine 0.1–0.15 mg/kg is given to provide analgesia at arousal. Alternate or adjunctive methods of postoperative analgesia, including transversus abdominis plane blocks (Chapter 5) can be used.

The Extubation Phase

If a woman has eaten recently or has gastric stasis (e.g., a diabetic patient with autonomic neuropathy), passing a large bore orogastric tube to suction the stomach should be considered during anesthesia. As surgery ends, inhalational anesthetics are reduced and ceased, aiming for end-tidal values of 0.1 MAC as quickly as possible.

- If neuromuscular function requires reversal (train-of-four ratio < 0.9) then neostigmine 20–50 mcg/kg and either glycopyrrolate 10 mcg/kg or atropine 20 mcg/kg (or after rocuronium or vecuronium, in the future possibly sugammadex) should be given.
- Extubation is safest if conducted with the woman in the left lateral position (to prevent aspiration after regurgitation).

- Extubation should be delayed until the patient is breathing adequately, has functioning airway reflexes, and responds to command.
- Supplemental oxygen should be given post-extubation.

Management of Complications of General Anesthesia

Aspiration

Characteristics

Aspiration pneumonitis is a rare complication that is thought to be more common in pregnancy as a result of the gastrointestinal changes that predispose to regurgitation (Chapter 2). Hormonal relaxation of the lower esophageal sphincter begins in the first trimester, and reflux symptoms are very common in late pregnancy, exacerbated by the effect of the expanding abdominal contents on the angle and function of the gastro-esophageal sphincter.

- Many cases of aspiration now occur outside the immediate perioperative period (e.g., in sedated or unconscious women in the intensive care unit, or after collapse or seizure).
- The rate of regurgitation during general anesthesia for cesarean delivery is 1 in 100–200.
- The rate of significant aspiration associated with general anesthesia is very low (estimate 1 in 600–2,000) but is twice as likely at non-elective cesarean delivery. This low incidence of clinical aspiration has been attributed to:
  - the predominant use of regional anesthesia
  - the use of rapid sequence induction for general anesthesia
  - pharmacological aspiration prophylaxis
- Improved critical care has led to a falling mortality rate (estimated < 5%).

Prevention of Aspiration

A number of measures to prevent aspiration are appropriate (Table 4.10 and Figure 4.15):

- Fasting
  - Guidelines such as ASA's *Practice Guidelines for Obstetric Anesthesia* and ACOG's *Committee Opinion on Oral Intake during Labor* describe accepted practice for oral intake in parturients. Labor is unpredictable, however, and the need to deliver takes precedence over fasting status.

- Pregnancy per se does not alter gastric emptying, but pain during labor and opioid analgesia markedly impair emptying (women entering labor may retain solids for many hours).
- Reduction of gastric acidity (gastric content of pH > 3 is much less likely to cause lung injury)
- Prevention of regurgitation into the hypopharynx on induction of anesthesia by effective application of cricoid pressure.

Management of Aspiration

Whenever consciousness or airway reflexes are significantly impaired or lost, airway protection by intubation is warranted. Despite a lack of

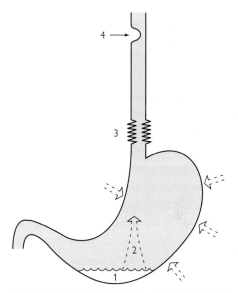

Figure 4.15 Measures directed at preventing aspiration pneumonitis associated with obstetric anesthesia. (1) Emptying of solids from the stomach and reduction of gastric fluid volume and acidity. (2) Prevention of sudden increases in intragastric pressure. (3) Prevention of fall in lower esophageal sphincter pressure and reflux. (4) Cricoid pressure to prevent regurgitation into the pharynx; and maintenance of active upper airway and laryngeal reflexes to prevent aspiration into the trachea. With kind permission from Springer Science: *Canadian Journal of Anesthesia*, The stomach: factors of importance to the anaesthetist, vol. 37, 1990, p. 902, Davies JM.

evidence for outcome benefit, cricoid pressure should be used until the lungs are isolated. Both induction and extubation are times of regurgitation risk, so safe patient positioning and timing of extubation are important.

If regurgitation is witnessed and aspiration is suspected, the airway should be assessed for soiling. If possible and appropriate, suctioning of both the upper airway and tracheobronchial tree, preferably under bronchoscopic vision, should be performed prior to controlled ventilation.

- The gastric fluid pH should be checked if feasible (for prognostic purposes).
- Patient assessment includes physical examination of the chest and observation for postoperative dyspnea, cough, and fever.
- Respiratory function should be closely monitored, with assessment of oxygenation (pulse oximetry, arterial blood gas analysis). A chest X-ray looking for evidence of infiltrates or consolidation should be done (though signs may not appear for several hours).
- A decision should be made as to whether controlled ventilation is required and, if so, what ventilatory support strategies, increased inspired oxygen, and respiratory care are needed.

The best environment for continuing respiratory care will be dependent on each facility's resources; this may be the labor ward, the postnatal unit, or the intensive care unit.

- Antibiotics are given based on microbiological evidence of infection.

Failed Intubation

Despite the infrequent use of general anesthesia for cesarean section, complications of airway management comprise a large proportion of "closed claims" and are the leading cause of anesthesia-related maternal death. There is some evidence that the incidence of the latter is falling, and epidemiological data shows that general anesthesia for cesarean delivery can be exceptionally safe. Nevertheless, airway assessment and management planning are anesthetic priorities whenever professional contact is made with a pregnant woman.

During pregnancy, the incidence of difficult intubation is much higher because of anatomical changes (fat deposition in the face, neck and chest, mucosal edema of the upper airway and occasionally larynx, and difficulty in optimizing the position of the patient).

- Maternal outcomes associated with difficult intubation are affected by the parturient's higher oxygen consumption and lower oxygen reserve, as well as concurrent medical conditions and obesity (obesity may be independently associated with a greater risk of difficult airway management).
- General anesthesia is often required for nonelective cesarean delivery when time pressure is great, and failed intubation occurs more frequently in urgent cases conducted by less experienced anesthesiologists.

Dealing safely with the airway is of primary importance. Concern has been raised that training and experience (which has fallen with the decreased use of general anesthesia in most developed countries) may be insufficient. This has increased the importance of simulation training and "failed intubation drills."

Case series and cohort studies suggest that 1 in 15–20 women will be assessed as likely to be difficult, and 1 in 20–50 will prove difficult to intubate.

- The incidence of abandoned ("failed") intubation at general anesthesia is 1 in 250–3000 (most cases being a grade 3 view at direct laryngoscopy), the incidence varying according to the experience and familiarity of the attending anesthesiologists.
- The incidence of "can't intubate, can't ventilate" situations during general anesthesia for cesarean delivery is estimated as 1 in 5,000–10,000.
- Regurgitation may be associated with difficult airway management and occurs in 1 in 100–200 general anesthetics for cesarean delivery.
- Severe hypoxemia occurs in 1 in 50, and other airway complications (bronchospasm, laryngospasm) in 1 in 100, general anesthetics.

Assessment and Planning

Management of the difficult airway starts with assessment (Table 4.9) and planning. Obstetricians must be encouraged to refer women who are of known or predicted difficulty. Early epidural catheterization during labor is a wise strategy. When difficulty is predicted, regional anesthesia is the best option, but preparedness for general anesthesia remains essential in case of high or failed block. Awake fiberoptic intubation may be required if regional anesthesia is contraindicated, and some obstetricians have the expertise to perform the surgery under local anesthesia.

Specific Equipment

An array of special devices and equipment must be available to the anesthesiologist in the operating area. This might include:

- Short-handle, Bullard or videolaryngoscopes (e.g., the Pentax Airway Scope AWS-S100, the Glidescope®, the AirTraq®)
- A fiberoptic laryngoscope
- Stylettes, bougies, small (e.g., 6.0 mm) internal diameter tracheal tubes, tube exchange catheters
- An intubating (Fastrach®) laryngeal mask, ProSeal® laryngeal mask, other supraglottic airway devices or a Combitube®
- Cricothyrotomy devices and percutaneous tracheostomy sets

A variety of awake intubation techniques have been described, but all require expertise and may be time-consuming. When possible, give pre-procedural aspiration prophylaxis and optimize topical anesthesia of the airway with lidocaine gels and spray.

- Consider mild sedation (e.g., remifentanil or midazolam) and drying of secretions with an anticholinergic (glycopyrrolate, which has minimal placental transfer).
- Use the oral route if possible to avoid nasal trauma and epistaxis.

Dealing with a Difficult Intubation

When difficult intubation occurs after induction of anesthesia, the plan must focus on:

- Oxygenation (oxygen desaturation will always occur before spontaneous ventilation resumes).
- Prevention of airway trauma.

A number of practice guidelines (e.g., the ASA) exist for nonobstetric patients, but are not specific to obstetric patients and situations, which are complicated by the considerations pertaining to the fetus. An example of a very simplified approach for a situation in which there is an immediate threat to the life of the fetus, based on two pathways, representing adequate mask ventilation versus inadequate ventilation, is outlined in Table 4.23.

- Attention to optimal patient positioning is paramount, especially in obese women, including elevation of the head and shoulders above the chest (Figure 4.13). Also, head support is helpful to prevent displacement as a result of left table tilt.
- Incorrectly applied cricoid pressure (Figure 4.12) can worsen the laryngoscopic view; so adjust it early (e.g., by requesting less

Table 4.23 Simplified Unanticipated Failed Intubation Management Algorithm

Grade 3 or 4 laryngoscopic view on induction

Provided patient is still well oxygenated, the most experienced anesthesiologist should make a second attempt to intubate under optimal conditions
- Adjust head or neck position
- Adjust cricoid pressure
- Apply thyroid cartilage pressure
- Change laryngoscope
- Intubate with a bougie and smaller tracheal tube

Declare failed intubation and call for help
- Maintain cricoid pressure and left pelvic tilt
- Do not give more neuromuscular blocking drug
- Oxygenate
- Ventilate via face mask
  - use two hands to open the airway, maximize jaw thrust and seal, insert an oral airway and get a second person to "bag"
- Insert and ventilate using LMA, Proseal LMA, Intubating LMA, i-gel
  - maintain cricoid pressure unless impeding placement of airway device or ventilation

Decide whether to:

Wake the patient (change to combined spinal epidural anesthesia or awake intubation)

or

Continue surgery (only if airway controlled and oxygenation satisfactory)
- Allow spontaneous ventilation to resume and maintain anesthesia with rapid onset/offset inhaled anesthetic in 100% oxygen

If unable to oxygenate / ventilate ("can't intubate, can't ventilate") use preferred cricothroidotomy technique
- Percutaneous needle / cannula technique with jet ventilation
- Scalpel, finger and bougie / tracheal tube technique
- Melker size 5.0 Seldinger airway technique

pressure, pushing to the right or higher on the thyroid cartilage) and release it completely if necessary—the first priority is effective ventilation and oxygenation.
- Call for help as soon as possible!
- Repeat doses of succinylcholine should not usually be given—maintaining spontaneous ventilation after control of a difficult airway is the safest option.
- A second, optimal attempt at intubation can be made, provided oxygenation is satisfactory and airway trauma can be avoided.

Nasal instrumentation and repeated impacts on the larynx are best avoided.

- A supraglottic airway device, such as the laryngeal mask, may prove easier to insert and allow oxygenation.
  - An intubating (Fastrach®) laryngeal mask allows subsequent blind or preferably fiberoptic-guided intubation.
  - The ProSeal® laryngeal mask adds protection against aspiration and is designed to allow intermittent positive pressure ventilation.
  - The i-gel airway has also been used.

If oxygenation can be achieved, then allowing the woman to wake is the safest approach; if oxygenation can be achieved but there is immediate danger to the life of the fetus, then continuing the operation using face or laryngeal mask ventilation, preferably with cricoid pressure still applied, can be considered.

If cricothrotomy is required because of severe hypoxemia, the method most familiar to the anesthesiologist should be attempted.

Awareness

Awareness refers to explicit recall of intraoperative events. The most commonly described events are sounds, conversation and tactile sensations (e.g., intubation), with visual and emotional memories and pain less frequent. As a result of the physiological changes of pregnancy and concern about fetal drug exposure, pregnant women having cesarean delivery represent a high-risk population (Table 4.24).

Awareness is reported at a rate of 1 in 150–400 (higher than the overall incidence in anesthesia of 1 in 500–1,000). It should be specifically discussed when obtaining consent for general anesthesia for cesarean delivery. If awareness occurs, it is likely to cause patient dissatisfaction.

- Some women have long-term psychological disturbance, with symptoms such as anxiety, phobia, sleep and mood disturbance.
- This "post-traumatic stress disorder" may lead to litigation.

Contributors to Awareness

Although awareness can occur despite the best of care, the main antecedents are:

- Human error, including inadvertent failure to administer anesthetic (e.g., a syringe swap of cephalosporin antibiotic for pentothal or of succinylcholine for fentanyl).
- Failure to provide adequate anesthetic agent, through inappropriate dosing or failure of drug delivery (e.g., an empty or turned off vaporizer).

Table 4.24 Reasons for Higher Risk of Awareness during General Anesthesia for Cesarean Delivery

High cardiac output during pregnancy
• rapid redistribution of intravenous anesthetic from effect sites and slower uptake of volatile anesthetic drugs
Uncertainty about intravenous drug dosing (based on pre-pregnancy or current body weight?)
Avoidance of intravenous opioids until after delivery
Higher rate of airway difficulty and thus delayed delivery of inhalational anesthetics
Limitation of volatile anesthetic delivery based on:
• concern about uterine myometrial relaxation and bleeding
• concern about maternal hypotension (especially in presence of antepartum hemorrhage or hemodynamic compromise)
• concern about neonatal effects

- Inadequate vigilance (e.g., failure to give more intravenous anesthetic during multiple attempts to establish a clear airway).
- Constrained drug administration (e.g., during severe hemodynamic compromise or in patients with poor cardiac reserve).
- Increased patient requirements for anesthesia, which may be genetic (e.g., past history of awareness during apparently uneventful anesthesia) or drug-related (e.g., chronic benzodiazepine use).

Prevention of Awareness

A number of practice changes and new technologies have been introduced with a view to reducing awareness. These address hastening the transition from intravenous induction to inhalational anesthetic maintenance, or means of detecting an inadequate depth of anesthesia. For general anesthesia for cesarean delivery these strategies include:

- More liberal use of opioids prior to delivery.
- Use of rapid uptake volatile anesthetics (e.g., sevoflurane, desflurane).
- Rapid uptitration of volatile anesthetic using agent monitoring ("overpressure" with high initial concentrations, to rapidly increase end-tidal concentration to at least 0.75 MAC after intravenous induction).
- Depth of anesthesia (brain function) monitoring (e.g., bispectral index [BIS]).
  - Pentothal (2–2.5 mg/kg) is being more widely used for intravenous induction, although an argument can be made that sodium pentothal 4–5 mg/kg more consistently achieves an adequate depth

of anesthesia. End-tidal anesthetic monitoring and BIS monitoring can reduce the risk of awareness but the number-needed-to-treat is high.

- To achieve BIS values within the range at which the chance of consciousness is very low (i.e., < 55–60) requires, for example, an end-tidal sevoflurane concentration of 1.5% in 50% nitrous oxide.

Management of the Patient Reporting Awareness

A patient reporting awareness needs consultation to ascertain exactly what has been recalled, using a structured series of questions (Table 4.25). If the story is convincing, or lack of adequate anesthesia has clearly occurred, frank discussion is warranted and clinical psychology services should also be used to support and counsel the patient and to organize ongoing review.

Venous Air Embolism

Mechanisms and Background

Air may enter the venous circulation whenever venous pressure at the site of surgery is near or below atmospheric pressure (gradients 2.5–5 cm water). This is the case when the surgical site is elevated compared with the heart and pertains at cesarean delivery in the supine position, when large venous sinuses are frequently open.

- Small air emboli occur most commonly between uterine incision and closure.
- The risk of air entrainment may be increased if the uterus is exteriorized (placing it well above the level of the heart).
- The incidence of subclinical air microemboli is approximately 90%–95% based on changes in end-tidal nitrogen and 40%–70% based on Doppler changes (detection of 0.1 ml bubbles).

Table 4.25 Patient Questionnaire to Evaluate Possible Awareness
Ask:
• What is the last thing you remember before going to sleep?
• What was the first thing you remembered when you woke up?
• Can you recall anything between?
• Did you have any dreams during your anesthetic?
If any evidence of awareness is encountered, obtain a narrative and decide whether awareness was unlikely, possible or probable.

- A large air embolus causing an air lock in the right heart (estimated volume > 100 ml), leading to cardiovascular collapse, is exceptionally rare.

The physiologic consequences depend on the volume of air and speed of entrainment, the amount of time air is trapped within the right atrium and ventricle (which may be up to 20 minutes), the degree of obstruction to the pulmonary circulation, and the patient's comorbidities. The cardiovascular response to embolized air includes:

- increased pulmonary and right heart pressures
- reduced or arrested cardiac output
- ventilation-perfusion mismatch and hypoxemia
- coronary artery ischemia.

Diagnosis

The detection of venous air embolism is based on monitoring and detection of its pathophysiologic consequences.

- Doppler ultrasound is very sensitive but not specific, often detecting turbulent flow. It is not clinically useful given the high frequency of microemboli.
- Central venous pressure or transthoracic/transesophageal echocardiography may reveal air bubbles, but are not indicated routinely.
- A small rise in ET-nitrogen concentration during gas monitoring is very sensitive but not likely to be of clinical relevance.
- A rapid fall in end-tidal carbon dioxide is an early feature of a large embolus that mandates immediate action.
- Oxygen desaturation will follow a clinically significant embolus.
- A "mill-wheel" murmur probably only develops with a large volume of air.

Depending on the size of the air embolus, cardiovascular changes may be absent, minor or severe (including cardiac arrest).

- Chest pain, dyspnea and loss of consciousness are manifestations during regional anesthesia.
- Seizures may result from cerebral hypoxia.
- Focal neurological deficits can result from paradoxical embolism through a patent foramen ovale, resulting in cerebral air emboli.

Management

The suggested plan of management of a large venous air embolus causing clinical compromise is shown in Table 4.26. Aspiration of air through a central venous catheter should be attempted in compromised

Table 4.26 **Management of Large Venous Air Embolism**
Stop air entrainment
• Advise the obstetrician of the suspected diagnosis
• Ask the obstetrician to flood the wound with saline and close any open vessels
• Consider placing the patient slightly head up
Supportive cardiorespiratory therapy
• Give 100% oxygen, cease nitrous oxide and ventilate if required
• Administer vasoactive drugs (metaraminol, phenylephrine, norepinephrine) to support the blood pressure
• If circulation is present, consider placing the patient in the left lateral position to float the air bubble away from the pulmonary inflow tract in the right ventricle
• If circulation is inadequate or absent, commence advanced life support, in particular external cardiac massage, to disperse the air lock from the right heart into the pulmonary circulation
Rapidly insert a central venous catheter
• Attempt aspiration of air from the right atrium and ventricle

patients, as the most rapid means of potentially restoring the circulation. The best position in which to place the patient is unknown and controversial. The lateral head-down position has been suggested to minimize pulmonary inflow obstruction, but reverse Trendelenburg position to lower the uterus below the level of the heart, and supine or slight head-up to prevent movement of gas into the pulmonary circulation and to aid aspiration from the right heart, have also been suggested.

Further Reading

1. Benhamou D, Wong C. Neuraxial anesthesia for cesarean delivery: what criteria define the "optimal" technique? (editorial) *Anesth Analg.* 2009; 109:1370-1373.

2. Levy DM. Emergency Caesarean section: best practice. *Anaesthesia.* 2006;61:786-791.

3. Reynolds F, Seed PT. Anaesthesia for Caesarean section and neonatal acid-base status: a meta-analysis. *Anaesthesia.* 2005;60:636-653.

4. Morgan P. Spinal anaesthesia in obstetrics. *Can J Anaesth.* 1995;42: 1145-1163.

5. Thompson KD, Paech MJ. The use of combined spinal epidural anaesthesia for elective caesarean section is a waste of time and money. *Int J Obstet Anesth.* 2001;10:30-35.

6. Cyna AM, Andrew M, Emmett RS, *et al.* Techniques for preventing hypotension during spinal anaesthesia for caesarean section. *Cochrane Database of Systematic Reviews 2006*, Issue 4. Art. No.: CD002251. DOI: 10.1002/14651858.CD002251.pub2.

7. Alonso E, Gilsanz F, Gredilla E, *et al.* Observational study of continuous spinal anesthesia with the catheter-over-needle technique for cesarean delivery. *Int J Obstet Anesth.* 2009;18:137-141.

8. Lipman S, Carvalho B, Brock-Utne J. The demise of general anesthesia in obstetrics revisited: prescription for a cure. (editorial) *Int J Obstet Anesth.* 2005;14:2-4.

9. MJ Paech, KL Scott, OM Clavisi, *et al.* and the ANZCA Trials Group. A prospective study of awareness and recall associated with general anaesthesia for caesarean section. *Int J Obstet Anesth.* 2008; 17:298-303.

10. NJ McDonnell, MJ Paech, OM Clavisi, *et al.* and the ANZCA Trials Group. Difficult and failed intubation in obstetric anaesthesia: an observational study of airway management and complications associated with general anaesthesia for caesarean section. *Int J Obstet Anesth.* 2008; 17:292-297.

11. Levy DM, Meek T. Traditional rapid sequence induction is an outmoded technique for caesarean section and should be modified. *Int J Obstet Anesth.* 2006;15:227-232.

Chapter 5

Post-Cesarean Analgesia

Craig M. Palmer, MD

Introduction

In 1979, Wang and colleagues reported that epidural morphine provided effective, long-lasting analgesia in patients suffering cancer pain. This report sparked a surge of innovation in our approach not only to post-cesarean analgesia, but also to most acute postsurgical pain control. The ensuing three decades have brought an enormous number of reports describing novel analgesic approaches following cesarean delivery, which continue to this day.

Cesarean delivery is the most frequently performed inpatient operation in the United States, and probably throughout the world. Given our understanding of postoperative pain management in this population, planning an anesthetic for cesarean delivery should also include planning for adequate postoperative analgesia.

For many years, intramuscular narcotics were the mainstay of analgesia after cesarean delivery; in some settings, they may still be used. Recent decades, however, have seen a major shift in methods of postoperative analgesia in obstetric patients, due to our improved understanding of CNS pharmacology, and improvements in technology.

Informing the Patient

Just as every elective anesthetic should begin with a discussion of options with the patient, parturients should be informed about options for postoperative pain management before their cesarean delivery is undertaken. While most practices tend to use a single form of postoperative pain control on all their cesarean patients, that method may not be appropriate for all women.

- It is important for anesthesiologists to be familiar with and maintain a number of options at their disposal.
- Each option discussed below may have differing advantages and disadvantages that patients should be informed about.
- Patients should be informed of the possibility of side effects, and the availability of supplemental analgesia if necessary.

Epidural Opioids

Epidural Morphine

As noted above, in 1979, the first reports were published showing that epidural morphine was effective for relief of cancer pain. Shortly thereafter, a number of studies reported epidural morphine to be effective for post-cesarean analgesia in doses ranging from 2 to 10 mg. Morphine is currently the most widely used epidural opioid for analgesia after cesarean section.

Analgesia following epidural morphine for post-cesarean pain relief follows a consistent dose-response relationship. As the dose of epidural morphine increases, analgesia improves, until the dose reaches about 4 mg (Figures 5.1 and 5.2). Increasing the dose beyond this level does not further improve analgesia, but does tend to increase side effects. A minimum volume of 5 to 6 ml should be used; most commonly, epidural morphine is administered at a concentration of 0.5 mg/ml. Some reports indicate improved analgesia with total diluent volumes of 10 to 12 ml.

The optimal dose of epidural morphine is approximately 4 mg, which provides 18 to 24 hours of good to excellent analgesia.

- As with any medication, there is interindividual variation, but for the most part, parturients respond remarkably consistently.
- If a patient does not have a good response to this dose of epidural morphine, an increased dose will usually not prove effective (assuming the first dose reached the epidural space).

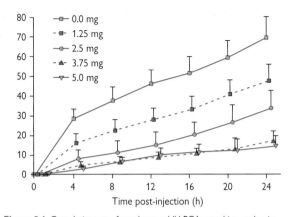

Figure 5.1 Cumulative use of supplemental IV-PCA morphine analgesia after increasing doses of epidural morphine. Reprinted with permission from Palmer CM, Nogami WM, Van Maren G, Alves D. Post-cesarean epidural morphine: a dose response study. *Anesth Analg.* 2000;90(4):887–891.

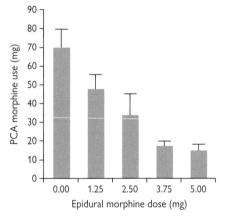

Figure 5.2 Cumulative 24-hour PCA morphine use with increasing dose of epidural morphine. As dose of epidural morphine increases from 0 to 5 mg, self-administered PCA morphine use for supplemental analgesia decreases until the dose reaches approximately 4 mg. Reprinted with permission from Palmer CM, Nogami WM, Van Maren G, Alves D. Post-cesarean epidural morphine: a dose response study. *Anesth Analg.* 2000;90(4):887–891.

- For failures of analgesia following epidural morphine, it is usually more efficacious to institute systemic analgesia, such as IV-PCA (see below).

Even at a dose of 4 to 5 mg, due to interindividual differences, some patients will require supplementation with other systemic analgesics. A higher failure rate (i.e., diminished analgesia) becomes apparent if the dose is reduced below 3 mg.

Side Effects of Epidural Morphine

While an effective analgesic, epidural morphine can have significant side effects.

Pruritus

Pruritus is the most consistently reported side effect after epidural morphine administration. In some series, the incidence approaches 100%. While not every parturient will volunteer the symptom, most will acknowledge it upon questioning (Figure 5.3).

- Pruritus associated with epidural morphine is usually mild.
- It occurs most often on the face or trunk, but may be generalized.
- Pruritus after epidural morphine is not significantly dose-related.

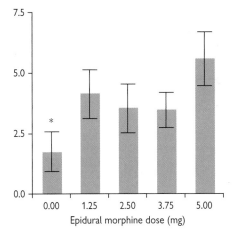

Figure 5.3 Cumulative 24-hour pruritus scores after varying doses of epidural morphine. The control group, Group 0, was significantly lower than the four epidural morphine groups, which were not significantly different from each other. Unpublished data from Palmer CM.

The exact mechanism by which epidural morphine causes pruritus is unknown. The available evidence indicates it to be more complex than a simple μ-receptor related phenomenon. The role of opioid receptors in pruritus may be primarily by facilitation of other excitatory neuronal pathways and protective reflexes. A full understanding of the phenomenon awaits further investigation.

Nausea and Vomiting

Nausea and vomiting are less frequent than pruritus after epidural morphine.

The reported incidence ranges from 11% to about 30%. Some series have indicated that nausea and vomiting after epidural morphine administration may not be different than placebo, and may actually be secondary to the surgery itself (see "Intrathecal Morphine" below).

Possible Mechanism

Epidural morphine can cause nausea and vomiting by stimulating the chemoreceptor trigger zone located in the base of the fourth ventricle of the brain. Morphine, which is highly hydrophilic, remains free (unbound) in the cerebrospinal fluid (CSF) for a significantly longer time than more lipophilic opioids (i.e., fentanyl or sufentanil).

Respiratory Depression

Shortly after the introduction of epidural morphine to clinical use, respiratory depression was recognized as a potentially serious complication. The risk at clinically used doses is quite low, however. A retrospective review of 4880 parturients receiving epidural morphine after cesarean delivery found a respiratory rate below 10 in only 12 patients, or 0.25%. A prospective study of 1000 parturients who received 5 mg epidural morphine reported 4 patients with a respiratory rate of below 10 (0.4%). Such reports indicate that the incidence of clinically significant respiratory depression after epidural morphine (at doses of 5 mg or less) in the obstetric population is at most 0.2%–0.3%.

Characteristics

Respiratory depression after epidural morphine is typically described as "late"; i.e., occurring 3–10 hours after administration.

- It is manifested as a gradual decline in respiratory rate, which leads to respiratory acidosis.
- Ventilatory support may be necessary if diagnosis is delayed, but it is readily reversed by naloxone.

The risk of respiratory depression likely increases with increasing dose (especially over 5 mg). Risk also increases significantly when other depressant medications are administered concurrently, such as:

- additional opioids
- anxiolytics
- sleep aids
- magnesium.

Concurrent conditions that may increase the risk of respiratory depression after epidural morphine include:

- obesity
- sleep apnea.

The characteristic "delayed onset" of respiratory depression after epidural morphine is due to slow cephalad migration within the CSF which can cause direct central depression of respiration. Morphine concentration in cervical CSF peaks 3–4 hours after injection (Figure 5.4).

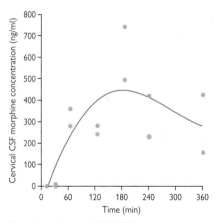

Figure 5.4 Cervical cerebrospinal fluid (CSF) morphine concentrations vs. time in patients after lumbar epidural administration of 10 mg epidural morphine. Reprinted with permission from Gourlay GK, Cherry DA, Cousins MJ. Cephalad migration of morphine in CSF following lumbar epidural administration in patients with cancer pain. *Pain*. 1985;23:317–326. This figure has been reproduced with permission of the International Association for the Study of Pain (IASP). The figure may not be reproduced for any other purpose without permission.

"Early" respiratory depression, within minutes after injection of epidural morphine, is also possible. This event probably arises from rapid systemic uptake or intravascular injection of the drug.

Treatment of Side Effects (Table 5.1)

Side effects of epidural morphine are generally mild. In most cases they do not require treatment.

Pruritus

Most cases of pruritus are mild and do not require treatment. When it becomes bothersome to the patient, options include:

- Diphenhydramine, 12.5–25 mg intravenously. The sedation associated with diphenhydramine may be as instrumental in providing relief as its antihistaminergic effect.
- Nalbuphine (5 mg intravenously) is an effective treatment for pruritus without significant side effects. At this dose, pruritus is effectively reversed, but analgesia is not affected.
- In rare cases, naloxone may be necessary to relieve severe pruritus (0.04–0.2 mg intravenously, followed by a continuous infusion—start at 0.4–0.6 mg/h and titrate as needed).
- Other treatments, including propofol, droperidol, and ondansetron, have been reported effective in treating pruritus, but are generally either too costly, or have significant side effects themselves.

Nausea and Vomiting

Treatment options for nausea and vomiting include antiemetics and opioid antagonists. As noted above, nausea and vomiting in this setting may be a consequence of the surgical procedure itself, *not* the epidural morphine, and conventional antiemetics are a better first option.

Table 5.1 Side Effects of Epidural Morphine			
Side effect	Incidence	Treatment	Comments
Pruritus	Up to 100%	Nalbuphine 5 mg IV or diphenhydramine 12.5–25 mg IV or naloxone 0.04–0.2 mg IV	Usually mild Naloxone rarely necessary
Nausea and vomiting	10–30%	Droperidol 0.625 mg IV or ondansetron 4 mg IV or nalbuphine 5–10 mg IV	Usually not related to epidural morphine
Respiratory depression	<0.25%	Naloxone 0.2–0.4 mg IV Assisted ventilation if necessary	Very rare in healthy parturients

- Intravenous ondansetron, 4 mg, or a similar antiemetic, is generally an effective treatment.
- Intravenous nalbuphine, 5–10 mg, or very low-dose naloxone, can relieve nausea and vomiting that is truly opioid-related.

Respiratory Depression

Early or late, the treatment of choice for respiratory depression is intravenous naloxone.

- Respiratory depression after epidural morphine does not have an abrupt onset. It is heralded by a gradual decrease in respiratory rate, and increasing somnolence. Monitoring protocols (in postoperative orders) are intended to detect this decline in respiratory rate and increased levels of sedation (see below). Such protocols are effective in identifying these infrequent patients early, when milder forms of treatment (supplemental nasal oxygen, encouragement to deep breathing) can be effective.
- Institute artificial or mechanical support of ventilation immediately if the patient is obtunded while waiting for naloxone to have effect.

Preemptive Therapy

Preemptive therapy to prevent the side effects of epidural morphine has been largely disappointing.

- While a number of treatments can prevent side effects, they generally also either decrease analgesia or cause side effects of their own.
- Intravenous naloxone and oral naltrexone can prevent side effects, but both decrease analgesia in a dose-dependent fashion.
- Epidural butorphanol modestly decreases side effects, but causes somnolence.
- Prophylactic transdermal scopolamine decreases the incidence of nausea and vomiting during the first 24 hours after cesarean delivery, but must be applied several hours in advance, and causes dry mouth.

Other Epidural Opioids

Fentanyl

Epidural fentanyl, 50–100 mcg, rapidly provides profound analgesia for up to 4 hours (Figure 5.5).

- Increasing the dose of epidural fentanyl beyond 100 mcg does not improve or prolong pain relief.
- Epidural fentanyl can cause all the same side effects as morphine, though in a shorter time frame.

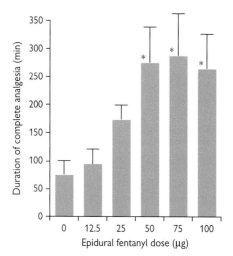

Figure 5.5 Duration of complete analgesia (visual analog pain score of 0) after doses of epidural fentanyl ranging from 0 to 100 mcg. Data are mean (standard error). Reprinted with permission from Naulty JS, Datta S, Ostheimer GW. Epidural fentanyl for post-cesarean delivery pain management. *Anesthesiology*. 1985;63(6):694–698.

- While useful as an intraoperative adjunct during epidural anesthesia for cesarean delivery (Figure 5.6), fentanyl's short duration limits its utility as a postoperative analgesic.

Sufentanil

Like fentanyl, the major advantage of epidural sufentanil over epidural morphine is its rapid onset.

- The incidence of side effects is comparable to, or higher than, equianalgesic doses of epidural morphine. Larger doses (up to 50 ug) provide analgesia for up to 4 hours.
- Little data is available to evaluate the risk of respiratory depression. When given intravenously at these doses, sufentanil can produce profound respiratory depression.

Others

- **Meperidine (pethidine).** The speed of onset and duration of analgesia from epidural meperidine (pethidine) increase as the dose increases up to about 25 mg, but further increasing the dose

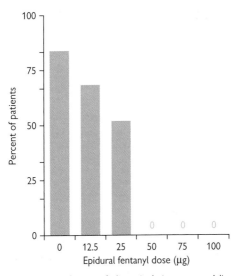

Figure 5.6 Percentage of patients feeling pain during cesarean delivery under epidural anesthesia vs. dose of epidural fentanyl. At doses above 50 mcg, no patient complained of pain. Reprinted with permission from Naulty JS, Datta S, Ostheimer GW. Epidural fentanyl for post-cesarean delivery pain management. *Anesthesiology.* 1985;63(6):694–698.

provides no additional benefit (Table 5.2). Pain relief lasts about 2.5 hrs, and while side effects are infrequent, clinical utility is limited by its short duration.

- **Hydromorphone** is a semisynthetic derivative of morphine. A dose of 1.0 mg provides analgesia comparable to 5 mg epidural morphine, but the duration of action is considerably shorter, about 12 hrs. The side effect profile is similar to morphine.
- **Methadone** has a more rapid onset than epidural morphine, but the duration of analgesia after 4 to 5 mg is only 5 to 6 hrs.
- **Diamorphine (heroin)** has been used as an epidural analgesic, but reports of the duration of analgesia are inconsistent, ranging from 5 to 15 hrs after 2.5 to 5 mg.

Mixed Agonist/Antagonist Opioids

- **Butorphanol** has a faster onset but a shorter duration than epidural morphine. The low incidence of pruritus after epidural

Table 5.2 Summary of Epidural Opioid Options			
Opioid	Dose	Reported duration (hours)	Comments
Morphine	3.5–4 mg	18–24	"Gold standard"
Fentanyl	50 mcg	Up to 4	Useful as an intraoperative analgesic
Sufentanil	10–20 mcg	Approx. 3	Also useful intraoperatively
Meperidine	25 mg	2–3	Local anesthetic effects
Hydromorphone	1.0 mg	Approx. 12	
Methadone	4–5 mg	5–6	
Diamorphine	2.5–5 mg	5–15	Heroin—not available in the USA

butorphanol is its major advantage, but the short duration and high incidence of somnolence are significant shortcomings.

- **Nalbuphine** is another mixed opioid agonist/antagonist. The duration of analgesia increases as the dose is increased from 10 mg to 30 mg, from about one hour to three hours. Its only significant side effect is somnolence, seen in up to 50% of patients after 30 mg. The safety of neuraxial nalbuphine has not been carefully evaluated, however, so its use cannot be recommended.

Extended-Release Epidural Morphine

In 2004, the U.S. Food and Drug Administration approved a new formulation of morphine for epidural use. The formulation consists of preservative-free morphine encapsulated in microscopic liposomes, which is injected as a suspension into the epidural space. In the epidural space, the liposomes degrade over time, slowly releasing the enclosed morphine. This has the effect of extending the duration of a single injection of morphine.

- The slow release of morphine into the epidural space results analgesia of the same quality as standard epidural morphine, but with a duration of approximately 48 hours.
- Side effects of extended release epidural morphine are comparable to those of standard epidural morphine.
- The recommended dose for post-cesarean analgesia is 10 mg.
- If unintentionally injected in the intrathecal space, the liposomes of the extended release formulation degrade much more rapidly, releasing the contained morphine more rapidly. The clinical effect would be that of an intrathecal morphine overdose.

- The unintentional intrathecal injection of an epidural dose of either standard or extended release morphine would result in a massive overdose, and significant side effects would result. These could include potentially life-threatening side effects such as respiratory depression and unconsciousness, as well as less critical effects like pruritus and nausea.
- Any patient suffering such an unintentional injection should be closely monitored in an ICU setting. A naloxone infusion will likely be necessary to counter the effects of the overdose. Temporary respiratory support, i.e., mechanical ventilation, may be necessary.

Non-Opioid Epidural Analgesics

Epinephrine

Epinephrine, a naturally occurring catecholamine with both α- and β-adrenergic agonist actions, has been used with a variety of epidural analgesics. The primary goal is to prolong analgesia, and secondary goals are to decrease the incidence of side effects and decrease systemic uptake.

- Alpha-2 agonism is likely responsible for most of epinephrine's intrinsic analgesic properties. Administered with lidocaine, epinephrine results in not only prolonged anesthesia, but also enhanced analgesia (Figure 5.7).
- In parturients, epinephrine may prolong the analgesic effects of shorter-acting opioids. This prolongation often comes at the expense of an increased incidence or severity of side effects.
- If used as a component of a continuous epidural infusion, epinephrine may reduce the infusion rate and total amount of opioid administered.

Clonidine

Clonidine is an α-adrenergic type-2 receptor agonist. After oral administration, it has significant antihypertensive actions. After epidural or spinal injection, it produces significant analgesia, most likely from activation of α-adrenergic receptors within descending inhibitory pathways of the spinal cord.

- In volunteers, the bolus administration of 700 mcg epidural clonidine results in significant sedation and decreased blood pressure.

At a dose of 150 mcg, epidural clonidine has been shown to modestly augment intrathecal morphine analgesia after cesarean section.

- In nonobstetric populations, the addition of clonidine to local anesthetic infusions improves postoperative analgesia, but at the cost of greater sedation and lower blood pressure.
- Due to a relatively short duration of action, for postoperative analgesia it is best administered via continuous infusion.
- Due to blood pressure and sedative effects, clonidine is not recommended for routine use in parturients.

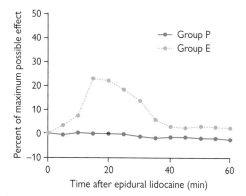

Figure 5.7 Epinephrine augmentation of epidural lidocaine anesthesia. When added to epidural lidocaine 1%, sensory block of an electrical stimulus was not merely prolonged, it was enhanced, illustrating epinephrine's intrinsic analgesic/anesthetic properties. (Group P, plain lidocaine 1%; Group E, lidocaine 1% with epinephrine 1:200,000).
Reprinted with permission from Sakura S, et al. The addition of epinephrine increases intensity of sensory block during epidural anesthesia with lidocaine. *Reg Anesth Pain Med.* 1999;24(6)541–546.

Summary of Epidural Analgesics

There are a variety of ways to provide epidural analgesia after cesarean delivery.

- Fentanyl, 50–100 mcg, mixed with the local anesthetic, enhances intraoperative comfort and provides early postoperative analgesia.
- Despite the occurrence of side effects, morphine is still the longest-lasting epidural opioid available, and is the mainstay of single-shot epidural postoperative analgesia. Immediately after delivery, administer

3.5 to 4 mg, in a volume of 8 to 10 ml. Because of a slow onset, 30 minutes or more are necessary for maximum effect.

- Both epidural fentanyl and epidural morphine are often used as part of the same anesthetic for maximum opioid effect. Fentanyl is administered with the induction dose of local anesthetic to enhance intraoperative analgesia; morphine is then administered via the epidural catheter for postoperative analgesia.

- Each parturient must be treated as an individual. While multiple studies have validated each of these medications and techniques as adequate for most patients, some women will fall outside the norms and may require additional analgesics.

- For the parturient who requires significant amounts of additional analgesics in the early postoperative period, options include:
  - PCA (intravenous)
  - Oral analgesics
  - As needed (PRN) intravenous analgesics

Postoperative Monitoring and Surveillance

Because of the theoretical risk of respiratory depression and the occurrence of side effects, standard postoperative orders are very useful (Table 5.3).

- Nurses should check and record respiratory rates hourly for 18 to 24 hours after epidural morphine. If respiratory rate falls below eight breaths per minute, the nurse should immediately inject naloxone and notify the anesthesiologist. In the absence of other sedatives or narcotics, respiratory depression of this degree is extremely uncommon.

Recognizing that respiratory depression after neuraxial opioid administration is a rare but preventable event, the American Society of Anesthesiologists convened a Task Force in 2007 to update recommendations for patient care. The *Practice Guidelines for the Prevention, Detection, and Management of Respiratory Depression Associated with Neuraxial Opioid Administration,* available on-line at www.asahq.org, outline specific precautions and management recommendations.

Some groups have advocated more intensive monitoring of all patients who receive neuraxial opioids. The Anesthesia Patient

Safety Foundation (APSF) in 2007 recommended continuous monitoring of both respiration (i.e., capnography) and oxygenation in all patients receiving epidural and PCA opioids, while others have recommended continuous pulse oximetry in the postoperative period. While this is a commendable goal, with current technology this is rarely practical outside the intensive care unit setting, and most obstetric anesthesiologists feel that the risk of serious respiratory complications is lower in the obstetric population than in the postsurgical population at large.

Table 5.3 Postoperative Neuraxial Opioid Orders

1.	Epidural/intrathecal _____, ___ mg, administered at ____ hours on _____ (date).
2.	No sedatives or narcotics administered except by order of anesthesiologist.
3.	One ampule naloxone at bedside at all times.
4.	Main IV access or heparin-lock at all times.
5.	Measure and record respiratory rate q 1 h; for respiratory rate <8/min, give naloxone, 0.2 mg IV slowly over 2 min; notify anesthesiologist.
6. Supplemental analgesia:	Morphine 2 mg IV q 1–2 h PRN or Ketorolac 15 mg IV q 6 h PRN or Ibuprofen 400 mg PO q 6 h PRN
7. For pruritus:	Nalbuphine, 5 mg IV q 4 h PRN itching.
8. For nausea/vomiting:	Ondansetron 4 mg IV q 6 h PRN nausea and vomiting.
9.	For pain, pruritus, or nausea/vomiting unresponsive to above, page anesthesiologist on call.
10.	This protocol covers 24 h after each dose of neuraxial narcotic.

Intrathecal Opioids

Morphine

Though hard data are not available, the resurgence of spinal anesthesia for cesarean delivery over the last several decades means that in the United States at least, the majority of cesarean deliveries are probably performed under spinal anesthesia. As the use of spinal anesthesia has increased, so has the use of intrathecal opioids for postoperative analgesia.

- Morphine is the mainstay of intrathecal post-cesarean analgesics. In parturients, intrathecal morphine produces excellent pain relief after cesarean section with surprisingly small doses. In studies, when self-administered PCA morphine is used to quantify analgesia, analgesia is not enhanced even when the dose of intrathecal morphine increases five-fold, from 0.1 to 0.5 mg (Figure 5.8).

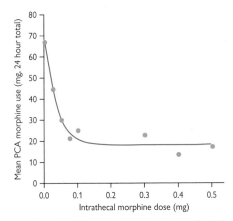

Figure 5.8 Mean 24-hour PCA morphine use after doses of intrathecal morphine from 0 to 0.5 mg in parturients after cesarean delivery. Data are mean (standard error). Reprinted with permission from Palmer CM, et al. Dose-response relationship of intrathecal morphine for post-cesarean analgesia. *Anesthesiology*. 1999;90(2):437–444.

> The fact that patients continue to self-medicate with PCA morphine at a fairly constant rate despite a five- to tenfold increase in the dose of intrathecal morphine suggests that optimal analgesia requires occupation of opioid receptors not only at the spinal level, but also elsewhere within the CNS; intrathecal morphine occupies spinal receptors, and parenteral systemic (PCA) morphine likely acts at supraspinal receptors. Support for this spinal-supraspinal receptor synergy can be found in animal models.

Side Effects of Intrathecal Morphine

- Side effects after intrathecal morphine are comparable to those seen after the administration of epidural morphine.
- Pruritus occurs in 40%–80% of patients and is somewhat dose-dependent (Figure 5.9).

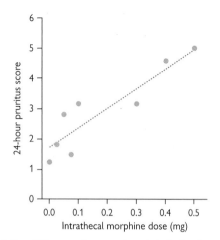

Figure 5.9 Mean 24-hour pruritus scores in parturients after doses of intrathecal morphine from 0 to 0.5 mg. Reprinted with permission from Palmer CM, *et al.* Dose-response relationship of intrathecal morphine for post-cesarean analgesia. *Anesthesiology.* 1999;90(2):437–444.

- Vomiting occurs rarely after low doses (0.1 mg) of morphine.
- Clinically significant respiratory depression is rare, but can occur.
  - In a review of over 1900 patients receiving 0.15 mg intrathecal morphine after cesarean delivery, only 6 had a recorded respiratory rate less than 10/minute, and only 1 required naloxone for decreased SaO_2.
  - At clinically relevant doses (<0.25 mg), the respiratory response to carbon dioxide challenge is not depressed.

Dosing

Based on the very steep dose response curve of intrathecal morphine, the optimal dose of intrathecal morphine for clinical use for post-cesarean analgesia lies between 0.1 mg and 0.2 mg, which should provide over 18–20 hours of good analgesia while avoiding excessive side effects.

- As with epidural morphine, standardized postoperative orders are very useful, and postoperative monitoring is essential.
- Also similar to epidural morphine, interindividual variation does occur, and a standardized dose of intrathecal morphine may not completely

eliminate the need for supplemental analgesics. The best way to insure optimal analgesia may be through a combination of intrathecal morphine and PCA supplementation.

Other Intrathecal Opioids

Fentanyl

Fentanyl is often used for analgesia at cesarean delivery; maximal clinical benefit occurs at very low doses.

- The duration of effective analgesia from intrathecal bupivacaine increases from 71.8 minutes without fentanyl to 192 minutes with 6.25 mcg of fentanyl (Figure 5.10), but 24-hour supplemental narcotic usage is not affected.
- In conjunction with lidocaine anesthesia, fentanyl has similar effects but the duration of effective analgesia is shorter.
- The relatively short duration of effective analgesia even at high doses limits the value of intrathecal fentanyl as a postoperative analgesic.
- As with epidural techniques, fentanyl and morphine are often combined in a single anesthetic, capitalizing on fentanyl's rapid onset and morphine's long duration for optimal effect.

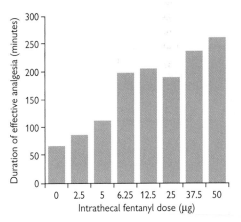

Figure 5.10 Duration of effective analgesia after fentanyl doses ranging from 0 to 50 mcg in parturients after cesarean delivery. Reprinted with permission from Hunt CO, *et al.* Perioperative analgesia with subarachnoid fentanyl bupivacaine for cesarean delivery. *Anesthesiology.* 1989;71(4):535–540.

- Pruritus occurs frequently with intrathecal fentanyl but rarely requires treatment; fentanyl can actually *decrease* the incidence of nausea and vomiting intraoperatively.

Others

- **Sufentanil** up to 10 mcg, has very similar analgesic properties to fentanyl. Like fentanyl, a short duration limits the usefulness of sufentanil as a postoperative analgesic.
- **Buprenorphine** 0.045 mg, also prolongs the pain-free interval after bupivacaine spinal anesthesia, perhaps as long as 6 to 7 hours; its only advantage would seem to be a lower incidence of pruritus.

Other intrathecal opioids that have been used in nonpregnant populations include methadone and oxymorphone.

- **Methadone** produces analgesia of shorter duration and less consistent quality than morphine, even at doses as high as 20 mg.
- **Oxymorphone** provides approximately 16 hours of analgesia when administered intrathecally, with predictable side effects of pruritus, nausea, and vomiting.

Table 5.4 Summary of Intrathecal Opioid Options for Post-Cesarean Analgesia

Opioid	Dose	Reported Duration
Morphine	0.1–0.2 mg	18–24 hours
Fentanyl	10–20 mcg	3–4 hours
Sufentanil	Up to 10 mcg	3–4 hours
Buprenorphine Methadone → Oxymorphone	Limited experience. Doses and durations not well characterized	

Non-Opioid Intrathecal Analgesics

While epinephrine can be added to intrathecal local anesthetics to prolong the duration of anesthesia, it does not augment intrathecal morphine postoperative analgesia. The addition of epinephrine to intrathecal morphine 0.2 mg does not increase the duration of postoperative analgesia or decrease the need for supplemental analgesics after cesarean delivery.

Summary

For single-shot spinal anesthesia for cesarean delivery, 0.1 to 0.2 mg of morphine (there is no evidence to suggest any increased benefit to a dose above 0.2 mg) and 10–15 mcg of fentanyl with either lidocaine or bupivacaine, remains the best choice of postoperative analgesic.

- Morphine provides 18 to 24 hours of good to excellent postoperative analgesia for most parturients, but if a patient is having significant discomfort, supplemental analgesia is appropriate. This may be IV-PCA morphine, but as many parturients are able to tolerate oral analgesics within hours after their surgery, oral pain medications can be equally effective.

- Fentanyl enhances intraoperative comfort and provides some early postoperative analgesia.

- Because of the very small volumes of opioids used with this technique, it is prudent to measure these drugs with a tuberculin (i.e., 1.0 ml) syringe to minimize the risk of accidental overdose.

- As with epidural morphine analgesia, close postoperative monitoring of patients is essential.

Continuous Intrathecal Analgesia

Continuous intrathecal analgesia can be used in those patients who have an intrathecal catheter in place.

Advantages

- Medications can be readily titrated to patient comfort.
- Additional boluses can be given for breakthrough pain.
- If necessary, the catheter can be used to rapidly induce surgical anesthesia.

Disadvantages

- Relatively few catheter options are available in most locales.
- There is a higher incidence of headache with larger diameter catheters.

Generally speaking, the highly lipid-soluble opioids, with their fast onset and relatively short duration of action, are the best-suited agents. When using continuous infusions containing fentanyl or sufentanil however, patients should be monitored in a higher intensity setting (such as an intensive care or step-down unit) with continuous with pulse oximetry.

- Sufentanil, 5 mcg/h (and often less), will provide adequate analgesia for most parturients after cesarean delivery.

- A combination of bupivacaine and fentanyl can also be used (fentanyl 15 mcg/h with bupivacaine 1.5 mg/h). This latter combination may be associated with greater motor block than the sufentanil infusion (Table 5.5).

Table 5.5 Continuous Intrathecal Infusion Therapy for Post-cesarean Analgesia

Medication	Initial Bolus	Infusion	Comments
Sufentanil	5 mcg	5–7.5 mcg/h	Mix as 1 mcg/ml infusion
Fentanyl/bupivacaine	Fentanyl 25 mcg with bupivacaine 2.5 mg	Fentanyl 15mcg/h Bupivacaine 1.5 mg/h	Mix infusion[a] with fentanyl 5 mcg and bupivacaine 0.5 mg/ml. Run at 3 ml/h

[a]To mix infusion: Begin with 50 ml normal saline; withdraw 15 ml; add 5 ml 0.5% bupivacaine and 5 ml fentanyl. **Note:** Most commercial infusion bags are slightly overfilled, therefore these numbers are very close approximations.

Non-Neuraxial Nerve Block

Peripheral nerve block has been used with mixed success for post-cesarean analgesia.

Ilioinguinal Nerve Block

- In patients who undergo cesarean delivery with a Pfannenstiel skin incision, bilateral ilioinguinal nerve block with 10 ml 0.5% bupivacaine has been shown to modestly reduce postoperative analgesic requirements compared to those receiving no block.
- When ilioinguinal block is combined with intrathecal morphine, 0.15 mg, postoperative analgesic requirements did not differ from patients not receiving the block.
- Using ultrasound guidance, catheters may be introduced into the plane between the transversus abdominus and internal oblique muscles anteriorly (the plane where the ilioinguinal nerves lie), allowing for continuous infusion of local anesthetics. When used in conjunction with oral ibuprofen on a fixed dosage schedule, supplemental postoperative morphine requirements were decreased.
- Ilioinguinal nerve block may be useful in patients who required general anesthesia or who have contraindications to neuraxial analgesics.

Transversus Abdominus Plane Block

As noted above, sensory innervation to the anterior abdominal wall runs between the transversus abdominus and internal oblique muscles. It is possible to introduce local anesthetics into this plane posteriorly, in the triangle of Petit via a loss of resistance technique, and block sensory innervation of the anterior abdominal wall.

- Used as part of a multimodal analgesic regimen that included oral acetaminophen, rectal diclofenac, and IV-PCA morphine (see below), supplemental morphine use was significantly lower in patients receiving the block (with ropivacaine 0.75% 1.5 mg/kg each side) than those who received sham injections. The majority of the benefit was in the first 12 hours after surgery.

Patient-Controlled Analgesia (PCA)

Intravenous PCA

Patient-controlled analgesia (PCA) is effective and has become popular in some practices for post-cesarean analgesia. Both intravenous (IV-PCA) and epidural (PCEA) PCA have been used for post-cesarean analgesia.

- While single injection epidural or intrathecal morphine analgesia was rated superior (by patients) to analgesia provided by IV-PCA morphine in one series, overall patient satisfaction with IV-PCA was equally high, probably because of the feeling of control that self-administered PCA provides parturients.
- Both IV-PCA and neuraxial morphine are markedly more effective than intramuscular injections.
- The choice of opioid for use with IV-PCA does not make any consistent difference in patient satisfaction or side effects, when equipotent doses are used.
- Use of a basal infusion does not change 24-hour opioid usage, but may decrease pain scores with movement. This minor advantage is offset by the fact that the incidence of nausea is higher when a basal infusion is used.
- PCA is an excellent choice to use in combination with neuraxial techniques (i.e., single-shot intrathecal or epidural morphine) for post-cesarean analgesia, and an effective way to titrate postoperative analgesia to individual requirements.

Patient-Controlled Epidural Analgesia (PCEA)

Patient-controlled epidural analgesia (PCEA) has a number of advantages in the post-cesarean patient:

- It gives the parturient a degree of control over her analgesia.
- It allows the use of local anesthetics, opioids, and other adjuncts (epinephrine) in multiple combinations.
- It may decrease the need for physician interventions in the postoperative period.

Compared to single bolus epidural morphine, use of opioid-only PCEA with fentanyl or sufentanil provides comparable analgesia, but the high total doses of opioid used by parturients raise the question of whether the analgesic effects are mediated primarily by systemic uptake rather than a true spinal mechanism.

- As with intravenous PCA, a basal (or "background") infusion does not significantly improve the quality of pain relief with PCEA.
- Background infusions *do* increase sedation.
- Background infusions generally increase total drug delivery.

When meperidine is used for PCEA, parturients use approximately 50% less opioid via the PCEA route than the IV-PCA route, and sedation scores are predictably higher in the IV-PCA group (Figure 5.11).

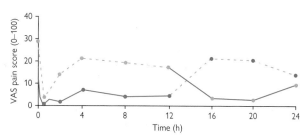

Figure 5.11 A comparison of pain scores between patient-controlled analgesia (intravenous PCA) and patient-controlled epidural analgesia (PCEA) after cesarean delivery. The solid line represents the period parturients received PCEA and the dashed line represents the period they received PCA. Pain scores were consistently lower in the PCEA group. Reprinted with permission from Paech MJ et al. Meperidine for patient-controlled analgesia after cesarean section. *Anesthesiology.* 1994;80:1268–1276.

Local anesthetics are frequently added to PCEA for post-cesarean analgesia.

- The concentration of local anesthetic must be low to avoid significant sensory or motor blockade, as many patients are ambulatory within hours of surgery.
- A concentration of bupivacaine as low as 0.03% has been reported to interfere with ambulation when used in combination with fentanyl or buprenorphine.
- A concentration of bupivacaine 0.01% does not interfere with ambulation, but epidural fentanyl consumption is comparable to PCEA fentanyl without added bupivacaine.
- It is unclear what benefit, if any, including dilute bupivacaine in a PCEA solution provides.

Other Adjuncts for PCEA

Clonidine and epinephrine (which both presumably activate α-2 adrenergic receptors) and neostigmine (which prevents the breakdown of synaptically released Ach) have also been used with PCEA.

- When combined with sufentanil PCEA, both epinephrine and clonidine significantly reduce epidural opioid use.
- Clonidine causes significant decreases in blood pressure and heart rate.
- Neostigmine, even at very low doses, significantly increases nausea and vomiting.
- Neither clonidine or neostigmine can be recommended for routine use with PCEA.

PCEA can be an effective technique for post-cesarean analgesia. Whether it offers distinct advantages over epidural or intrathecal morphine is a matter of dispute. A disadvantage is the necessity to maintain a functioning epidural catheter in the postoperative period. Further, in many practices cesarean delivery is likely to performed with a single-shot spinal anesthetic technique, without an epidural catheter inserted. PCEA remains a useful technique for selected patients and populations.

Nonsteroidal Agents (NSAIDs)

The NSAIDs are not potent enough in and of themselves to provide complete analgesia for most patients after a cesarean delivery. As adjuncts to neuraxial morphine, NSAIDs have shown inconsistent results.

While in some situations NSAIDs can decrease postoperative opioid use, at this point it is difficult to make a blanket recommendation for their use. Nevertheless, nonsteroidal agents (NSAIDs) may be of value in this population.

- Many patients who have had a cesarean delivery remain NPO for some period of time following delivery; during this period, a parenteral alternative to oral medications may be necessary.
- While unrestricted oral intake may not resume for up to 24 hours after delivery, many parturients are able to tolerate small amounts of fluids, and can take an oral NSAID as an adjunct to neuraxial or parenteral analgesics.

A number of NSAIDs have been used in the post-cesarean period. Various NSAIDs may be administered via the intravenous, intramuscular, or rectal routes.

- Ketorolac 30 mg IM is roughly comparable to meperidine 75 mg IM, but ketorolac is somewhat inconsistent and of short duration. Ketorolac has also been administered IV on a scheduled basis after cesarean delivery with mixed results.
- When administered via continuous intravenous infusion, diclofenac or ketoprofen decrease postoperative analgesic requirements by about 40% when compared to placebo.
- Propoacetamol is widely used in some parts of the world via rectal administration following cesarean delivery.

In general, the drawbacks to the use of an NSAID in conjunction with intrathecal or epidural opioids are minimal. When used, they should be administered on a scheduled basis rather than PRN ("as needed") dosing. The anesthesiologist must remain aware that while potentially helpful, NSAIDs will be ineffective adjuncts for many patients, and alternative therapy will be necessary.

Other Oral Agents

Tramadol is a synthetic 4-phenyl-piperidine analogue of codeine, which has a low affinity for mu opioid receptor. It inhibits serotonin and nore-pinephrine neuronal reuptake. Reported use as an oral analgesic in the post-cesarean population has been very limited, but it has been used as a "rescue" analgesic in combination with other analgesic modalities, or as an alternative to an oral opioid if a parturient is intolerant.

- A 25mg dose can be administered every 4 to 6 hours.
- Tramadol should probably be avoided in patients with seizure disorders or severe preeclampsia, as it has been shown to decrease seizure threshold.

Further Reading

1. Cohen SE, Desai JB, Ratner EF, *et al*. Ketorolac and spinal morphine for postcesarean analgesia. *Int J Obstet Anesth*. 1996;5:14-18.

2. Eisenach JC, Grice SC, Dewan, DM. Patient-controlled analgesia following cesarean section: A comparison with epidural and intramuscular narcotics. *Anesthesiology*. 1988; 68:444-448.

3. Gourlay GK, Cherry DA, Cousins MJ. Cephalad migration of morphine in CSF following lumbar epidural administration in patients with cancer pain. *Pain*. 1985;23: 317-326.

4. Helbo-Hansen HS, Bang U, Lindholm P, *et al*. Maternal effects of adding epidural fentanyl to 0.5% bupivacaine for caesarean section. *Int J Obstet Anesth*. 1993;2: 21-26.

5. McDonnell NJ, Keating ML, Muchatuta NA, *et al*. Analgesia after caesarean delivery. *Anaesth Intensive Care* 2009;37:539-551.

6. Paech MJ, Moore JS, Evans SF. Meperidine for patient-controlled analgesia after cesarean section. *Anesthesiology*. 1994; 80:1268-1276.

7. Paech MJ, Pavy TJG, Orlikowski CEP, *et al*. Postoperative epidural infusion: a randomized, double-blind, dose-finding trial of clonidine in combination with bupivacaine and fentanyl. *Anesth Analg*. 1997;84: 1323-1328.

8. Palmer CM. Continuous intrathecal sufentanil for postoperative analgesia. *Anesth Analg*. 2001;92: 244-245.

9. Palmer CM, Voulgaropoulos D, Alves D. Subarachnoid fentanyl augments lidocaine spinal anesthesia for cesarean delivery. *Reg Anesth*. 1995;20(5): 389-394.

10. Palmer CM, Emerson S, Voulgaropoulos D, *et al*. Dose-response relationship of intrathecal morphine for post-cesarean analgesia. *Anesthesiology*. 1999; 90:437-444.

11. Palmer CM, Nogami WM, Van Maren G, *et al*. Post-cesarean epidural morphine: a dose response study. *Anesth Analg*. 2000;90:887-891.

12. Wang JK, Nauss LA, Thomas JE. Pain relief by intrathecally applied morphine in man. *Anesthesiology*. 1979;50:149-155.

Chapter 6

Anesthesia for Surgery During and After Pregnancy

Michael J. Paech, FANZCA
Robert D'Angelo, MD
Laura S. Dean, MD

Anesthesia for Reproductive Technologies

Assisted reproductive technologies (ARTs) involve a sequence of hormonal stimulation of the ovaries followed by egg retrieval and subsequent embryo transfer. Depending on the timing of intervention, these procedures may involve transcervical, transabdominal or laparoscopic approaches, each of which has a number of anesthetic options.

Assisted reproductive technology results in a higher incidence of multiple gestation and ectopic pregnancies, both of which are associated with higher maternal morbidity and mortality than singleton pregnancy. Additionally, as ART success rates increase among women of advancing maternal age, preexisting comorbidities become more apparent. Pregnancy resulting from ART has a greater chance of preterm delivery and birth of babies that are small for gestational age.

Numerous ART procedures can be performed and are outlined:

- **Hormonal stimulation and oocyte retrieval**. Hormonal therapies encourage the production of multiple ovarian follicles per cycle, allowing for subsequent retrieval of multiple oocytes. Most oocytes are retrieved by ultrasound-guided vaginal aspiration, unless immediate transfer is planned.
- *In-vitro* fertilization. Following retrieval, oocytes are incubated and inseminated.
- **Embryo transfer**. Oocytes that were fertilized successfully are transferred into the fallopian tubes or into the uterine cavity, usually via a transcervical approach.
- **Gamete intrafallopian transfer (GIFT)**. Oocytes are retrieved and inspected. If mature, they are then injected with donor sperm directly into the distal fallopian tube via a laparosopic approach, after which fertilization occurs *in vivo*.
- **Zygote intrafallopian transfer (ZIFT)**. Oocytes are retrieved and inseminated. Fertilized eggs are transferred to the distal fallopian tube via laparoscopy.

Ovarian hyperstimulation syndrome can occur as a result of follicle stimulating hormone (FSH) and human menopausal gonadotropin therapy. The syndrome presents as ascites, pleural effusion, hemoconcentration, oligura, and thromboembolic events.

Anesthetic Implications

All patients should have a preoperative assessment. Assisted reproductive technologies rely on timing for success, so it very important for patients to follow fasting guidelines prior to surgery in order to avoid unnecessary, costly, and emotionally stressful delays. Some specific considerations should be considered.

- Unique to anesthesia for ART is the added goal of limiting interference with oocyte fertilization or embryo implantation. The optimal choice of anesthetic drugs and techniques is unclear, but maintenance of hemodynamic stability remains the primary concern regardless of anesthetic choice.
- Transvaginal oocyte retrieval is most commonly performed under intravenous sedation, but movement needs to be avoided at the time of actual retrieval, so progression to deep sedation or anesthesia may be necessary. Spinal anesthesia is also appropriate and minimizes the concentration of anesthetic in follicles.

- Transcervical embryo transfer can often be achieved without analgesia, although the same anesthetic options as those used for oocyte retrieval are suitable.
- Laparoscopic procedures are used for embryo transfer.
  - Trendelenburg positioning may reduce chest wall compliance.
  - Pneumoperitoneum is usually achieved with carbon dioxide, and a rare complication is carbon dioxide embolization.
  - Peritoneal and diaphragmatic irritation may cause postoperative pain.
  - General anesthesia is most commonly performed using intravenous induction agents, muscle relaxation, and either nitrous oxide or volatile inhalational anesthetics.

Anesthesia in Early Pregnancy

1%–2% of women will experience a condition requiring surgery during pregnancy. In the early to mid second trimester, procedures requiring anesthesia include insertion of cervical suture for incompetent cervix, and an array of nonobstetric operations and procedures (e.g., laparosocopy or laparotomy for acute appendicitis or cholecystitis or ovarian cyst accidents, neurosurgery for cerebrovascular events, operations for traumatic or other injury, and oncological operations). With embryo or fetal demise, evacuation of retained products of conception may be necessary.

Early pregnancy loss (mainly prior to 13 weeks gestation) is common (incidence 15%–20% of all pregnancies). Although not all women require evacuation of retained products of conception, this is a very common operation for which general anesthesia is usually provided. Termination of pregnancy is also a common procedure in some countries, but general anesthesia is used infrequently; sedation, with or without regional anesthesia (e.g., paracervical block), is often delivered by non-anesthesiologists.

Whenever continued fetal viability is desired, and particularly during initial embryo development and organogenesis (days 14 to 56), remember that:

- Drugs may have both direct (pharmacologic) and indirect effects on the fetus (e.g., vasoactive drugs may affect placental blood flow).
- Adequate uteroplacental perfusion must be assured by maintaining maternal blood pressure and cardiac output and avoiding peripheral vasoconstriction.

Anesthetic Principles and Management

Epidemiological studies suggest that the risk of loss of a viable pregnancy, and premature or low birth weight delivery, are increased by surgery but *not* influenced by anesthesia or anesthetic technique. Other factors that are likely more important are maternal illness and current disease, with fetal loss more likely after operations on the genital tract (e.g., cervical suture), abdomen, or pelvis.

During early pregnancy, the teratogenic and carcinogenic potential of anesthetic or sedative drugs assumes particular importance. The anesthesiologist must understand potential effects of anesthetic and analgesic drugs on pregnancy, so that sound decisions can be made and so that informed consent can be obtained from the patient. A joint statement on *Non-obstetric surgery during pregnancy* by the American College of Obstetricians and Gynecologists and the American Society of Anesthesiologists notes: "No currently used anesthetic agents have been shown to have any teratogenic effects in humans when using standard concentrations at any gestational age."

- Midazolam, opioids (e.g., IV fentanyl or remifentanil), propofol and the inhalational anesthetic agents are popular and appear safe.

The primary concern during nonobstetric surgery during pregnancy is always the safety of the mother.

- Aspiration prophylaxis should be considered based on the gestational age; prior to 16 weeks gestation, the risk of aspiration probably does not differ greatly from nonpregnant patients.

- Aortocaval compression is a possibility after the uterus rises out of the pelvis at approximately 20 weeks gestation (or earlier if multiple pregnancy).

- The effect of anesthesia on the fetus remains a prime consideration, both up to the time of viability (23–24 weeks gestation) and in the weeks thereafter, when premature delivery has substantial morbidity and mortality implications (see Chapter 11); preterm delivery potentially involves costly health care, severe parental psychological stress, and sometimes lifelong impact on the child's health.

- Whenever possible, elective surgery should be postponed until after pregnancy. (Though never demonstrated in humans, drugs have potential nonteratogenic effects on developing fetal organ systems, especially the central nervous system.)

- Essential but nonurgent surgery should be deferred until after fetal viability (although inevitably, urgent surgery will be mandated by surgical and medical emergencies).

Fetal monitoring should be considered on a case-by-case basis. Prior to viability, at 22–24 weeks estimated gestational age, ascertaining the fetal heart rate prior to and after surgery is sufficient. If the fetus is considered viable and the situation allows, expert advice should be sought but simultaneous electronic fetal heart rate and contraction monitoring can be performed before and after the procedure to assess fetal well-being and the absence of contractions.

Intraoperative electronic fetal monitoring may be appropriate when the following apply:

- The fetus is viable.
- It is physically possible to perform intraoperative electronic fetal monitoring.
- A provider with obstetrical surgery privileges is available and willing to intervene during the surgical procedure for fetal indications.
- The woman has given informed consent to emergency cesarean delivery.

Loss of beat-to-beat variability and fetal bradycardia are effects of anesthetic drugs and hypothermia, so interpretation of fetal heart rate patterns requires special expertise.

After fetal death *in utero*, a coagulopathy may develop over time but does not usually become clinically relevant for 3–4 weeks.

Although not evidence-based, the core principles of anesthesia are listed in Table 6.1 and a management plan outlined in Figure 6.1.

Table 6.1 Key Principles of Anesthesia from Early to Term Pregnancy
Communicate with the surgeon regarding the urgency of surgery
Postpone elective surgery until after pregnancy
If possible, defer non-elective surgery until after fetal viability (22–24 weeks)
During assessment, be aware of the changes resulting from pregnancy and the exposure of the fetus to radiation during imaging
Avoid drugs with potential for fetal harm
Avoid drugs that stimulate uterine contractility
Maintain normal pregnant physiology
Consider the merit of continuous intraoperative fetal monitoring
If suitable, use regional anesthesia whenever possible (to minimize maternal risks and fetal drug exposure)
Provide effective postoperative analgesia

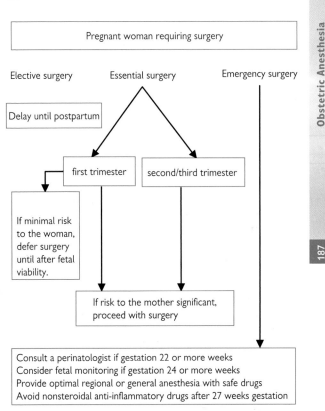

Figure 6.1 Management plan for a pregnant woman requiring surgery.

Anesthesia for Removal of Retained Products of Conception

This is an occasion of considerable emotional disturbance for many women, so general anesthesia is normally preferred. Rapid discharge from hospital can usually be achieved as quickly or more quickly than after sedation or spinal anesthesia.

When providing anesthesia for this procedure, be compassionate and tactful.

- Be aware that drugs used for cervical ripening (e.g., prostaglandin E2) may cause preoperative pelvic pain, nausea, and fever.

- Most women will benefit from preoperative or preinduction anxiolysis.
- IV anesthetic requirements at induction may be increased and their duration of effect shorter because of rapid redistribution as a result of high sympathetic activity and cardiac output.
- Decisions about aspiration risk must be made based on gestational age and patient symptoms, although in most cases a supraglottic airway (LMA) device is appropriate.
  - Rapid sequence induction and tracheal intubation is reserved for patients with symptomatic reflux, and is most often used after the mid second trimester.
- Spontaneous ventilation is usually suitable.
- Opioid analgesic requirements are variable but often minimal, as the procedure is not usually associated with prolonged postoperative pain. Nonsteroidal anti-inflammatory drugs (NSAIDs) such as IV ketorolac or parecoxib intraoperatively, or one of the many oral NSAIDs postoperatively, decrease "cramping" discomfort (uterine visceral pain) and provide good analgesia.

Anesthesia in Later Pregnancy

In providing anesthesia for women in whom the pregnancy is expected to continue, the principles considered in Chapter 4 apply when choosing between general and regional anesthesia. Fetal monitoring is discussed in detail in Chapter 12. Regional anesthesia has the advantages of:

- Avoiding the risks associated with difficult airway management.
- Avoiding issues related to certain anesthetic and analgesic drugs.

If spinal anesthesia is chosen:

- Local anesthetic dose requirements are reduced (by approximately 30%) from the first trimester.
- Hypotension should be managed aggressively.
- Plain ropivacaine is an option (at least 15 mg, with fentanyl 10–20 mcg) to achieve a less intense motor block of shorter duration compared with spinal bupivacaine, thus promoting rapid postoperative recovery (hyperbaric lidocaine is no longer used in many countries because of transient lumbar pain and neurotoxicity issues).
- Patients should be informed about post-discharge post-spinal headache, and provided with advice on how to seek follow-up.

Anesthesia for Laparoscopic Surgery

Complex laparoscopic surgery with carbon dioxide pneumoperitoneum has been performed safely in many pregnant women. Outcomes are generally very good, and better than after laparotomy, although physiological derangements such as hypoxemia, hypercarbia, and hypotension need management. The typical physiologic changes are similar to nonpregnancy:

- An increase in cardiac output postinduction.
- A fall in cardiac output secondary to increased systemic vascular resistance and mean arterial blood pressure at the time of establishing the pneumoperitoneum.
- An increase in end-tidal (ET)-carbon dioxide with pneumoperitoneum that may require increased minute ventilation to normalize.

The decrease in placental blood flow as intra-abdominal pressure rises is usually well tolerated by the fetus. Nevertheless, occasional cases of severe fetal bradycardia are reported in the presence of good maternal oxygenation and blood pressure.

In general, surgery should be deferred until the second trimester if possible.

- Use low pressure pneumoperitoneum and maintain maternal normocarbia (approximately 30–32 mmHg) if possible, using adequate ventilation and alveolar recruitment strategies.
- As far as possible, shield the fetus from radiation.
- Keep maternal oxygenation normal or high.
- Provide prophylaxis against postoperative venous thromboembolism.

Pharmacological Considerations During Pregnancy

Considerations relevant to common anesthetic and analgesic drugs are shown in Table 6.2. No anesthetic drug has proven to be teratogenic in humans, but a number of anesthetic and analgesic drugs have not been adequately evaluated during pregnancy, making this area of practice and pain management challenging and controversial.

In general:

- Single doses of a benzodiazepine appear safe throughout pregnancy.
- Ketamine increases uterine tone, which is undesirable and may decrease uteroplacental flow. This myometrial effect diminishes in

later pregnancy when ketamine is effective and safe for general anesthesia for cesarean delivery.

- Propofol has been extensively used in early and later pregnancy and has not been reported to cause problems. It has also been widely used during reproductive technology techniques involving embryo transfer, without apparent affect on fertilization or pregnancy rate. In some countries it was released with the caveat "Should not be used during pregnancy," which creates off-label use issues.
- Sodium Pentothal (sodium thiopental or thiopentone) is safe.
- The inhalational anesthetics are tocolytic (usually a useful effect) and cause no known direct fetal hazards.
- The safety of nitrous oxide is unclear, but it can easily be omitted.

Nitrous oxide inhibits methionine synthase after a couple hours of administration, resulting in raised homocysteine concentrations and reduced thymidine synthesis; this has potential effects on deoxyribonucleic acid (DNA) formation and cell division. Despite no evidence of teratogenicity or fetotoxicity in humans, these actions raise concerns about a potential effect on the developing fetus, as placental transfer is rapid. High levels of occupational exposure to nitrous oxide during early pregnancy appear associated with fetal loss, but exposure within scavenged environments appears safe.

- Neuromuscular blocking drugs do not cross the placenta in significant amounts.
- The acute administration of vasoactive drugs such as β-blockers and nitroglycerin (glyceryl trinitrate [GTN]) appears safe.
  Among common analgesic drugs:
- Acetaminophen (paracetamol), opioids, and local anesthetics are considered safe. Like opioids, tramadol has reversible adverse effects but no evidence of teratogenesis, so appears safe.
- NSAIDs in early pregnancy are associated with spontaneous abortion, and in late pregnancy with fetal renal toxicity, necrotizing enterocolitis, neonatal intracranial hemorrhage, and pulmonary hypertension due to premature closure of the ductus arteriosis, especially after 32 weeks gestation. They are ideally avoided after 27 weeks estimated gestational age.

- Data on cyclooxygenase2-specific inhibitors (coxibs) and gabapentinoids (e.g., gabapentin, pregabalin) are insufficient to allow firm recommendations, although no specific concerns have been reported. Parecoxib and celecoxib appear safe for short-term administration during breastfeeding.

Radiological Exposure

Radiation exposure during early pregnancy is a concern due to the potential hazards of:

- embryo damage and failure to implant
- death or congenital malformations (especially brain, eye and skeletal) after exposure during organogenesis (second to eighth gestational weeks)
- death, growth restriction, and postnatal neoplasia after post-organogenesis exposure.

Nevertheless, radiology is a diagnostic modality that is critical to optimal maternal evaluation and safe care, so it should not be withheld based on potential fetal hazards.

In general the risk of hazard depends on:

- the fetal estimated gestational age
- the radiation dose (but there are only risk thresholds for some hazards and others may be "all or nothing," especially in the first trimester)
- the radiation dose rate.

Table 6.2 Anesthetic and Analgesic Drugs of Potential Concern During Pregnancy

Nonsteroidal anti-inflammatory drugs
- best avoided in the first trimester due to association with pregnancy loss in population studies
- best avoided after 27 weeks gestation and contraindicated after 32 weeks gestation because of potential fetal effects:
  - necrotizing enterocolitis
  - renal damage
  - premature closure of the ductus arteriosis
  - intracranial hemorrhage

Midazolam, diazepam, temazepam and other benzodiazepines
- chronic use in the first trimester associated with cleft palate
- appear safe with short-term use (i.e., perioperative) or single dose

Nitrous oxide
- probably safe with short duration use (< 2 hours)
- easily avoided

The radiation exposure of the fetus (dose absorbed) varies with different equipment, techniques, maternal size and with shielding of the fetus with a lead apron. When many maternal exposures are required over time a thermoluminescent dosimeter attached to the patient can serve as a guide to total exposure. In general, X-ray beams aimed more than 10 cm from the fetus are not dangerous, and the radiation doses of various procedures are shown in Table 6.3.

If the fetus is exposed to less than 50–100 mGy (a milliGray is equivalent to a milliSievert [mSv] or to 100 millirads [mrad]) then there is a 99% chance it will not develop childhood cancer. The risk of any abnormality increases from a baseline nonexposure rate (60 per 1000) by 30 per 1000 for each 10 mGy (1000 mrad) of exposure. At greater than 150–200 mGy (15,000–20,000 mrad) exposure there is a 5% risk of mental retardation and 3% risk of neonatal or childhood cancer.

Anesthesia for Fetal Surgery

Advances in diagnostic techniques have improved detection of fetal anomalies that may be amenable to surgical intervention prior to delivery. However, fetal surgery has many social, ethical, legal and monetary constraints. This discipline of medicine continues to evolve and is beginning to address some of these difficult issues.

Depending on the fetal ultrasound diagnosis, interventions may be performed as:

- minimally invasive endoscopic approaches
- open intrauterine approaches
- ex utero intrapartum therapy (EXIT)

Table 6.3 Estimated Radiation Exposure to the Shielded Fetus

Imaging	Exposure (mrad/mGy)
Head & cervical spine	0.02
Chest X-ray	2/< 0.01
Pelvic X-ray	350/20
Intravenous pyelogram	500
CT head	50
CT chest	1000
CT abdomen	3000/25

Mrad = millirads. mGy = milliGray

Indications for surgical intervention include those anomalies that have significant morbidity and are correctable *in utero*. Examples include:

- obstructive uropathies
- congenital diaphragmatic hernia
- congenital cystic adenomatoid malformation
- sacrococcygeal teratoma
- myelomeningocele
- complications of monochorionic twins (twin-twin transfusion syndrome)
- congenital heart defects
- congenital pleural effusions
- fetal chylothorax
- fetal cardiac arrhythmias

Surgical concerns unique to this subspecialty include the necessity for complete uterine relaxation to assure continued placental circulation, but tight closure of the uterus to prevent subsequent amniotic fluid loss.

Anesthetic Implications

Most minimally invasive endoscopic procedures can be performed with local or neuraxial anesthesia, whereas open intrauterine procedures typically require general anesthesia with uterine relaxation. Anesthetic goals for nonobstetric surgery during pregnancy apply to this patient population—specifically maternal safety, avoidance of teratogenic drugs, and prevention and detection of preterm labor. Additional fetal considerations are intraoperative monitoring and *in utero* fetal analgesia and anesthesia.

Anesthesia for Endoscopic Fetal Surgery

The principles are:

- The patient should be fasted; administer a nonparticulate antacid, and ensure left uterine displacement if appropriate.
- Local anesthesia should be used on the abdominal wall, with maternal and fetal sedation (e.g., IV remifentanil infusion, midazolam), for percutaneous minimally invasive procedures.
- Administer direct umbilical venous or fetal intramuscular injection of neuromuscular blocking and analgesic drugs if warranted.

Neuraxial (spinal or epidural) anesthesia appears beneficial for more extensive ultrasound-guided endoscopic procedures.

Anesthesia for Open Fetal Surgery

The principles are:

- The patient should be fasted; administer a nonparticulate antacid, and ensure left uterine displacement if appropriate.
- Consider a neuraxial procedure for postoperative analgesia.
- A rapid sequence induction is indicated for general anesthesia.
- For maintenance, inhalational anesthetics provide useful uterine relaxation.
- Hysterotomy is performed with staples to avoid uterine hemorrhage.
- Medications for fetal anesthesia and immobility are given to the surgeons for intramuscular administration within the sterile field.
- Additional tocolytics (IV nitroglycerin or magnesium sulfate) are often necessary to achieve full uterine relaxation and may be continued postoperatively, watching for pulmonary edema.
- Close monitoring of fetal heart rate and uterine activity is necessary for 2–3 days postoperatively. It should be noted that urgent cesarean delivery may be necessary in the event of uterine rupture.

Anesthesia for *Ex Utero* Intrapartum (EXIT) Procedures

The principles are:

- The patient should be fasted; administer a nonparticulate antacid, and ensure left uterine displacement if appropriate.
- Consider a neuraxial procedure for postoperative analgesia.
- A rapid sequence induction is indicated with general anesthesia.
- For maintenance, high-concentration inhalational anesthetic provides uterine relaxation.
- Hysterotomy is performed with staples to avoid uterine hemorrhage.

The fetus is given intramuscular analgesia and the head and shoulders of the fetus are delivered; intubation is accomplished and fetal surgery (a range of surgical procedures) is commenced.

- When the umbilical cord is clamped following fetal surgery, uterine relaxation is immediately reversed to avoid uterine atony.
- An option for less extensive fetal surgery is neuraxial maternal anesthesia, using high doses of IV nitroglycerin (100–500 mcg) for uterine relaxation.

Anesthesia for Postpartum Sterilization

Postpartum tubal ligation (PPTL) is a common procedure in the immediate hours following vaginal delivery. The most appropriate timing of this elective surgery and the choice of anesthesia are somewhat controversial. The American Society of Anesthesiologists (ASA) Practice Guidelines for Obstetric Anesthesia suggest that postpartum tubal ligation during the first eight hours after delivery does *not* increase maternal complications.

The advantages of immediate postpartum sterilization are:

- lower cost
- avoidance of inconvenient further hospitalizations
- enhanced surgical exposure of the enlarged uterine fundus
- poor patient compliance may prevent return for delayed sterilization.

However, delaying the procedure 6 weeks after delivery gives the woman more time to consider her decision and for the assessment of the newborn to be completed.

Anesthetic Implications

The postpartum period is a time of altered maternal physiology. The patient may have lost a significant volume of blood during labor and delivery, so careful assessment of hemodynamic status is required before anesthesia and surgery.

The risk of aspiration must be considered.

- There is no difference in gastric volume or gastric pH in postpartum patients at any time interval after delivery when compared to nonpregnant controls, but those receiving opioids for labor analgesia may have delayed gastric emptying during the early postpartum period.
- Lower esophageal sphincter tone is decreased during pregnancy, but the incidence of reflux normalizes approximately 24 hours or more following delivery.

To reduce risk of gastric aspiration, for immediate postpartum tubal ligation:

- The patient should be fasted for 6 hours prior to surgery.
- Administer a nonparticulate antacid within 30 minutes of surgery.
- Consider using metoclopramide or an H2-receptor antagonist in women with symptomatic reflux.

- Neuraxial anesthesia is usually preferred for all immediate post-partum procedures.

Anesthetic Techniques

The ASA guidelines state that neuraxial anesthesia for postpartum tubal ligation (PPTL) is likely to reduce risk when compared with general anesthesia. Local anesthesia for tubal ligation is used in some countries, but in the United States, neuraxial anesthesia is preferred. In practice, the timing of the procedure in relation to delivery and the choice of anesthesia is determined on an individual basis and takes into account the patient's preferences, the presence of an epidural catheter, underlying medical concerns, and anesthetic risks factors.

Neuraxial Anesthesia

Either epidural or spinal techniques are suitable for postpartum tubal ligation.

- The primary advantage of an epidural technique exists when a functioning epidural catheter is already present.
- The disadvantages of epidural anesthesia include an increased failure rate with increasing time from delivery, and the need for large volumes of local anesthetic, increasing the potential for toxicity and time consuming dosing.

For an epidural technique:

- Confirm IV access.
- Consider avoiding IV opioids if immediate postpartum tubal is planned, because of delayed gastric emptying.
- Reconfirm correct location of the labor epidural catheter by sub-arachnoid and intravenous test doses.
- Extend the sensory block to dermatomes T_4–T_6 with short acting local anesthetic in incremental doses (i.e., 3% 2-chloroprocaine or 2% lidocaine with epinephrine [adrenaline]).
- Administer sedatives for patient comfort as required.

Advantages of spinal techniques include a reliable, dense block and predictable sensory levels.

- Spinal block for PPTL is efficient, simple, and has a quick onset.
- Small volumes of local anesthetic eliminate toxicity concerns.
- A high quality block can be achieved, especially when labor epidural analgesia was inadequate or the procedure is delayed (a higher risk of epidural failure).

The disadvantages of spinal anesthesia are relatively minor:

- a low risk of post-dural puncture headache
- the increased risk posed by an additional procedure.

For a spinal technique:

- Confirm IV access.
- Choose a small gauge (< 24 gauge) pencil point spinal needle.
- Administer intrathecal bupivacaine 7.5–10 mg (with fentanyl 10–20 mcg).

General Anesthesia

General anesthesia offers the advantage of efficiency and avoids an additional regional procedure in women who no longer have an epidural catheter in place. The primary issues associated with use of general anesthesia for PPTL include the risk of aspiration and possibility of difficult airway management.

A suggested technique includes:

- Standard ASA monitoring.
- Rapid sequence induction with tracheal intubation.
- Inhalational anesthetic concentration should be minimized to decrease uterine blood loss in the postpartum period, especially for women with or at risk of postpartum hemorrhage.
- Low doses of both depolarizing and nondepolarizing neuromuscular blocking drugs should be used only as necessary, as both have a prolonged duration in postpartum patients.

Further Reading

1. Vlahos NF, Giannakikou I, Vlachos A. Analgesia and anesthesia for assisted reproductive technologies. Vitoratos N. *Int J Gynaecol Obstet.* 2009;105:201-205.

2. Tsen LC. Anesthesia for assisted reproductive technologies. *Int Anesthesiol Clin.* 2007 Winter; 45:99-113.

3. De Buck F, Deprest J, Van de Velde M. Anesthesia for fetal surgery. *Curr Opin Anaesthesiol.* 2008;21:293-297.

4. Gaiser RR, Kurth CD. Anesthetic considerations for fetal surgery. *Semin Perinatol.* 1999;23:507-514.

5. Shaver SM, Shaver DC. Perioperative assessment of the obstetric patient undergoing abdominal surgery. *J Perianesth Nurs.* 2005;20:160-166.

6. Mhuireachtaigh RN, O'Gorman DA. Anesthesia in pregnant patients for nonobstetric surgery. *J Clin Anesth.* 2006;18:60-66.

7. Sanders RD, Weimann J, Maze M. Biologic effects of nitrous oxide: A mechanistic and toxicologic review. *Anesthesiology.* 2008;109:707-722.

8. Practice Guidelines for Obstetric Anesthesia. An updated Report by the American Society of Anesthesiologists Task Force on Obstetric Anesthesia. *Anesthesiology.* 2007;106:843-863.

9. Gin T, Cho AMW, Lew JKL, *et al.* Gastric emptying in the postpartum period. *Anaesth Intensive Care.* 1991;19:521-524.

10. Wong CA, Loffredi M, Ganchiff JW,*et al.* Gastric emptying of water in term pregnancy. *Anesthesiology.* 2002; 96:1395-1400.

Chapter 7

Pregnancy Induced Hypertension and Preeclampsia

Kenneth E. Nelson, MD
Robert D'Angelo, MD

Introduction

Blood pressure decreases somewhat during a normal pregnancy, and an elevated blood pressure is always considered abnormal. Hypertension during pregnancy is a condition that leads to a marked increase in both maternal and fetal morbidity and mortality. "Hypertensive disorders of pregnancy" includes both pregnancy-induced hypertension (PIH) and chronic hypertension that persists into the puerperium. Although the classic triad of preeclampsia includes hypertension, proteinuria and edema, the American College of Obstetricians and Gynecologists (ACOG) has established specific criteria defining both preeclampsia and severe preeclampsia (Table 7.1).

Despite these "classic" definitions, the clinical presentation of preeclampsia can be highly variable from one individual to another. Eclampsia is the condition defined by a seizure as a complication of preeclampsia. With an understanding of this condition, the anesthesia care provider can have an impact by increasing the safety of anesthesia.

Table 7.1 Criteria for the Diagnosis of Mild and Severe Preeclampsia*

- **Mild Preeclampsia:**
  - Hypertension: SBP ≥ 140 or DBP ≥ 90 mmHg or
  - Proteinuria: 24 hr collection ≥ 300 mg protein or
    1–2+ protein with urine dipstick
- **Severe Preeclampsia:**
  - Hypertension: SBP ≥ 160 mmHg or DBP ≥ 110 mmHg
  - Proteinuria: ≥ 5g in 24 hour collection
    3–4+ protein with urine dipstick
  - Evidence of End-Organ Involvement
  - Cerebral: Headache, scotomata, altered level of consciousness
  - Pulmonary: Pulmonary edema, cyanosis
  - Hepatic: Increased liver function tests
    Epigastric or right upper quadrant pain
  - Renal: Oliguria, elevated creatinine
  - Hematologic: Thrombocytopenia
  - HELLP Syndrome: <u>H</u>emolysis, <u>E</u>levated <u>L</u>iver Enzymes, <u>L</u>ow <u>P</u>latelets

* Source: the ACOG Practice Bulletin #33. Diagnosis and management of preeclampsia and eclampsia. *Obstet Gynecol.* 2002; 99:159–167.

The anesthetic implications of preeclampsia are summarized briefly in Table 7.2.

Pathophysiology

The exact cause of preeclampsia remains unknown. In normal pregnancy, both thromboxane and prostacyclin levels increase, but the balance favors prostacyclin and thus vasodilation. In PIH, thromboxane levels increase markedly while prostacyclin levels are abnormally low, an imbalance that favors vasoconstriction. It remains unknown if this imbalance causes PIH or, rather, is an effect of other pathophysiologic changes of preeclampsia.

Additional indicators implicated as having a role in preeclampsia include:

- elevated endothelin
- reduced nitric oxide
- lack of normal increases of renin, angiotensin II, and aldosterone
- increased capillary permeability.

Preeclampsia is a multisystem disorder that can affect every major organ system including but not limited to the brain, lungs, heart, liver, and kidneys. The combination of a constricted vasculature and

Table 7.2 Anesthetic Implications of Preeclampsia

- **Blood Pressure Control:**
  - Especially important with GA to blunt the exaggerated response to laryngoscopy
  - <u>Baseline control</u> with:
    - <u>Hydralazine</u> 5 mg IV q20 min up to 20 mg
    - <u>Labetalol</u> 5 mg IV, double dose q10 min up to 300 mg total dose
  - Titrate to DBP 90–100 mmHg
  - <u>Acute control with nitroglycerine, magnesium, opioids</u>
- **Thrombocytopenia:**
  - Especially important to assess when using regional anesthesia to reduce the risk of epidural hematoma
  - <u>Recent Platelet Count</u> – usually within 6 hours of regional block
  - Start with threshold of 100,000/mm^3 (consider modifying as low as 75,000/mm^3 if contraindications to GA)
- **Magnesium:**
  - No reduction of <u>succinylcholine</u> dose for rapid sequence induction, but expect increased sensitivity
  - Use <u>nondepolarizing relaxants</u> sparingly and titrate to effect
- **Airway:**
  - Exaggerated edema
  - Anticipate difficult intubation
  - Consider smaller tracheal tube (6.0–6.5mm)
  - Avoid nasal intubation
- **Eclampsia:**
  - Be aware of potential seizure regardless of severity of preeclampsia
  - Magnesium for prophylaxis and treatment
  - Benzodiazepines or barbiturates for seizures unresponsive to magnesium

"leaky capillary membranes" leads to intravascular hypovolemia, as water moves from the intravascular space into other body compartments.

Pulmonary

Approximately 3% of patients with severe preeclampsia will develop pulmonary edema. This can be attributed to a reduction in plasma oncotic pressure and increased vascular permeability. Large fluid boluses in patients with severe preeclampsia, especially those administered magnesium sulfate, can increase the risk of acute respiratory distress syndrome.

Cardiovascular

Although elevated blood pressure is the hallmark of the disease, a progressive increase typically starts in the second to third trimester.

Preeclamptic parturients may exhibit:

- An exaggerated response to exogenous catecholamines. When necessary, vasopressors should be administered cautiously.
- An exaggerated hypertensive response to laryngoscopy. Close blood pressure control is required to prevent complications such as pulmonary edema and intracranial hemorrhage.

Blood volume, CVP, and PCWP can vary markedly from patient to patient.

Coagulation

Thrombocytopenia (i.e., platelet count below 150,000/mm^3) occurs in up to 30% of patients with preeclampsia, yet the platelet count falls below 100,000/mm^3 in less than 10% of patients presenting with severe preeclampsia. The degree of thrombocytopenia is generally related to the severity of disease.

- Although the mechanism of thrombocytopenia in preeclampsia is unknown, damage to the endothelium has been implicated.
- This causes thromboxane and serotonin to be released by activated platelets.
- A platelet consumption cascade ensues.

Renal

Proteinuria is a marker for renal dysfunction. Although chronic renal failure is rare, urine output should be monitored closely to help prevent complications. The degree of proteinuria increases with the severity of disease, as capillary permeability of the glomerulus increases.

- Glomerulopathy is correlated with the severity of the preeclampsia.
- Oliguria may occur with severe preeclampsia.
  - Careful balance in hydration between maintaining adequate renal preload and avoiding overload must be maintained, or the patient can develop pulmonary edema.
  - Urine output less than 0.5 ml/kg/h despite apparently adequate intravascular volume may necessitate pulmonary arterial pressure monitoring, or other monitors to assess preload and cardiac function.

Complications

Severe Preeclampsia

The morbidity and mortality that occurs with preeclampsia is proportional to the severity of disease. It is characterized by progressive deterioration of maternal and fetal well-being, and significantly increases neonatal and maternal morbidity and mortality. Preeclampsia includes objective measures of hypertension and proteinuria and becomes severe when additional objective criteria are met (Table 7.1).

HELLP Syndrome

HELLP is an acronym for <u>h</u>emolysis, <u>e</u>levated <u>l</u>iver enzymes, and <u>l</u>ow <u>p</u>latelet count. Although usually considered to be a type, or subset, of severe preeclampsia, the syndrome has been described in the absence of hypertension and proteinuria. Signs and symptoms associated with the syndrome are outlined in Table 7.3. Patients with HELLP should be closely monitored and delivery is usually indicated when there is evidence of progressive severity of disease.

Obstetric Management

Obstetric management of patients with preeclampsia will depend on the individual clinical situation, and can change abruptly.

Factors used to determine obstetric management include:

- severity of the hypertension
- presence of complications such as thrombocytopenia and oliguria
- fetal condition.

Conservative management involves controlling hypertension in the outpatient setting, with the goal of vaginal delivery nearer to term. With more severe cases, inpatient control is required, using IV antihypertensives and seizure prophylaxis (magnesium is used for seizure prophylaxis in the United States, while benzodiazepines and barbiturates are more often used outside the United States). If preeclampsia

---

Table 7.3 Signs and Symptoms Associated with HELLP Syndrome

- Malaise
- Epigastric or right upper quadrant pain
- Nausea and vomiting
- Thrombocytopenia
  - Platelet count can fall precipitously
  - Maternal morbidity increases significantly as the platelet count falls below 50,000/mm^3
- Regional anesthesia may be contraindicated
  - Develop plan for general anesthesia

cannot be controlled, or if fetal distress occurs in spite of medical management, cesarean delivery may be the best option to ensure well-being of both the mother and fetus.

Pharmacologic Agents

Magnesium

Magnesium sulfate raises the seizure threshold. In the United States, it is used prophylactically in patients with severe preeclampsia or rapidly progressing disease, or as treatment to reduce the morbidity associated with eclampsia. Although it transiently decreases blood pressure, it is not effective as an antihypertensive.

The recommended dosing schedule for magnesium sulfate is:

- 4–6 gm loading dose administered over 20 minutes followed by a 1–2 gm/h infusion.
- An additional 2–4 gm administered over 10 minutes is recommended for recurrent seizures.
- Magnesium has a narrow therapeutic index.
- Blood levels should be monitored.
- Clinical signs of toxicity such as sedation and loss of patellar deep tendon reflexes must also be monitored.

Magnesium administration has significant implications for the anesthesiologist, especially when managing a general anesthetic (Table 7.4). Muscle relaxation must be carefully monitored, and special care should be taken to avoid accidental rapid infusion of the magnesium sulfate during surgery.

Antihypertensives

Blood pressure control is a major goal of the management of preeclampsia, and may be accomplished with any of several pharmacologic agents. Common agents utilized include:

Alpha methyldopa (Aldomet)

- First-line agent used to treat mild preeclampsia during outpatient therapy
- Administered orally
- Indirectly inhibits dopaminergic and adrenergic neurotransmission by inhibition of dopamine formation

Hydralazine

- Administered intravenously during hospitalization
- Direct acting arterial and arteriolar vasodilator

Table 7.4 Anesthetic Implications of Magnesium Sulfate

- Mild sedation
- Mild reduction in blood pressure
- Possibly small increase in intraoperative blood loss during cesarean delivery
- Potentiates effects of both depolarizing and nondepolarizing muscle relaxants via both pre- and postsynaptic mechanisms
  - Time to recovery from succinylcholine is prolonged, although reduction of succinlycholine dose is not recommended during rapid sequence induction
  - Long duration of succinylcholine potentially complicates difficult intubation scenario
  - The dose of nondepolarizing muscle relaxants should be significantly reduced, if used at all, and the effect monitored using a nerve stimulator
- Inadvertent rapid infusion of magnesium during cesarean delivery can lead to life-threatening cardiovascular collapse
  - Hold the infusion during cesarean delivery if being administered prophylactically to prevent eclampsia
  - Continue the infusion on a separate IV pole with separate IV tubing during cesarean delivery if being administered as treatment for eclampsia

---

- Onset after IV administration takes several minutes, and up to 45 minutes for full effect
- May cause reflex tachycardia

Labetalol

- Administered intravenously during hospitalization
- Nonselective beta and alpha blocker (beta:alpha effect 3:1 orally, 7:1 intravenously)
- Onset after IV administration takes several minutes, has a half-life of 5–8 hours, eliminated via hepatic metabolism

All intravenous antihypertensives must be carefully titrated to avoid hypotension and subsequent reduction of uteroplacental blood flow. The goal is generally to achieve a diastolic blood pressure of 90–100 mmHg but the fetal status must be monitored.

- Usually the fetus tolerates the reduction in maternal blood pressure, but in a small number of cases, the reduction in uterine perfusion accompanying blood pressure reduction may not be tolerated by the fetus.

The anesthetic implications of antihypertensive agents in this population include the possibility of an exaggerated sympathectomy with induction of regional anesthesia, resulting in hypotension.

Similarly, during general anesthesia, intravenous induction agents and volatile inhalational agents may cause an exaggerated reduction in SVR.

- The risk of a hypertensive response to laryngoscopy and intubation must always be considered, and usually requires additional antihypertensive medications prior to or during induction.

Anesthetic Management

General Considerations

Volume Status

Although the plasma volume can vary significantly in patients with severe preeclampsia, important factors should be kept in mind when caring for these parturients:

- Hypotension from regional anesthesia ranges from profound to nonexistent. A subset of patients will remain severely hypertensive even during high, dense spinal anesthesia.
- Crystalloids should be used with caution due to the risk of volume overload causing pulmonary edema. This risk may be exaggerated in patients administered high doses of labetalol and magnesium sulfate.
- Vasopressors such as phenylephrine or ephedrine should be initially used with caution, due to risk of an exaggerated response.

Coagulation

As noted above, 30% of patients with preeclampsia develop thrombocytopenia. The platelet count at which neuraxial anesthesia becomes contraindicated cannot be defined. Trauma to epidural veins is impossible to prevent during epidural or spinal placement, but normally does not present a problem. In the patient with preeclampsia complicated by thrombocytopenia, uncontrolled bleeding could result in an expanding epidural hematoma, which if not recognized and treated promptly, could lead to permanent neurologic injury. Recommendations for the anesthetic management of the preeclamptic patient with thrombocytopenia are outlined in Table 7.5.

Airway

General anesthesia carries increased risk specific to the pregnant patient. Weight gain, breast engorgement, upper airway edema, and airway mucosa friability combine to make endotracheal intubation more difficult. This technical difficulty is further complicated by a

Table 7.5 Anesthetic Management of the Preeclamptic Patient with Thrombocytopenia

- Platelet count should be obtained before performing a regional block
  - In patients with thrombocytopenia, a platelet count should be obtained within 6 hours of the regional procedure, because a precipitous decline can be associated with severe disease
  - In patients with a normal platelet count, the likelihood of a platelet count < 100,000/mm^3 within 24 hours is negligible
- Epidural hematoma is rare but potentially neurologically devastating
  - Risk is probably higher with epidural techniques than with single-shot spinal techniques
- Platelet level at which risk of epidural hematoma increases is unknown
  - In absence of other confounding factors, risk is negligible with a platelet count over 100,000/mm^3
  - After considering benefits of regional anesthesia in the individual patient and other patient factors, such as airway classification and patient weight, using a threshold of 75,000/mm^3 is reasonable
- The role of thromboelastography remains unknown but may be another factor to consider when the platelet count falls between 50–75,000/mm^3
- Few experts would recommend a regional anesthetic, under almost any circumstance, in a patient with a platelet count < 50,000/mm^3

decreased FRC and increased oxygen consumption present in all pregnancies. All of these factors can be further exaggerated by preeclampsia, making regional anesthesia an especially attractive alternative when feasible. However, when a fetal emergency arises, leaving little time for regional anesthesia, or when regional anesthesia is contraindicated, a general anesthetic may be unavoidable. In these cases, full preparation must be made for a difficult intubation. In all cases, preparations for management of the difficult airway must be made (Table 7.6).

Anesthetic Options

An aggressive approach to providing regional anesthesia in patients presenting with severe preeclampsia should always be considered in an attempt to reduce overall risk (Table 7.7).

Labor and Vaginal Delivery

Regional Analgesia

Epidural analgesia is considered ideal for the management of labor pain in the preeclamptic because it:

- reduces catecholamine levels
- reduces hyperventilation

Table 7.6 Suggested Equipment for Difficult Airway Management Cart*

- Assorted laryngoscopes and blades
- Assorted endotracheal tubes and stylettes
- Assorted laryngeal mask airways or supraglottic airway devices (e.g., Intubating LMA or Proseal® LMA)
- Endotracheal tube guides (assorted intubating or lighted stylettes, manipulation forceps)
- Flexible fiberoptic intubation equipment
- Retrograde intubation equipment
- Emergency noninvasive airway ventilation devices such as an esophageal-tracheal Combitube or a hollow jet ventilation stylet
- Cricothyrotomy kit with or without jet ventilation
- Exhaled CO_2 detector
- Emergency tracheostomy kit
- Difficult Airway Algorithm readily posted on cart and in operating rooms

* Source: the Practice guidelines for management of the difficult airway: an updated report by the ASA task force on management of the difficult airway. *Anesthesiology.* 2003; 98:1269–1277.

- allows flexibility for varying labor analgesia needs
- allows the ability to dose for anesthesia when C/S is required.

"Early" epidural placement in the patient with severe preeclampsia is recommended to reduce risk and increase safety by reducing the need for general anesthesia should urgent cesarean section become necessary. Further, if severe thrombocytopenia develops, the risk of developing an epidural hematoma is probably less with an indwelling epidural catheter than attempting the procedure in a patient with severe thrombocytopenia.

After obtaining informed consent, the epidural catheter should be inserted and tested. If bilateral analgesia is observed, the catheter is secured and additional local anesthetics are administered when the patient requests labor analgesia.

Table 7.7 Reducing Anesthetic Risks in Patients with Severe Preeclampsia

- **Early epidural catheter placement** and testing whenever possible (technique is described in detail in Chapter 9)
- **Spinal anesthesia** for cesarean section when the patient presents without an existing epidural catheter and without contraindications to regional anesthesia
- **General anesthesia** only when regional anesthesia is contraindicated
  - Emphasis on blood pressure reduction and blunting the hypertensive response to laryngoscopy

Systemic Analgesia

When regional anesthesia is contraindicated in the patient with preeclampsia, systemic analgesia might become the only safe option. However, side effects from analgesics may be more likely in patients receiving magnesium sulfate. Alternative labor analgesics are discussed in Chapter 3.

Cesarean Section

Epidural Anesthesia

Traditional teaching has encouraged epidural over spinal anesthesia for patients with severe preeclampsia requiring cesarean section. Though most of these assumptions have never been rigorously investigated in randomized controlled trials, epidural anesthesia has been seen as preferable for the following reasons:

- These patients can present with extreme intravascular volume depletion.
- The gradual-onset sympathectomy, which can be achieved through incremental dosing, was thought necessary to avoid precipitous drops in maternal blood pressure and uterine perfusion pressure.
- The technique improved blood pressure control.
- Vasopressor requirements were lower.
- Intravenous fluid volume requirements were lower.
- The technique is easier to adapt for longer surgical duration.

Many of these traditional, non-evidenced-based assumptions have been called into question in recent years in a number of randomized clinical trials.

Spinal and Combined Spinal Epidural

Recent data have confirmed the safety of spinal anesthesia for cesarean section (C/S) in the patient with severe preeclampsia (Figure 7.1). With severe hypovolemia, spinal anesthesia potentially causes a rapid sympathectomy and uncontrollable hypotension; however, the hypertension and resulting indirect hypovolemia associated with preeclampsia is not entirely sympathetically mediated. For this reason, the drop in blood pressure observed during sympathectomy is less in a patient with severe preeclampsia than might be observed in patients with hypovolemia secondary to causes such as hemorrhage. The degree of hypotension and amounts of vasopressor required does not differ when comparing spinal and epidural anesthesia in patients with severe preeclampsia. Further, a spinal needle is theoretically safer than an

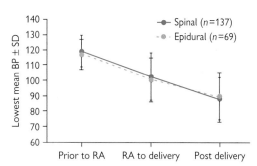

Figure 7.1 The illustration represents 206 patients with severe preeclampsia presenting for cesarean section and administered regional anesthesia (RA). The data are presented as the lowest mean arterial blood pressure recorded in mmHg and do not differ between groups. "Prior to RA" is the blood pressure recorded 20 min before induction, "RA to Delivery" is the lowest blood pressure recorded between induction and delivery and "Post Delivery" is the lowest blood pressure recorded from delivery to the end of surgery. Figure based on internal data and adapted from Hood DD. Anesthesiology 1999; 90: 1276-1282.

epidural needle in a patient with "borderline" coagulopathy as it is less likely to cause epidural vein trauma.

Doses of medications for spinal anesthesia in the preeclamptic are generally the same as would be used in a nonpreeclamptic patient.

A combined spinal epidural (CSE) anesthetic may be more appropriate than a spinal anesthetic when prolonged surgical time is anticipated due to:

- Morbid obesity
- Multiple gestation
- Multiple prior C/S
- Prior pelvic or abdominal surgery

General

General anesthesia should be considered for patients with severe preeclampsia only when regional anesthesia is contraindicated. Preeclampsia increases the difficulties encountered during airway management because of increased extravascular fluid causing engorgement of the upper airway. The following recommendations are relevant when general anesthesia cannot be avoided (Table 7.8):

- Two anesthesia providers should be present if at all possible.
- Thoroughly preoxygenate/denitrogenate with a tight mask seal whenever possible, as five minutes of tidal volume breathing offers a greater safety margin over five vital capacity breaths alone.

Table 7.8 General Anesthesia for Cesarean Section: Recommended Technique

- **Preparation:**
  - Antihypertensive pretreatment prior to anesthesia to achieve DBP 90–100 mmHg if time allows
  - Standard monitors
  - Left uterine displacement
  - Limit intravenous fluid administration
- **Airway:**
  - Prepare for difficult intubation
  - Preoxygenate for 5 min (4–6 vital capacity breaths in emergency)
  - 6.5 or 7.0 mm tracheal tube
- **Induction:**
  - Rapid sequence induction
    - Cricoid pressure until breath sounds identified and positive ETCO$_2$
    - Minimum 4 mg/kg thiopental (up to 7 mg/kg if necessary for BP control)
    - 1–1.5 mg/kg succinylcholine
    - Consider fentanyl 100–150 mg and lidocaine 100 mg IV
    - Nitroglycerine (GTN) 200 mcg (100 mcg bolus during induction and 100 mcg bolus during laryngoscopy)
  - Awake intubation
    - When difficult intubation is anticipated
- **Maintenance:**
  - 50/50 O$_2$/N$_2$O prior to delivery
  - 0.5 MAC volatile agent prior to delivery
  - Nondepolarizing muscle relaxant titrated to effect (reduced dose in patients administered magnesium sulfate)
  - Opioids and other agents as needed after delivery
  - Consider additional antihypertensives for extubation (e.g., esmolol, GTN)

- Prevent hypertension during laryngoscopy and intubation to reduce potential complications such as pulmonary edema and intracranial hemorrhage. Consideration should be given to use of higher than normal doses of induction agent (i.e., sodium pentothal up to 7 mg/kg).
- Pharmacologic agents which may be used prior to airway manipulation in addition to standard rapid sequence induction agents include:
  - Hydralazine: at least 20 min prior to induction
  - Labetalol: at least 10 min prior to induction
  - Esmolol: up to 2 mg/kg bolus immediately prior to induction
  - Nitroglycerine: 50–100 mcg boluses immediately prior to and during induction as needed
  - Sodium nitroprusside: infusion initiated at 0.5 mcg/kg/min prior to induction and titrated to effect

- Fentanyl: 100–150 mcg bolus immediately prior to induction
- Remifentanil: 1 mcg/kg bolus immediately prior to induction
- Lidocaine: 100 mg during induction

Summary

Patients with severe preeclampsia usually have multisystem involvement, and are at increased risk for significant obstetric and anesthetic complications. Anesthetic risks can be reduced by:

- assessing platelet count when appropriate
- early epidural catheter placement whenever possible
- utilizing spinal anesthesia for urgent cesarean section when preexisting catheter is not present
- reserving general anesthesia for when regional anesthesia is contraindicated
- controlling blood pressure, especially during general anesthesia
- preparing for difficult airway management.

Further Reading

1. Diagnosis and management of preeclampsia and eclampsia. ACOG Practice Bulletin #33. *Obstet Gynecol.* 2002;99:159-167.

2. Practice guidelines for management of the difficult airway: an updated report by the ASA task force on management of the difficult airway. *Anesthesiology.* 2003;98:1269-1277.

3. Hood DD, Curry R. Spinal versus epidural anesthesia for cesarean section in severely preeclamptic patients: a retrospective survey. *Anesthesiology.* 1999;90:1276-1282.

4. Horlocker TT, Wedel DJ, Benzon H, *et al.* Regional anesthesia in the anticoagulated patient: defining the risks. *Reg Anesth Pain Med.* 2003; 28:172-197.

5. Huda SS, Freeman DJ, Nelson SM. Short and long term strategies for the management of hypertensive disorders of pregnancy. *Expert Rev Cardiovasc Ther.* 2009;7:1581-1594.

6. Norris MC, Dewan DM. Preoxygenation for cesarean section: a comparison of two techniques. *Anesthesiology.* 1985;62:827-829.

7. Polley LS. Chapter 45: Hypertensive Disorders. In Chestnut DH, Polley LS, Tsen LC, Wong CA, eds. *Chestnut's Obstetric Anesthesia Principles and Practice 4th Ed.* Philadelphia, PA: Mosby Elsevier. 2009:975-1008.

8. Sibai BM. Diagnosis, prevention, and management of eclampsia. *Obstet Gynecol.* 2005;105:402-410.

9. Sibai BM. Hypertension (Chapter 28). In Gabbe SG, Niebyl JR, Simpson JL, eds. *Obstetrics: Normal and Problem Pregnancies, 4th Ed.* Churchill Livingstone 2002: 945-1004.

Chapter 8

Obstetric Hemorrhage

Craig M. Palmer, MD

Introduction

Hemorrhagic complications can arise at almost any point during pregnancy, labor or delivery, quickly turning an uneventful pregnancy into an emergent situation requiring prompt, aggressive treatment to ensure the health and well-being of mother and infant. Several series have confirmed that hemorrhage remains one of the leading causes of maternal mortality.

Understanding the causes of maternal hemorrhage and treating it effectively require an understanding of the normal anatomy of the uteroplacental unit and its physiologic adaption to the birth process.

Uteroplacental Anatomy and Normal Delivery

The human uterus is an extremely plastic organ.

- A nonpregnant, parous uterus weighs only about 70 g.
- At term, the uterus weighs well over a kilogram.

- The increase in size of the myometrium occurs in response to both steroid hormones produced during pregnancy, and distention due to the developing fetus, placenta, and amniotic fluid volume.

Along with this increase in size and weight, there is a corresponding increase in blood flow to the uterus and placenta. At term, maternal blood flow to the uterus may be well over 15 percent of cardiac output.

- The primary maternal blood supply is from the uterine arteries, which arise as a branch of the anterior trunk of the internal iliac arteries.
- The ascending branch of the uterine artery supplies the major portion of the body of the uterus and the placental bed.
- A variable portion of the blood supply to the placenta may come from the ovarian arteries.
- In the placental bed, small endometrial (or spiral) arteries carry the actual blood supply to the placenta.

The maternal blood supply to the placenta is unique, in that maternal blood actually leaves the maternal circulation, circulates through the intervillous space lined by placental trophoblastic syncytium rather than endothelium, and returns to the maternal circulation (Figure 8.1).

- Maternal arterial pressure provides the driving force that circulates maternal blood into the intervillous space to bathe the chorionic villi, which contain the fetal capillaries. Oxygen and nutrient exchange occurs, and maternal blood is drained back into the maternal circulation through openings in the basal plate of the placenta to the endometrial veins.
- On the fetal side, deoxygenated blood is delivered to the placenta by the paired umbilical arteries, which branch into capillaries within the chorionic villi. Oxygen and nutrient exchange occurs in the capillaries, and blood returns to the fetus via the umbilical vein.

The decidua is a specialized form of endometrium, which forms the boundary between the mother and fetus.

- At delivery, the placenta separates from the placental bed, leaving behind in the uterus the basal zone of the decidua that ultimately gives rise to new endometrium.
- With separation, the myriad small endometrial arteries that supplied the placenta are torn: in the absence of a mechanism to halt blood loss, they would continue to spurt blood into the now empty uterine cavity. Two mechanisms normally prevent ongoing blood loss:

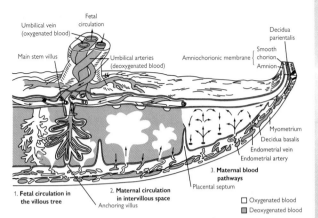

Figure 8.1 Schematic cross-section of the anatomy of a normal human placenta. Deoxygenated blood from the fetus enters the placenta and flows through capillaries in the villi where oxygen and nutrient exchange occurs, before returning to the fetal circulation via the umbilical vein. Maternal blood enters via the endometrial arteries, circulates through the intervillous space and returns to the maternal circulation through the endometrial veins. Reprinted with permission from Cunningham FG, Macdonald PC, Gant NF, et al. *Williams Obstetrics, 19th ed,* pp. 165–207. 1993, McGraw-Hill.

- the elasticity of the arterioles allows them to retract and constrict;
- contraction of the myometrium physically compresses the disrupted vessels.

Obstetric hemorrhage most often results from impaired myometrial contraction.

Assessment of the Bleeding Parturient

While there are a number of well-described causes of bleeding in the parturient, recognizing that the patient may have suffered significant blood loss is the crucial first step in management. Regardless of the cause, symptoms of hemorrhage generally reflect the amount of bleeding and degree of hypovolemia.

- In many cases, there may be little external evidence of bleeding. Recognition and diagnosis of the problem will begin with physical examination of the patient and assessment of vital signs.

- Most parturients are young and in relatively good health. Even with blood loss of one liter or more, systemic blood pressure tends to be maintained, though tachycardia to varying degrees may be apparent. Though there are a number of causes of tachycardia, hemorrhage should be excluded as a cause even if blood pressure is normal.
- While there is some overlap between categories, the causes of obstetric hemorrhage can be generally classified as occurring prepartum, intrapartum, or postpartum.

Prepartum Hemorrhage

Placental Abruption

Definition

Placental abruption refers to the premature partial separation of a normally implanted placenta; in rare instances the separation may be complete.

- This may occur either prepartum or intrapartum.
- The reported frequency of abruption depends on the criteria used for diagnosis, but the incidence has been estimated to be between 1 in 77 and 1 in 86 deliveries.

Risk Factors

While there is no single cause for abruption, a number of conditions have been associated with a higher incidence of abruption (Table 8.1).

Table 8.1 Factors Associated with Increased Risk of Placental Abruption
Pregnancy-induced hypertension (PIH)
Chronic hypertension
Premature rupture of membranes
External trauma
Cigarette smoking
Cocaine abuse
Uterine leiomyoma
Increased parity
Increased age

Implications

Abruption has both maternal and fetal implications. Uterine bleeding associated with delivery is usually limited by myometrial contraction, as discussed above; in abruption, placental separation is not followed by myometrial contraction. The uterus does not empty; therefore, effective myometrial contraction cannot occur, and ongoing maternal blood loss usually results. For the fetus, the decrease in placental surface area may result in asphyxia.

- Abruption is severe enough to be fatal to the fetus in about 1 in 750 deliveries, and accounts for about 15% of third trimester stillbirths.
- When abruption occurs, perinatal mortality is approximately 10%.
- Severe neurologic damage may occur even in surviving neonates.

Symptoms and Presentation

The most common symptom of abruption is vaginal bleeding, usually associated with uterine tenderness or back pain. Other signs include fetal heart rate abnormalities, preterm labor or uterine hypertonus, and infrequently, fetal demise (Table 8.2).

Table 8.2 Signs and Symptoms of Placental Abruption	
Sign/symptom	Frequency (percent of cases)
Vaginal bleeding	78
Uterine tenderness or back pain	66
Fetal distress	60
Increased uterine tone/contractions	34
Preterm labor	22
Fetal demise	17

Reprinted with permission from Hurd WW, Miodovnik M, Hertzberg V, and Lavin JP. Selective management of abruptio placentae: A prospective study. *Obstet Gynecol*. 1983;61(4):467–473.

Clinical Course

Up to 90% of abruptions will be either mild or moderate, without fetal distress, maternal hypotension or coagulopathy.

- It is important to note that the amount of visible vaginal blood loss usually markedly underestimates the actual maternal blood loss (Table 8.3).
- While some vaginal bleeding is usually apparent, up to 3000 ml of blood can be sequestered behind the placenta in a "concealed"

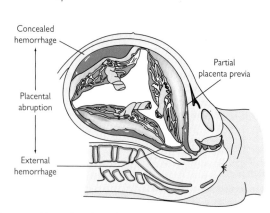

Figure 8.2 Hemorrhage from placental abruption and placenta previa. External (vaginal) bleeding is usually apparent in both conditions, although up to 3 liters of blood may be lost in a concealed hemorrhage without evidence of external blood loss. Reprinted with permission from Cunningham FG, Macdonald PC, Gant NF, *et al. Williams Obstetrics, 19th ed,* pp. 165–207. 1993, McGraw-Hill.

hemorrhage without external bleeding. This may occur when the placenta remains circumferentially adherent around a central area of abruption (Figure 8.2).

In severe cases, maternal coagulopathy can occur.

- Abruption is the most common cause of disseminated intravascular coagulation (DIC) during pregnancy.
- This is manifested as thrombocytopenia, hypofibrinogenemia, and decreased levels of Factors V and VIII; fibrin-split products appear in the maternal circulation, and clinical oozing may become apparent.

Two possible mechanisms for the development of this coagulopathy have been proposed:

- activation of circulating plasminogen, or
- alternatively, placental thromboplastin may trigger activation of the extrinsic clotting pathway.

Anesthetic Management (Figure 8.3)

If abruption is suspected, blood should be drawn immediately to check:

- hemoglobin and hematocrit;
- platelet count;

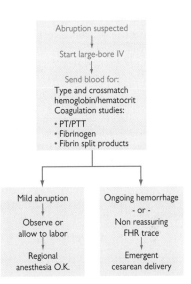

Figure 8.3 Management of the parturient with suspected placental abruption.

- fibrinogen;
- fibrin-split products.
- Blood should also be sent for type and crossmatch.

Subsequent management depends on the severity of the situation.

Labor may be induced with continuous fetal monitoring assuming:

- no ongoing blood loss;
- no evidence of maternal hypovolemia;
- no evidence of coagulopathy;
- the presence of a reassuring fetal heart rate.

Regional anesthesia can also be safely employed in these patients, assuming there is no evidence of uncorrected maternal hypovolemia and the platelet count is stable and roughly 75,000 or higher.

- Regional anesthesia should be avoided if the mother is hypovolemic, if there is ongoing hemorrhage, or if there are significant fetal heart rate abnormalities.

With a severe abruption (i.e., with ongoing blood loss, coagulopathy, or a nonreassuring fetal heart rate), emergent cesarean delivery may be necessary, with general anesthesia usually indicated for these reasons.

Most obstetric anesthesiologists will accept a platelet count as low as 70,000 when performing a neuraxial anesthetic, and sometimes lower, if there are strong maternal indications for using a regional anesthetic. The decision to employ regional anesthesia in such patients is simply a risk-benefit analysis. The benefits of a regional anesthetic, either an epidural catheter for labor or a spinal anesthetic for cesarean delivery, can be considerable for some parturients. The risk is that of theoretically causing an epidural hematoma and additional morbidity; in most cases this risk is very low. See also Chapter 3.

Table 8.3 Clinical Signs and Symptoms of Blood Loss in the Parturient

Amount of blood loss		Clinical finding
Mild bleeding	15% of blood volume (up to 1000 ml)	Mild tachycardia
		Normal blood pressure and respiration
		Negative tilt test
		Normal urine output
Moderate bleeding	20%–25% of blood volume (up to 1600 ml)	Tachycardia (heart rate 110–130)
		Decreased pulse pressure
		Moderate tachypnea
		Positive capillary blanching test
		Positive tilt test
		Urine output <1 ml/kg/h
Severe bleeding	30%–35% of blood volume (up to 2400 ml)	Marked tachycardia (heart rate 120–160)
		Cold, clammy, pallid skin
		Hypotension
		Tachypnea (respirations > 30/min)
		Oliguria
Massive bleeding	40% of blood volume (over 2400 ml)	Profound shock
		Mental status changes/disorientation
		Systolic blood pressure <80 mmHg
		Peripheral pulses absent
		Marked tachycardia
		Oliguria or anuria

Reprinted with permission from Ferouz F. Peripartum hemorrhage and maternal resuscitation. In: Norris MC, *Obstetric Anesthesia, 2nd ed.* 1998, Lippincott, Williams & Wilkins.

- Once the decision to proceed to cesarean delivery has been made, the first anesthetic consideration should be maternal volume status. A healthy term parturient can lose 10 to 15 percent of circulating blood volume without any change in vital signs (Table 8.3).
- If a parturient is tachycardic, hypotensive, or oliguric, she is likely severely volume depleted. Adequate intravenous access is essential; at least one (ideally two) large-bore IV (16 gauge or larger) should be in place.

General Anesthesia in the Hypovolemic Parturient (Table 8.4)

In addition to routine precautions for cesarean delivery (Chapter 4), the hypovolemic parturient presents additional considerations.

Because **sodium pentothal** is a vasodilator, it is not an appropriate induction agent. **Propofol** is a myocardial depressant, which can also significantly decrease maternal blood pressure. **Ketamine**, which supports blood pressure through sympathetic stimulation, is the agent of choice.

Table 8.4 General Anesthesia in the Hypovolemic Parturient
Adequate IV access
Routine precautions • Aspiration prophylaxis—oral sodium citrate • Denitrogenation • Assistance available
Anesthetic agents • Induction: ketamine, 1–1.5 mg/kg • Relaxation: succinylcholine relaxant of choice
Maintenance (pre-delivery) • Nitrous oxide (with ongoing fetal stress, 100% O_2 indicated for fetal oxygenation) • Inhalational agents: 0.5 MAC or less if maternal blood pressure tolerates
Maintenance (post-delivery) • Continue relaxation (follow train-of-four) • Inhalational agent: isoflurane 0.2% or sevoflurane 0.5% for amnesia • Nitrous oxide (up to 70%) if tolerated • Opioid—fentanyl
Monitoring • Routine: ECG, BP, PO, ET-CO_2 and Foley • Invasive? Consider arterial line

- After induction but before delivery, support of the fetus is critical; despite clear evidence of benefit, in the setting of potentially decreased placental perfusion, delivery of 100% oxygen will maximize oxygen delivery to the fetus.

After delivery, up to 70% nitrous oxide may be used if the maternal SaO_2 remains adequate, and conversion to a "nitrous/narcotic" anesthetic allows use of minimal concentrations of inhaled anesthetic; all the inhaled anesthetic agents cause dose-related uterine relaxation, which can contribute to blood loss.

- If aggressive fluid resuscitation fails to restore adequate maternal blood pressure, additional "stat" labs should be sent to check hematocrit, coagulation status, and acid-base balance (arterial blood gas analysis).

- In the unstable parturient, serious consideration should be given to placement of an arterial line for continuous blood pressure monitoring and repeated blood draws for lab work.

Even following delivery, be prepared for massive blood loss. Blood infiltrating the myometrium may result in a "Couvelaire" uterus, preventing adequate uterine contraction and inhibiting hemostasis.

- In addition to oxytocin, other uterotonic agents may be necessary for adequate uterine contraction (see below).

- In rare situations, internal iliac artery ligation or hysterectomy may be necessary to stop hemorrhage.

> Once hemorrhage is controlled, coagulation should return to normal within several hours, but getting control of the bleeding may require aggressive treatment of the coagulopathy, utilizing not only PRBCs but also fresh-frozen plasma, platelet concentrates, and even cryoprecipitate. Use of these blood products is ideally based on laboratory evidence of derangements, but clinical judgment may be the only tool available in a rapidly changing, emergent situation.

Placenta Previa

Definition

Placenta previa refers to an abnormal implantation of the placenta, over or close to the cervical os. It can be classified as complete, partial, or marginal (Figure 8.4). The incidence of placenta previa at term is about 1 in 200–250 deliveries.

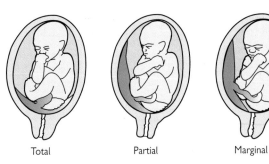

| Total | Partial | Marginal |

Figure 8.4 Classification of placenta previa.

- Routine prenatal ultrasonography generally identifies a higher percentage of previa in early gestation, but most of these resolve by the third trimester, as enlargement of the gravid uterus carries the implantation site away from the cervical os.
- Previa is more common in the multipara, particularly those with prior cesarean delivery (see Chapter 11), or a history of prior previa.

Implications

With the onset of labor the cervical os begins to dilate; in the presence of placenta previa, the placenta over the os will detach and maternal hemorrhage will ensue. As with abruption, bleeding will continue until the uterus can contract effectively, i.e., once the uterus is empty after delivery. Further, the lower uterine segment where the placenta is implanted has fewer contractile elements than the corpus, where normal placental implantation occurs. Because neither the mother nor the fetus can tolerate the blood loss or the loss of placental surface area, respectively, once diagnosed, delivery will always be via cesarean section.

Signs and Symptoms

The undiagnosed placenta previa usually presents as painless vaginal bleeding in the third trimester; for this reason, all vaginal bleeding in the third trimester should be considered placenta previa until proven otherwise. Bleeding due to previa may stop spontaneously if the area of disruption is small, but it may be sudden and severe. The diagnosis can be made or confirmed readily with transabdominal ultrasonography.

In the not-so-distant past, the definitive diagnosis of placenta previa was made by direct examination of the cervical os with a vaginal speculum exam. Because this exam can provoke brisk, even torrential hemorrhage, the exam was performed as a "double set-up"—the parturient was placed in lithotomy position for the speculum exam in the operating room, but with her abdomen prepped and draped in preparation for an immediate cesarean delivery. Today, the widespread use and availability of ultrasonography, and its excellent accuracy in diagnosis, have all but eliminated the need for the double set-up.

Anesthetic Management

Management of the diagnosed previa depends on the stage of gestation and clinical presentation.

- In the face of ongoing bleeding, expeditious cesarean delivery is indicated. With rapid or massive blood loss, general anesthesia is usually necessary, as it is the most rapid way to deliver the infant and stabilize the mother—blood loss will continue until infant and placenta are delivered.
- If the initial bleeding episode has stopped spontaneously, regional anesthesia can be employed following careful assessment of maternal volume status (heart rate, blood pressure, urine output); maternal hypovolemia is a strong relative contraindication to the use of regional anesthesia.

When diagnosed prior to about 32 weeks gestation, obstetric management is "expectant"—primarily, bed rest and hope (that the patient won't start bleeding).

Due to the increased risk of bleeding near term, after about 32 weeks gestation, fetal maturity is assessed (usually by amniocentesis), and elective cesarean delivery undertaken once maturity is confirmed.

Intrapartum Hemorrhage

Uterine Rupture

Definition

Uterine rupture may occur prepartum, intrapartum, or even postpartum, but is most commonly an intrapartum event, as uterine contractions increase in force. While the associated maternal mortality is usually low (about 0.1% in the United States), it can be catastrophic for both the mother and infant. See also "Anesthetic considerations for vaginal birth after cesarean delivery" (VBAC) in Chapter 11.

Risk Factors (Table 8.5)

By far, the most common cause of uterine rupture is separation of a previous uterine scar, from a prior C-section.

- A scar from a classical (vertical) uterine incision is more likely to dehisce during labor than a low-transverse segment scar.
- The classical incision extends well into the myometrium, whereas the low-transverse segment incision is primary through connective tissue; this lower incision heals much more solidly than an incision through uterine muscle.
- The risk of uterine rupture is 3 to 15 times greater for VBAC patients than those without a uterine scar, and if rupture occurs, neonatal mortality is increased by a factor of 10.
- Maternal mortality is higher if there is no prior uterine scar, or the rupture is traumatic.

Table 8.5 Causes of Uterine Rupture
Previous uterine scar (prior cesarean section: "VBAC")
External trauma
Excessive oxytocin stimulation
Grand multiparity
Fetal malpresentation
Uterine distention (macrosomia, hydramnios)
Internal trauma: • Forceps, vacuum use • Curettage • Internal version • Manual exploration

Signs and Symptoms

Symptoms of rupture include vaginal bleeding, severe uterine or abdominal pain, shoulder pain, the disappearance of fetal heart tones, and/or hypotension (Table 8.6). In a parturient with obvious hypotension or shock, general anesthesia is indicated to rapidly deliver the infant and explore the abdomen to control hemorrhage.

Table 8.6 **Signs and Symptoms of Intrapartum Uterine Rupture**
Fetal heart rate abnormalities/fetal stress
Vaginal bleeding
Abnormal labor pattern or uterine hypertonus
Hypotension
Atypical abdominal pain (not associated with uterine contractions)
Abdominal tenderness

Postpartum Hemorrhage

While technically, any vaginal or uterine bleeding within 6 weeks after delivery is considered postpartum hemorrhage, truly significant blood loss usually occurs immediately after delivery, or within one to two hours.

- Postpartum hemorrhage is the most common cause of serious blood loss in obstetrics.

Retained Placenta

Definition

If the uterus does not empty completely after delivery, it will not be able to fully contract, and arteries of the decidua basalis will continue to bleed. Retained placenta occurs in about 1% of deliveries, and usually requires manual exploration of the uterus.

Anesthetic Management

Anesthetic management of retained placenta must take into account two factors: uterine relaxation and analgesia.

In order to manually explore the uterus, it is usually necessary to relax the uterus:

- Traditionally, the inhalational agents (halothane, isoflurane) have been used for this—at inhaled concentrations well over 1 MAC, they are very effective uterine relaxants. Use at these concentrations means inducing a general anesthetic, however, with all the associated concerns of aspiration risk, airway management, maternal volume status, etc.
- Nitroglycerin has been shown to be an effective alternative for uterine relaxation, which does not require induction of general anesthesia (Table 8.7). Bolus intravenous administration of 100–200 mcg nitroglycerin will produce uterine relaxation within 30–45 seconds

that lasts only 60–90 seconds due to its short half-life. Due to systemic vasodilation, maternal hypotension can be significant, but this should be a short-lived side effect.

Nitroglycerin does not provide analgesia, however, so other measures may need to be taken. If a parturient has an epidural catheter in place from labor, this can be used for analgesia but again, careful consideration must be paid to maternal volume status before dosing the epidural and potentially vasodilating the patient.

Table 8.7 Clinical Use of Nitroglycerin (Glyceryl Trinitrate) for Uterine Relaxation
Prepare appropriate dilution
• NTG supplied as 50 mg/10 ml vial (5 mg/ml)
• Add to 500 ml normal saline
• Result: 100 mcg/ml
Administration: bolus dosing
• Begin with 100 mcg bolus
• Increase by increments of 100 mcg until desired effect (i.e., uterine relaxation)
Action
• Onset 30–45 seconds
• Duration 60–90 seconds
Side effects: hypotension
• R_x with phenylephrine bolus IV as necessary

Uterine Atony

Definition

Uterine atony occurs in varying degree following 2% to 5% of deliveries, and is the most common cause of serious blood loss in obstetrics. With 15% or more of maternal cardiac output at term going to the gravid uterus, a completely atonic uterus can easily lose 2 liters of blood in 5 minutes.

Risk Factors

A number of factors, listed in Table 8.8, have been shown to increase the risk of uterine atony.

Anesthetic Management

- Initial management of uterine atony is medical.
- Fluid resuscitation
  - This should always be the initial intervention, as maternal blood loss is often underestimated. Volume resuscitation can be lifesaving.

Table 8.8 Conditions Associated with Uterine Atony
High parity
Dysfunctional labor
Uterine distention   • Multiple gestation   • Polyhydramnios   • Macrosomia
Retained placenta
Infection   • Chorioamnionitis
Medications   • Prolonged oxytocin use during labor   • Tocolytic agents   • Inhalational anesthetics

- Oxygen supplementation (high flows via face mask)
- External uterine massage
- Use of uterotonics
- These steps may allow avoidance of operative intervention (see below).

Use of Uterotonics

The initial management of uterine atony is with uterotonic agents, which increase uterine contractility and tone and allow the normal process of postdelivery hemostasis to occur. Three classes of uterotonics are currently available for clinical use: oxytocin, ergot alkaloids, and prostaglandins (Table 8.9).

- **Oxytocin** is usually the initial therapy—up to forty IU/l may be infused as rapidly as possible; increasing the dose beyond this does not offer any benefit.
  - Oxytocin is a naturally occurring neurohypophyseal hormone for which specific receptors exist in the myometrium.
  - Systemically, oxytocin is a vasodilator, and may aggravate hypotension if administered rapidly; if both rapid volume infusion and rapid oxytocin infusion are necessary concurrently, consider using two intravenous lines.
- **Methylergonovine** (Methergine®), a commercially available ergot alkaloid, is a second-line agent for the treatment of uterine atony, and is particularly effective for producing a sustained increase in uterine tone.

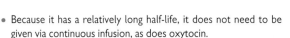

- Because it has a relatively long half-life, it does not need to be given via continuous infusion, as does oxytocin.
- Methylergonovine is administered intramuscularly at a dose of 0.4 mg; if two doses do not restore appropriate uterine tone, other therapy should be instituted.
- Systemically, methylergonovine can cause hypertension, likely due to α-adrenergic stimulation; systemic hypertension is a relative contraindication to its use.

> The ergot alkaloids have been used in obstetrics for over 400 years; they are derived from a fungus that grows upon grain, particularly rye. Ingestion of contaminated grain can cause intense vasoconstriction and even gangrene. During the Middle Ages, outbreaks of "ergotism" were named "St. Anthony's Fire" because of the burning sensation sufferers felt in their extremities.

- **Carboprost** tromethamine is a third uterotonic option. Carboprost is a stable analog of the naturally occurring prostaglandin, Pg-F$_{2\alpha}$.
  - It is given at a 0.25 mg dose IM, or can be injected directly intramyometrially. Total dose should probably not exceed 0.75 to 1.0 mg.
  - Carboprost is an extremely effective uterotonic, but it has significant systemic side effects; it should never be administered intravenously.
  - Carboprost is a potent systemic and pulmonary vasoconstrictor, and bronchoconstrictor. Intravenous administration can be associated with severe bronchospasm, and systemic and pulmonary hypertension. Intramyometrial administration should also be used with caution, as rapid uptake by uterine venous sinuses can have the same effect as intravenous administration.
  - Due to its propensity to cause bronchospasm, carboprost should be used with caution in asthmatics; the urgency of the need to increase uterine tone should be weighed against the severity of the patient's asthma.

Misoprostol is also a prostaglandin analog (PGE$_1$). Unlike oxytocin and carboprost, it is thermostable and does not require refrigeration. For this reason, while not usually as effective as oxytocin, it is sometimes used to treat uterine atony in the developing world.

Table 8.9 Uterotonic Agents

Medication	Class	Administration	Dosing	Side effects	Comments
Oxytocin	Neurohypophyseal hormone	Infusion	Up to 40 IU/l	Hypotension with rapid infusion	Initial therapy
Methylergonovine	Ergot alkaloid	Intramuscular	0.4 mg IM; repeat once	Hypertension	Sustained increase in uterine tone
Carboprost	Prostaglandin	Intramuscular Intramyometrial	0.25 mg IM repeat up to 1.0 mg total	Systemic and Pulmonary hypertension, bronchospasm	Never administer intravenously

Placenta Accreta

Definition

Placenta accreta (and variants placenta increta and placenta percreta) refers to abnormal development and implantation of the placenta without the decidua basalis layer. The decidua basalis forms the normal interface and cleavage plane between the placenta and the uterus; in its absence, the placenta implants directly onto (placenta accreta) the myometrium.

- Placenta increta refers to a placenta that invades into the myometrium,
- Placenta percreta occurs when the placenta actually invades through the myometrium, and may implant on other intra-abdominal structures.

With any of the variations, separation of the placenta after delivery disrupts the myometrium and can result in severe bleeding; complete separation of the placenta is not possible, and continuing blood loss results.

Risk Factors

The overall incidence of placenta accreta is about 1 in 2500 deliveries or less, but it is not usually diagnosed until after delivery, when prompt action becomes necessary.

- In the absence of placenta previa, and without a uterine scar (i.e., no previous cesarean delivery), the risk of placenta accreta is only 1 in 22,150.
- One patient population is known to have a predictably higher incidence of placenta accreta: patients with known placenta previa. Risk increases even further in those with both placenta previa and a prior C-section: as the number of prior C-sections increases, the risk also increases. In patients with a placenta previa and 2 or more prior C-sections, the incidence has been reported to be over 33% (Table 8.10).

Table 8.10 Risk of Placenta Accreta and Previous Cesarean Delivery

Number of prior C/S	Risk of placenta accreta (%)
0	3.4
1	14.7
2 or more	33.7

Reprinted from the *American Journal of Obstetrics and Gynecology*, Vol. 177 Issue no. 1, Miller DA, *et al.* Clinical risk factors for placenta previa-placenta accrete, pp. 210–214, Copyright (1997), with permission from Elsevier.

- Advanced maternal age, >35 years, further increases risk for placenta accreta in the presence of placenta previa.

Non-Operative Interventions for Management of Obstetric Hemorrhage

In some situations, non-operative interventions to decrease blood loss may be effective.

- **Radiologic interventions**. Interventional radiologists have proven helpful in management of obstetric hemorrhage in two situations:
  - *Placement of preoperative iliac balloon catheters.* When a patient is confirmed to be at significant risk of hemorrhage *prior* to cesarean delivery, such as a confirmed diagnosis of placenta accreta, placement of balloon catheters in the internal iliac arteries bilaterally before surgery has been reported helpful in controlling blood loss. Immediately after delivery of the infant, the balloons can be inflated, halting blood flow to the uterus, which allows the surgeon to perform the indicated procedure.
  - *Postpartum embolization.* Infrequently, despite optimal medical management following delivery (vaginal or cesarean), less vigorous bleeding may occur. In such situations, radiologically guided selective catheter embolization of the offending vessels has been reported effective. It should be noted that this is rarely an option for treatment of acute, severe hemorrhage.
- **Intrauterine tamponade**. Intrauterine placement of a Sengstaken-Blakemore tube has been reported for the control of uterine bleeding secondary to uterine atony. Such catheters are more commonly used for control of bleeding esophageal varices. Inflation of the intrauterine balloon with 400 ml saline for 24 hours has been reported up to 80% effective for control of bleeding.

Anesthetic Management: Peripartum Hysterectomy

On infrequent occasions, significant hemorrhage secondary to problems such as placenta accreta may be controlled with noninvasive options. More often, surgical intervention is necessary, usually hysterectomy. As noted above, maternal blood flow to the uterus at term is substantial, and the major vessels are located deep in the pelvis;

control of these vessels is the major obstacle facing the obstetrician, and is rarely accomplished without substantial blood loss.

Once the decision to perform a hysterectomy is made (or even considered), the anesthesiologist should anticipate a difficult case with major ongoing blood loss.

- The first priority should be to establish large-bore intravenous access for fluid resuscitation. It is important to try to do this before major blood loss has occurred, because once the patient has become hypovolemic, vasoconstricted, and cold, it becomes very difficult to place peripheral IV lines.

- With regard to monitoring, an arterial cannula is extremely useful, as blood pressure swings can be rapid, unpredictable, and extreme; the arterial line also provides a convenient method to draw blood for serial determinations of hemoglobin, hematocrit, and coagulation profile.

- Anticipating the likelihood of the need for transfusion, type and crossmatched blood should be brought to the operating room; if crossmatched blood is not available, "emergency release" type O-negative blood should be requested.

- Even if the delivery has been performed with an adequate regional anesthetic, if the maternal airway can be readily secured, conversion to a general anesthetic and intubation of the patient should be strongly considered. The wide swings in blood pressure that often occur usually make for a very uncomfortable, nauseous patient, and it is difficult to attend to the patient and aggressively volume-resuscitate her at the same time.

- A second pair of hands (i.e., someone to assist you) to help in these cases is almost essential.

The primary goal during a peripartum hysterectomy is to maintain circulating blood volume. Depending on the degree of blood loss, transfusion with packed red blood cells is usually necessary. The degree of blood loss will also dictate the need to support maternal coagulation status: with substantial blood loss, fresh-frozen plasma and platelet transfusion are often necessary.

Fetal Hemorrhage

Vasa Previa

Definition

Vasa previa differs from the problems discussed previously, in that the blood loss is fetal, not maternal. Vasa previa is present when placental blood vessels overlie the internal os of the cervix in advance of the fetal presenting part. They are unsupported by the umbilical cord or other placental tissue. The condition may develop as a result of a velamentous insertion of the umbilical cord, or as a remnant of the resolution of a partial placenta previa as gestation progresses.

Risk Factors

The incidence of vasa previa in the general obstetric population is about 1 in 2500 deliveries, but it may be as high as 1 in 300 if the pregnancy was the result of *in vitro* fertilization techniques and reimplantation.

Implications

With the onset of labor, cervical dilation causes the disruption of the overlying blood vessels, with rapid hemorrhage. If the diagnosis is not made immediately and surgical delivery of the infant accomplished promptly, fetal exsanguination and death often result.

* The perinatal mortality of vasa previa is as high as 60%.

Symptoms and Presentation

Vasa previa should be considered any time rupture of membranes is accompanied by bleeding and fetal heart rate decelerations and bradycardia.

Anesthetic Management

Once the diagnosis is entertained, surgical (cesarean) delivery should be accomplished as rapidly as safely possible, usually with a general anesthetic technique.

Transfusion in Obstetrics

The need for transfusion in the obstetric population is not uncommon, but there is often reluctance on the part of anesthesiologists to employ it, due to the perceived risks. A considered decision to employ transfusion therapy must take into account not only the risks, but also the benefits of the therapy.

Risks of Transfusion

The risks associated with transfusion can be classified as infectious and noninfectious. Noninfectious risk includes those most often due to human error, i.e., incompatible transfusion and circulatory overload.

- An ABO incompatible transfusion occurs about 1:12,000 transfused units, but is fatal in only a small number of cases (estimated at 19 per year in the United States). Errors resulting in an incompatible transfusion can occur at any step of the transfusion process, from collection of blood from the donor, through blood banking procedures, to administration to the recipient.
- Acute lung injury, also known as TRALI (transfusion related acute lung injury) is probably the most common cause of death from transfusion. While the incidence is unknown, it is often cited to occur once per 5000 plasma-containing components. The mechanism likely involves transfusion of leukocyte antibodies. The mortality rate is probably in the range of 5%–10%.
- Circulatory overload should occur less frequently in the obstetric population than most populations requiring transfusion, and should cause less morbidity and no long-term sequelae.

Infectious risks, i.e., acquiring a viral infection from a transfusion, can also occur, but infrequently.

- Fear of acquiring HIV is common, but the risk of acquiring HIV via transfusion is actually quite low; with current screening technology, only about 1 unit in 2 million are potentially infectious.
- Hepatitis B is more common, with about 1 in 200,000 units potentially infectious. Only about 1 in 10 patients infected will develop long-term sequelae, however.
- Like HIV, the risk of hepatitis C is about 1 in 2 million units potentially being infectious. It can take decades to develop clinically apparent disease after infection with hepatitis C, but the young age of the obstetric population means that once infected, most will live long enough to become symptomatic. Though our understanding of this disease is still evolving, some experts believe that almost all patients infected will eventually develop chronic disease, either cirrhosis or chronic active hepatitis.

Benefits of Transfusion

The obvious benefits of transfusion include:

- increased oxygen-carrying capacity of the blood (resulting in increased tissue delivery of oxygen);
- restoration of circulating blood volume;
- elevation of clotting factors.

In practice, few parturients will require transfusion with a hemoglobin level of 7.0 g/dl or greater, assuming appropriate volume replacement has been provided. Complete (albeit slow) recovery has been reported in parturients who refused transfusion despite hemoglobin levels below 3.0 g/dl.

> The critical level of oxygen delivery is probably in the range of 300 to 330 ml/min/m^2 of body surface area (BSA). In a hypothetical "average" parturient with a BSA of 1.7 m^2, cardiac output of 6 l/min, and hemoglobin of 6.0 g/dl, calculated oxygen delivery will be only 277 ml/min/m^2. Such a situation should be unusual, however: the normal response to blood loss is to increase cardiac output to compensate, increasing oxygen delivery proportionately. Increasing cardiac output by one-third, to 8 l/min, (within reason for almost all parturients) will increase oxygen delivery to over 350 ml/min/m^2.

Use of blood products other than PRBCs is most common in the setting of massive blood loss (>150 ml/min, or loss of over 50% of circulating blood volume in 3 hours).

- The most common (earliest) derangement in this setting is thrombocytopenia.
  - Platelet transfusion should infrequently be necessary with a stable platelet count over 50,000/μL.
  - In the average (70–80 kg) parturient, each unit of platelets should raise the platelet count by 5,000–10,000/μL.
  - A unit of plasmapherized platelets is equivalent to 5–8 single donor units.
- Acutely, massive blood loss and rapid replacement is also likely to require replacement of circulating clotting factors with FFP.
- Cryoprecipitate should be used to specifically raise fibrinogen levels.

Obstetric Massive Transfusion Protocol

In areas of clinical practice such as trauma anesthesia, the use of "massive transfusion protocols" has been found very helpful in potentially life-threatening situations. Obstetrics is no different, as the potential for rapid, life-threatening blood loss exists for every parturient. Establishment of an obstetric massive transfusion protocol with the help of blood banking specialists in each institution can provide a mechanism to more rapidly alert the blood bank to a problem and obtain the necessary blood products without multiple orders, phone calls, and delays. Such protocols will alert the blood bank to send to the operating room blood products in preset fixed ratios, optimizing the possibility of controlling hemorrhage and maintaining hemostasis.

These protocols need not be complicated. As an example, in the event of unexpected bleeding, necessary steps would include:

- control of the bleeding by the operating obstetrician or surgeon;
- restoration of circulating blood volume, initially with crystalloid infusion.

Once a certain level of estimated blood loss is reached, if bleeding is not yet controlled, blood products should be administered in fixed ratios:

- Packed red blood cells (PRBCs) and fresh-frozen plasma (FFP) in a 1:1 ratio. The goal should be to maintain the PT within 1 to 1.5 times the normal level, in addition to maintaining adequate circulating hemoglobin levels.
- Platelet transfusion once blood loss has reached roughly 1.5 times the parturient's estimated blood volume.
- Cryoprecipitate or fibrinogen concentrate to maintain the parturient's measured blood level above 100mg/dl.

Blood Storage and Salvage

In recent years, new strategies to reduce the need for homologous transfusion have been applied to the obstetric population; these include autologous donation of blood, and intraoperative blood salvage.

Autologous Donation

Autologous donation has been found to be safe for pregnant patients and their fetuses, assuming the parturient does not have a preexisting anemia (hgb < 11g/dl).

- The limitation of autologous donation is in identifying appropriate candidates; the low incidence of the need for transfusion in the overall obstetric population does not make autologous donation practical or cost effective for routine use.
- Autologous donation may have a place in the management of certain high-risk patients, such as those with placenta previa or accreta, women with known abnormal antibodies, or those undergoing scheduled cesarean hysterectomy.

Blood Salvage

Blood salvage has recently been shown to be a viable option in the obstetric population. Initial fears that autologous transfusion during cesarean delivery might induce amniotic fluid embolism have proven unfounded, using published red cell salvage protocols.

- As with autologous donation, the low incidence of the need for transfusion at cesarean delivery does not make it cost effective for routine use. In those settings where major blood loss can be anticipated, it is an excellent option. Table 8.11 lists several situations where the reported incidence of transfusion exceeds 10% of patients.

Table 8.11 Clinical Scenarios where Planned, Prospective use of Cell Salvage may be Helpful		
Diagnosis at cesarean delivery	Reported incidence of transfusion: Primary C/S	Reported incidence of transfusion: Repeat C/S
HELLP Syndrome	15%	7%
Abruption	14%	14%
Placenta previa	15%	32%
Pre-op hematocrit < 25%	36%	28%

Recombinant Factor VIIa

Recombinant factor VIIa (RFVIIa) is a vitamin K-dependent glycoprotein that is structurally similar to human plasma-derived Factor VIIa. In the presence of tissue factor, factor VIIa facilitates the conversion of factor IX to factor IXa, and factor X to factor Xa, facilitating coagulation. RFVIIa is FDA approved only for the treatment of hemophilia and some specific factor-deficiency syndromes.

A number of recent reports suggest that RFVIIa may be effective in controlling obstetric hemorrhage that is unresponsive to conventional surgical approaches and restoration of clotting factors and blood volumes. In a review of its use in treating primary postpartum hemorrhage in northern Europe, respondents to a survey reported a response rate of 80% to a single dose of RFVIIa.

- RFVIIa should only be used in conjunction with standard resuscitation and treatment protocols for obstetric hemorrhage.

- A consensus conference convened by the manufacturer of RFVIIa recommended an initial dose of 90 mcg/kg rapidly infused intravenously after failure of standard blood product therapy to control bleeding (Table 8.12).
- While RFVIIa is currently very expensive (about $1 US per microgram), its cost should be weighed against potential savings in other blood products, medications, and operating room and intensive care unit costs.

Table 8.12 Protocol for use of Recombinant Factor VIIa

Exhaust all medical treatment, then use blood component therapy
- 4u packed RBCs, 4u FFP, Platelets...repeat!
- Then consider rFVIIa 90 mcg/kg IV over 3–5 min
- If no response: Correct temp, pH, s. Ca++, platelets, fibrinogen...then consider 2nd dose

If still bleeding > hysterectomy

RBCs = red blood cells. FFP = fresh frozen plasma

Approach to the Jehovah's Witness Patient

On occasion, religious or moral beliefs may be at odds with the rationalism of modern medicine, as is the case with the Jehovah's Witness. Witnesses' religious beliefs are based on a literal interpretation of the Bible, and include a prohibition against receiving blood products, even in life-threatening situations. This prohibition is derived from scriptural passages such as Genesis 9:4 and Leviticus 17:10:

- "But flesh with the life thereof, which is the blood thereof, shall ye not eat."
- "And whatsoever man there be of the house of Israel, or of the strangers who sojourn among you, who eateth any manner of blood, I will even set My face against that soul who eateth blood and will cut him off from among his people."

When counseling the Jehovah's Witness prior to labor, delivery, or planned surgery, it is important to not make the discussion a challenge of the parturient's beliefs. Rather, the anesthesiologist should try to determine exactly what therapies the individual would accept (and which they would refuse), and make sure they are aware of the consequences of their actions.

Examples of practices which *may* be acceptable to some Witnesses include:

- use of cell-salvage during surgery, with or without a continuous loop to the patient's circulation
- use of plasma products other than PRBCs
- albumin infusion
- platelet transfusions.

Individual acceptance of various therapies varies widely, which reinforces the need to discuss options with the individual.

In the cases of severe anemia, synthetic erythropoietin has been used to stabilize and improve hematocrit levels. Unfortunately, in difficult cases, care of the Jehovah's Witness can also prove challenging to the moral beliefs of their care providers.

Further Reading

1. Alfirevic Z. Elbourne D. Pavord S, et al. Use of recombinant activated factor VII in primary postpartum hemorrhage: the Northern European registry 2000-2004. *Obstet Gynecol.* 2007;110:1270-1278.

2. Allam J, Cox M, Yentis M. Cell salvage in obstetrics. *Int J Obstet Anesth.* 2008;17:37-45.

3. Waters JH, Biscotti C, Potter PS, et al. Amniotic fluid removal during cell salvage in the cesarean section patient. *Anesthesiology.* 2000;92:1531-1536.

4. Clark SL, Belfort MA, Dildy GA, et al. Maternal death in the 21st century: causes, prevention, and relationship to cesarean delivery. *Am J Obstet Gynecol.* 2008;199:36.e1.

5. Grobman WA, Lai Y, Landon MD, et al. Prediction of uterine rupture associated with attempted vaginal birth after cesarean delivery. *Am J Obstet Gynecol.* 2008;199:30.e1-30.e5.

6. Karalapillai D, Popham P. Recombinant factor VIIa in massive postpartum haemorrhage. *Int J Obstet Anesth.* 2007;16:29-34.

7. Macones GA, Alison GC, Stamilo DM, et al. Can uterine rupture in patients attempting vaginal birth after cesarean delivery be predicted? *Am J Obstet Gyn.* 2006;195:1148.

8. Miller DA, Chollet JA, Goodwin TM, et al. Clinical risk factors for placenta previa–placenta accrete. *Am J Obstet Gynecol.* 1997;177:210-214.

9. Riley, ET, Flanagan, B, Cohen, SE, et al. Intravenous nitroglycerin: a potent uterine relaxant for emergency obstetric procedures. Review of literature and report of three cases. *Int J Obstet Anesth.* 1996;5:264-268.

10. Thachil J, Toh CH, *et al.* Disseminated intravascular coagulation in obstetric disorders and its acute haematological management. *Blood Reviews.* 2009;23:167-176.
11. Welsh A, McLintock C, Gatt S, *et al.* Guidelines for the use of recombinant activated factor VII in massive obstetric haemorrhage. *Aust N Z J Obstet Gynecol.* 2008;48:12-16.

Chapter 9

Obesity

Robert D'Angelo, MD
Medge D. Owen, MD

Introduction

Obesity is a condition of excess body fat that is reaching epidemic proportions and becoming a worldwide public health problem. Obesity has joined underweight, malnutrition, and infectious diseases as major health problems threatening the developing world.

- In 2006 the World Health Organization estimated that worldwide 1.7 billion people were overweight, 312 million were obese, and 155 million children were either overweight or obese.
- In developed countries, including Europe and the United States, obesity affects more than 30% of the population and is primarily associated with poverty. In contrast, in developing countries, affluence carries a higher risk.

Obesity results in an increased utilization of health care resources. In obstetric patients, obesity may be the most common high-risk problem seen by the anesthesiologist.

- In the United States, approximately 40% of obstetric patients have a body mass index (BMI) >30kg/m^2 and 10% have BMIs that exceed 40kg/m^2.

Many criteria have been used to define obesity, without agreement, and there is no accepted definition of obesity in pregnancy. Most commonly, BMI is used to define obesity (Table 9.1) but a simpler definition is 200% of ideal body weight. Morbid obesity is generally defined by a BMI >40kg/m^2.

Pathophysiology

Obesity during pregnancy increases the risk of maternal and fetal morbidity and mortality. Obesity exaggerates the normal physiologic changes of pregnancy, creating more work for an already stressed cardiorespiratory system, and affects the body's most vital organ systems. The most significant pathophysiologic changes with anesthetic implications occur in the pulmonary, cardiovascular, and gastrointestinal systems (Table 9.2).

Pulmonary

Increased body size increases energy requirements, causing oxygen consumption and carbon dioxide production to increase in proportion to weight. To meet the added energy demands, minute ventilation must also increase, but a large body habitus makes this difficult.

Significant Pulmonary Effects

- Increased chest wall weight decreases lung compliance, requiring even greater energy expenditure to lift the chest during inspiration.
- Abdominal mass further restricts diaphragmatic movement, making breathing more difficult, especially in the supine or Trendelenburg position.

Table 9.1 Weight Classification by BMI*	
• Normal	18.5–24.9
• Overweight	25.0–29.9
• Obesity I	30.0–34.9
• Obesity II	35.0–39.9
• Obesity III	> 40
• Morbid Obesity	> 40

*BMI = Body mass index = $\dfrac{\text{Weight (kg)}}{\text{Height (m)}^2}$.

Table 9.2 **Pathophysiologic Changes Associated with Obesity**

- Systemic
  - $\uparrow$ Energy requirements
  - $\uparrow$ O_2 consumption
  - $\uparrow$ CO_2 production
- Pulmonary
  - $\downarrow$ FRC
  - V/Q mismatch
  - Chronic hypoxemia
  - Pulmonary hypertension
- Cardiovascular
  - $\uparrow$ Cardiac output
  - Chronic hypertension
- Gastrointestinal
  - Hiatal hernia
  - Delayed gastric emptying
  - Insulin resistance

- Lung volumes and capacities are reduced, and functional residual capacity (FRC) may become less than closing capacity, resulting in airway closure during tidal ventilation.
- Abdominal and chest wall weight also promote airway closure in dependent parts of the lung, shifting ventilation to the more compliant, nondependent lung areas.
- Since pulmonary blood flow preferentially occurs in the dependent lung segments, ventilation/perfusion mismatch and hypoxemia can result.
- Airway resistance and diffusion capacity usually remain normal.

Cardiovascular

Morbid obesity increases demands on the cardiovascular system.

- Pulmonary hypertension is relatively common, and can develop from the increased pulmonary blood flow, chronic hypoxemia, or both.
- Obesity is associated with a threefold increase in hypertension that can lead to left ventricular hypertrophy and abnormal diastolic function.
- There is a clear relationship between obesity and death due to cardiovascular causes, including ischemic heart disease, coronary artery disease, and cardiac arrhythmias.
- In obese young adults 25–34 years of age, a twelvefold increase in the risk of death from cardiovascular disease has been reported.

Gastrointestinal

Obese patients have an increased prevalence of hiatal hernia and delayed gastric emptying and, during pregnancy, the risks of aspiration are increased. Even when fasting:

- Most obese patients will have a gastric volume more than 25 ml with a gastric pH less than 7.25, putting them at risk of aspiration pneumonitis.
- All obese parturients should be considered to have a full stomach.
- A nonparticulate oral antacid prior to surgery should be considered.

Pregnancy and Obesity

In some instances, pregnancy may offer a degree of protection to the obese patient. Frequent shallow respirations are more efficient for obese patients, but during pregnancy, hormone-induced increases in tidal volume produce higher PaO_2 levels compared with nonpregnant obese patients. This increased ventilation accounts for similar $PaCO_2$ values seen in both obese and non-obese pregnant patients. Although FRC is decreased in both pregnancy and obesity, the conditions are not additive.

Obstetric Complications

Obesity increases the risk of anesthesia, obstetric, and fetal/neonatal complications. Numerous obstetric problems have been associated with obesity and occur throughout the puerperium.

Antepartum

Obesity associates with an increased risk of antepartum complications.

- Obese mothers tend to be older and more parous than non-obese mothers, which may account for some of the coexisting medical problems.
- Independent of medical problems, obesity alone places the parturient in a "high risk" category and can complicate the obstetric course (Table 9.3).
- Obesity prior to pregnancy, weight gain during pregnancy, and the higher incidence of gestational diabetes in the obese parturient can lead to fetal macrosomia, a problem that can dramatically alter the course of labor and delivery.

Table 9.3 Antepartum Obstetric Complications Associated with Obesity

- Early miscarriage
- Recurrent miscarriage
- Congenital anomalies
  - Neural tube defects
  - Omphalocele
- Intrauterine fetal demise
- Insulin resistance syndrome
- Gestational diabetes
- Gestational hypertension
- Chronic hypertension
- Preeclampsia
- Hyperlipidemia
- Obstructive sleep apnea

Because obesity increases obstetric risk, it is recommended that obese patients lose weight before becoming pregnant. Although a combination of diet and exercise can be effective, making the lifestyle changes necessary for sustained weight loss is difficult for obese patients and many pregnancies are unplanned.

Alternatively, nearly 50,000 premenopausal women undergo bariatric surgery each year in the United States. Although obstetric risks associated with obesity may be reduced following weight loss, women that undergo bariatric surgery are at increased risk of malabsorption and intestinal obstruction during pregnancy.

Peripartum

Obese parturients are at lower risk for premature labor compared to non-obese controls, but are at greater risk for late or failed spontaneous onset of labor (Table 9.4). For this reason, medical induction of labor frequently occurs. Fetal macrosomia may lead to complicated

Table 9.4 Peripartum Obstetric Complications Associated with Obesity

- ↓ Spontaneous onset of labor
- ↑ Failed induction of labor
- ↑ Instrumental delivery
- ↑ Cesarean delivery
- ↑ Operative blood loss
- ↑ Operative time

vaginal delivery, but more likely results in cephalopelvic disproportion (CPD) and arrest of labor necessitating cesarean section.

- Induction of labor, fetal macrosomia, and obesity are independent risk factors for cesarean section.
- The incidence of cesarean section is increased twofold in patients with a BMI >35kg/m^2.
- The incidence of cesarean section increases further as BMI increases.
- Approximately 60% of patients weighing over 300 pounds (135 kg) require cesarean section; half of these will be for urgent or emergent indications.
- Prolonged surgical duration and increased blood loss should be anticipated.

Postpartum

Obesity increases the risk of postoperative complications (Table 9.5).

- Postsurgical wound infection is related to larger incisions, protracted surgical time, excess operative traction causing tissue trauma, and the inability of adipose tissue to resist infection secondary to decreased blood flow.
- Diabetes mellitus also increases the risk of wound infection.
- Restoration of normal pulmonary function may take several days following abdominal surgery, and atelectesis may lead to pneumonia.
- With the obesity-related increase in deep vein thrombosis and pregnancy-related hypercoagulability, obese patients are at an increased risk for pulmonary thromboembolism.

Table 9.5 Postpartum Obstetric Complications Associated with Obesity

- Hemorrhage
- Thrombophlebitis
- Deep vein thrombosis
- Pulmonary embolus
- Pneumonia
- Urinary tract infection
- Wound infection
- Wound dehiscence
- Prolonged hospitalization
- ↑ Cost of medical care
- Sudden death

- The increased risk of obstructive sleep apnea in obese patients may increase the risk of sudden death. Obstructive sleep apnea is discussed below.

Fetal Complications

Fetal complications associated with obesity are listed in Table 9.6.

- Newborns are at increased risk for complications, admission to the neonatal intensive care unit, and death.
- Prenatal fetal anomalies may be undiagnosed because ultrasonographic visualization is impaired with morbid obesity.
- Macrosomia is positively correlated with birth trauma, shoulder dystocia, and asphyxia.
- Neonatal hypoglycemia can alter newborn thermoregulation and decrease cardiac output.

Anesthetic Considerations

In obese parturients, the lack of an anesthetic plan can be disastrous. Since as many as 30% of morbidly obese parturients require an urgent or emergent cesarean section, an anesthetic plan is essential for optimizing medical management and should include early consultation by the anesthesiologist.

- The American College of Obstetricians and Gynecologists (ACOG) recommends antenatal anesthesia consultation for morbidly obese patients.
- Evaluation of the airway and a thorough review of coexisting medical problems is paramount.

Table 9.6 Fetal Complications Associated with Obesity
• Congenital anomalies
• Intrauterine demise
• Macrosomia
• Multiple gestation
• Breech presentation
• Shoulder dystocia
• Birth asphyxia
• Birth trauma
• Neonatal hypoglycemia
• ↑ NICU admission

- A previous uneventful anesthetic may be irrelevant if there has been significant weight gain since the previous anesthetic, or during pregnancy.
- A history of obstructive sleep apnea may suggest the potential for mechanical airway obstruction when the level of consciousness is decreased. It is important to discuss anesthetic interventions in advance, particularly regional anesthesia techniques and awake fiberoptic intubation.

Equipment

Appropriately sized hospital beds, stretchers, wheelchairs, and operating tables must be available to accommodate the obese patient's size and weight. Many older operating tables are only rated for 500 lbs (227 kg), which may be insufficient for morbidly obese patients, especially if the table is articulated.

Recommendations

- An operating table rated for 1,200 lbs (545 kg) unarticulated and 800 lbs (364 kg) articulated is recommended.
- Left uterine displacement may create an unstable situation. The patient must be well secured to the operating table because the abdomen may shift markedly when the patient is tilted leftward.
- In rare cases it may be necessary to either use the labor bed as an operating table, or two side-by-side operating room tables.
- Extra personnel are essential to safely transport the patient, especially if she is immobilized due to regional anesthesia.

Problems include monitoring and occasional difficult intravenous access:

- A standard blood pressure cuff will give falsely high measurements when placed on a large, funnel shaped arm. The width of the blood pressure cuff should cover at least half the length of the upper arm. As an alternative, a standard sized cuff may also be placed on the forearm if the forearm is positioned at the level of the heart.
- Despite increased amounts of subcutaneous fat, establishing intravenous access is generally not difficult, due to an expanded blood volume.

Positioning in the Labor Unit

Proper positioning of the obese parturient can facilitate oxygenation and reduce the likelihood of complications.

- The semi-recumbent or lateral position displaces the panniculus off the abdomen and improves lung expansion. It helps minimize cardiovascular stress by reducing intra-abdominal pressure, and allows greater diaphragmatic excursion during respiration.
- Elevation of the head of the bed also reduces premature airway closure, thus reducing hypoxemia.
- Oxygen administration is helpful and may provide a margin of safety to the mother and fetus.
- The supine position should be avoided because aortocaval compression may be exacerbated by the weight of a large panniculus. Airway obstruction and circulatory changes such as hypotension and elevated pulmonary occlusion pressures can occur, and cardiac arrest has been reported when morbidly obese patients have been placed in the supine position.

Analgesia for Labor and Delivery

Parenteral analgesics during labor, supplemented with pudendal block and perineal local infiltration at delivery, may be appropriate for some obese patients. More often, they are ineffective and increase the risk of complications, including opioid-induced respiratory depression. Since the potential is higher in obese patients for complicated vaginal or surgical delivery requiring profound anesthesia, regional anesthesia is preferred whenever possible.

Epidural Analgesia

In obese parturients, the most appropriate anesthetic technique for labor pain relief is epidural analgesia.

Benefits of Epidural Analgesia

- Decreased oxygen consumption
- Decreased work of breathing
- Improved oxygenation
- Decreased catecholamine secretion that may increase blood pressure and cardiac output
- Most importantly, epidural analgesia allows for controlled drug administration that can be utilized for surgical anesthesia should cesarean section be required.

Ideally, morbidly obese parturients should be identified and seen by an anesthesiologist upon admission, informed consent obtained, and an epidural catheter inserted and tested even before the onset of active labor. A commitment from the obstetric team for delivery during the current hospitalization is required for early epidural catheter placement. The catheter can be tested if the patient is not in active labor, and then reactivated later when the patient requests labor analgesia. Patients invariably consent to early epidural catheter placement when the risks and benefits are presented in clear, understandable terms.

Reasons for Early Epidural Catheter Placement in Obese Parturients

- It may take longer to position the patient and place the catheter.
- Catheter placement before active labor minimizes patient movement and improves cooperation, thus increasing the chance for success.
- Block placement can be technically challenging due to obscured anatomical landmarks.
- Most importantly, this technique minimizes overall risk by maximizing the likelihood of a successful regional anesthetic should an urgent cesarean section be required.

The sitting position usually provides easier identification of midline, although locating an interspace is not guaranteed. A recommended technique for epidural catheter placement is listed in Table 9.7.

Important Points When Placing an Epidural Catheter in an Obese Patient

- When landmarks cannot be palpated insert the epidural needle in the midline, perpendicular to the skin at an imaginary point anchored

---

Table 9.7 Recommended Technique for Epidural Catheter Placement in the Morbidly Obese Parturient

- Early epidural catheter placement
- Sitting position
- Low midline approach (Figure 9.1)
- >6 cm catheter insertion length
- Secure catheter with patient in lateral position
- Test catheter with 10 ml 2% lidocaine (2 + 5 + 3 ml)
- For:
  - <u>Adequate analgesia:</u> administer additional local anesthetics when patient requests analgesia
  - <u>Inadequate analgesia:</u> withdraw catheter 2–3 cm and administer additional lidocaine 5 ml
  - <u>Persistent inadequate analgesia:</u> remove epidural catheter and replace
- Maintenance of labor analgesia: dilute local anesthetic with opioid (0.0625%–0.125% bupivacaine + fentanyl 2 mcg/ml)

horizontally by the first skin crease above the gluteal fold and vertically by an imaginary line drawn from the C_7 spinous process to the gluteal fold (Figure 9.1).

- The increased depth to the epidural space contributes to a high failure rate by exaggerating minor directional errors and increasing the chance of identifying the lateral epidural space (Figure 9.2). Ultrasound guidance may also facilitate epidural catheter placement but familiarity with the technique is essential for success.

- In cases of difficult placement, the patient can assist by reporting any left or right sided discomfort. Directing the epidural needle hub towards the discomfort will direct the needle tip in the opposite direction and back towards the midline.

- Even in the morbidly obese patient, the inability to identify the epidural space is more likely misdirection rather than inadequate needle length. Although a standard 3.5 inch (89 mm) epidural needle is almost always sufficient, a longer needle may occasionally be required. For this reason, a stock of 5–6 inch (127–152 mm) disposable epidural needles should be readily available.

- Once the epidural space is identified, the epidural catheter should be inserted at least 6 cm within the epidural space to minimize the

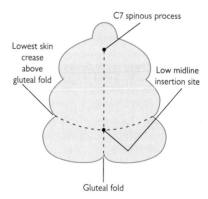

Figure 9.1 Approach to epidural catheter insertion in the morbidly obese parturient. With the patient in the sitting position, insert the epidural needle in the midline perpendicular to the skin at a point anchored horizontally by the first skin crease above the gluteal fold and vertically by an imaginary line drawn from the C_7 spinous process to the gluteal fold.

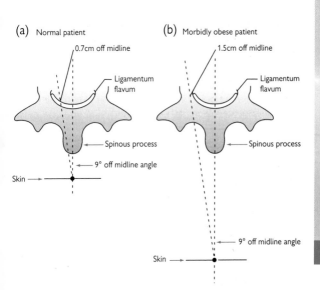

(a) Normal patient

0.7cm off midline

Ligamentum flavum

Spinous process

9° off midline angle

Skin

(b) Morbidly obese patient

1.5cm off midline

Ligamentum flavum

Spinous process

9° off midline angle

Skin

Figure 9.2 Increased skin-to-epidural space depth in obese patients exaggerates minor directional errors during epidural needle insertion and increases failure rate. As drawn, a 9° off-midline angle at the skin translates into an approximate 0.7 cm deviation from midline when entering the epidural space in the normal patient with a 4 cm skin-to-epidural space distance, versus an approximate 1.5 cm deviation from midline in the morbidly obese patient with a 9 cm skin-to-epidural space distance.

risk of subsequent catheter dislodgement because of the potential for increased movement of tissues between the skin and the epidural space.

- Ultrasound guidance may also facilitate epidural catheter placement but familiarity with the technique is essential for success.
- Move the patient to the lateral position before securing the epidural catheter, since the sitting position decreases the skin-to-ligamentum flavum distance. The epidural catheter can move inwards as much as 4 cm in a morbidly obese patient when assuming the lateral position. Once secured, record the length of catheter in the epidural space and the catheter marking at the skin in the anesthesia record.
- Administer enough local anesthetic (usually 10 ml of 1%–2% lidocaine) to fully test the catheter. If the patient develops bilateral analgesia and the catheter was inserted early, no additional

local anesthetics are administered until the patient requests pain relief.

- For inadequate analgesia, the epidural catheter is manipulated or replaced until a well-functioning epidural catheter is established.
- Although initial epidural catheter failure may be over 40% in obese parturients, eventual success rates comparable to non-obese controls can be obtained.

Initiating Labor Analgesia

- Local anesthetics alone or with minimal opioid should be used to establish catheter function.
- Opioid administration by any route produces some degree of pain relief and may theoretically mask a malpositioned catheter. Once the catheter function is proven and a bilateral block as been established, epidural opioids can be administered.
- Although local anesthetic requirements may be reduced with obesity (due to a reduction in epidural volume by fatty infiltration or engorged epidural veins), epidural analgesic requirements generally remain similar to those of non-obese parturients.

Combined Spinal Epidural (CSE)

The use of CSE analgesia in obese parturients is not routinely recommended.

- The CSE technique delays recognition of a poorly functioning epidural catheter that may become problematic should an emergency cesarean section be required.
- The incidence of epidural catheter failure with CSE in the obese patient population remains unknown. Although it has been suggested that a successful CSE improves subsequent catheter function (since obtaining cerebrospinal fluid indicates likely midline epidural needle position), adequate epidural anesthesia can not be guaranteed.
- The benefit of faster onset labor analgesia does not outweigh the risk of epidural catheter failure should emergency cesarean section be required.

Continuous Spinal Analgesia

A subarachnoid catheter can be dosed incrementally or by continuous infusion for labor analgesia. As with epidural analgesia, the block can be quickly augmented in the event of cesarean section, but unilateral blockade is less likely. However, the technique is not recommended for routine use because of the following theoretical concerns:

- During a long course of labor, tachyphylaxis may develop to intrathecal local anesthetics, making assessment difficult.
- Catheter lengths inserted more than 4 cm into the spinal space increases the risk of spinal cord penetration or spinal nerve root impingement.
- With 4 cm or less of subarachnoid catheter, patient movement may dislodge the spinal catheter.
- Most importantly, an indwelling spinal catheter on the labor unit is a safety concern. As multiple anesthesia providers are typically involved in the care of the labor patient, a spinal catheter may be mistaken for an epidural catheter and doses of local anesthetic intended for epidural administration may be injected. These larger doses may increase the risk of high spinal blockade in the uncontrolled setting of the labor ward.

Recommendations for Continuous Spinal Anesthesia

- Urgent situations when difficult tracheal intubation is anticipated
- Inadvertent wet tap during difficult epidural catheter placement
- Inadvertent wet tap with anticipated imminent delivery

Spinal catheter management is outlined in Table 9.8.

Table 9.8 Technique for Spinal Catheter Placement and Management in the Morbidly Obese Parturient

- Sitting position
- Low midline approach (Figure 9.1)
- 4 cm catheter insertion length
- Secure catheter with patient in lateral position
- Labor Analgesia:
  - <u>Intermittent dosing</u>: routine CSE boluses (1.75–2.5 mg bupivacaine + fentanyl 15–25 mcg)
  - <u>Continuous Dosing</u>: routine epidural solutions (0.0625%–0.125% bupivacaine + fentanyl 2 mcg/ml) @ 1–2 ml/hour
- Anesthesia for Cesarean Section:
  - <u>Initiation</u>: 5mg 0.5% plain bupivacaine + fentanyl 15–20 mcg (wait at least 5 min before administering additional dose)
  - <u>Additional boluses</u>: 1.25–2.5 mg plain bupivacaine until desired sensory level achieved

Anesthesia for Cesarean Delivery

During cesarean delivery, obesity increases the risk of maternal mortality. In obese patients most anesthesia-related maternal deaths occur secondary to airway problems encountered during general anesthesia or in the recovery period. For this reason, general anesthesia should be avoided if at all possible.

Positioning in the OR

As discussed previously, care must be taken when positioning any morbidly obese patient, since left uterine displacement may markedly shift the abdomen and create an unstable situation. The large panniculus may make surgical exposure difficult.

Techniques to Facilitate Surgical Exposure

- Retraction of the panniculus cephalad onto the chest using Montgomery straps; however, in rare cases, the massive weight of the panniculus on the chest may compromise both pulmonary and cardiac function resulting in hypoxia and hypotension.
- The panniculus can either be lifted and tethered to reinforced ceiling hooks, or to an orthopedic lift device. Utilization of these techniques must be planned in advance and require the placement of sterile rods or hooks through the panniculus by the surgeons.
- In massively obese patients with supine aortocaval compression-related symptoms, consider utilizing reverse Trendelenburg positioning during surgery as dictated by patient symptoms (Figure 9.3). This technique requires coordination of the obstetric and anesthesia teams since a supra umbilical vertical skin incision and a classical uterine incision is necessary. Further catheter facilitated regional techniques (epidural, CSE, or spinal) allow additional local anesthetic administration to maintain a dense T_4 sensory during prolonged surgeries.

Obese patients may be at increased risk of developing a high spinal block from exaggerated spread of local anesthetic for several reasons.

- Difficulty in identifying interspaces may lead to a higher than anticipated block placement.
- Cerebral spinal fluid volume may be decreased.
- Gluteal adipose tissue may place the vertebral column in a relative Trendelenburg position when the patient is supine.

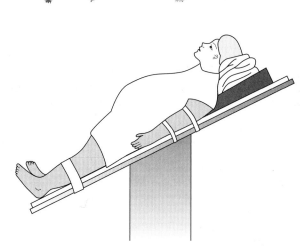

Figure 9.3 Positioning the morbidly obese patient with supine hypotensive syndrome using reverse Trendelenburg positioning to reduce the weight load against the chest, which could further augment symptoms of aortocaval compression. Reverse Trendelenburg positioning will necessitate a vertical skin incision, a classical uterine incision, and coordination by the anesthesia and obstetric teams.

Recommended techniques that reduce the likelihood of high spinal block in an obese parturient include:

- Slight elevation of the head to minimize cephalad spread when administering hyperbaric local anesthetic.
- Shoulder and neck rolls in addition to the elevated headrest.
- Utilization of reverse Trendelenburg positioning to "level" the spinal column in patients with significant amounts of gluteal adipose tissue.

Despite utilization of techniques to minimize risks, high spinal blocks can still occur, and the anesthesia provider must be prepared to emergently secure the airway.

Epidural Anesthesia

Epidural anesthesia is an excellent choice for cesarean delivery in morbidly obese patients, whether presenting for elective surgery or coming from the labor ward.

- If a preexisting epidural catheter is in place, epidural local anesthetics may be administered in the labor room, obviating failure should the catheter become dislodged during transport to the operating room.

- If anesthesia appears to be inadequate for a surgical incision while dosing in the labor room, it may be prudent to move the patient to the operating room table, withdraw the epidural catheter so that 3–4 cm remains within the epidural space, and then administer additional local anesthetics.

- Should inadequate surgical anesthesia persist, consideration should be made for replacing the epidural catheter in the operating room.

Although it has been suggested that epidural local anesthetics requirements are reduced by approximately 20% in obese parturients, individual patients have varying requirements.

- If the block exceeds the desired sensory level, a slight head-flexion of the operating table lessens patient complaints without adversely affecting the surgery.

Other benefits of epidural anesthesia include potentially better hemodynamic control compared to spinal anesthesia, and the flexibility to administer opioid and local anesthetic solutions for postoperative analgesia.

- In an emergency, a well-functioning labor epidural can usually be quickly extended for surgical anesthesia, but establishing a block *de novo* may take too long and a spinal technique may be preferable.

Spinal Anesthesia

Spinal anesthesia is an option for cesarean section, but as with other regional techniques in obese patients, placement can be difficult.

- Fatty deposits about the hips can lead to false identification of the superior iliac crests. This may result in inadvertently high needle placement, possibly leading to spinal cord damage if the needle is inserted above L_2 spinous process. The increased risk of high spinal block secondary to adipose tissue distribution was previously discussed.

- Because of excessive abdominal and chest wall mass, even the usual mid-thoracic sensory levels required for cesarean section may cause inadequate ventilation in obese patients.

- When prolonged surgical durations are anticipated, a continuous spinal or CSE anesthetic may be more appropriate choices than a one-shot spinal. These techniques similarly provide rapid anesthesia but allow for subsequent dosing if necessary.

General Anesthesia

In obese parturients, general anesthesia for cesarean section should be used only in patients with contraindications to regional anesthesia.

Any discussion of general anesthesia in the obese parturient must begin with special emphasis on airway evaluation.

- Difficult intubation has been reported in 33% of obese parturients having cesarean section, compared to 13% in nonpregnant obese patients undergoing abdominal surgery.
- A large tongue and airway soft tissue engorgement can further complicate intubation efforts.
- In the obese patient, the complexity of intubation coupled with the propensity for rapid desaturation can be disastrous.

Whenever possible, two anesthesia providers should be present for induction, since maintaining the airway may be complicated and the primary anesthesia provider can fatigue quickly.

- Assorted laryngoscope blades, a variety of endotracheal tubes, a gum elastic bougie, standard and intubating laryngeal mask airways, and equipment for transtracheal ventilation should be immediately available.
- A short-handled laryngoscope is also useful because limited extension of a short, thick neck and pendulous breasts often hamper insertion with a standard length handle.

In obese parturients, swift intubation is important because rapid desaturation may occur despite adequate preoxygenation, due to the decreased FRC and increased oxygen requirements.

- Hypoxemia and hypercarbia can precipitate sudden pulmonary hypertension and cardiac arrhythmias.
- If mask ventilation becomes necessary, airway obstruction and high abdominal pressure can impede ventilation. In this scenario, insufflation of the stomach may occur and increase the risk of aspiration.
- Obesity impairs identification of the cricoid ring, making it difficult to properly apply cricoid pressure and to perform cricothyrotomy in an emergency.

If a difficult intubation is anticipated, and regional anesthesia is contraindicated, an awake intubation is recommended. Topical anesthesia consumes time, and in the presence of fetal distress, an anesthesiologist may feel compelled to proceed with rapid sequence induction. In this situation, the risk of a failed intubation and potential catastrophic maternal outcome must be weighed against the risk of fetal compromise by delaying surgery to secure the airway.

Positioning recommendations that may facilitate tracheal intubation:

- Proper "sniffing position" is vital (Figure 9.4).
- Adipose tissue on the upper back ("buffalo hump") can elevate the chest in relation to the skull, which may misalign the oroglottic axis and make vocal cord visualization difficult.
- Utilize shoulder and neck rolls before attempting tracheal intubation. Ideally, after proper positioning, an imaginary line drawn between the external auditory meatus and the sternal notch should be parallel with the floor (Figure 9.4).
- Be aware that when the head is positioned midline and the body tilted leftward, visualization may be obscured.

Technique for Inducing General Anesthesia

- 30 ml of a nonparticulate antacid should be administered within 60 minutes of surgery.
- Preoxygenate with 100% oxygen using a tight fitting mask for at least 3 minutes, with 4 vital capacity breaths taken immediately prior to induction.
- Rapid sequence induction with cricoid pressure (Sellick manuever).
- Sodium pentothal 500 mg. This is less than the usual 4 mg/kg recommended dose, because larger doses may prolong awakening in case of failed intubation.
- Succinylcholine 1–1.5 mg/kg of actual body weight up to 200 mg.

A balanced anesthetic technique is used once the airway is secured.

- Atracurium, mivacurium, and rocuronium are preferred nondepolarizing relaxants because metabolism is not organ dependent. Regardless of the agent utilized, neuromuscular blockade must be carefully monitored to minimize the risk residual weakness and in airway obstruction following extubation.
- Fentanyl elimination is similar in obese and non-obese patients, making it more predictable. In contrast, sufentanil and alfentanil may have longer elimination times in the obese patient.
- While isoflurane has limited biotransformation, time to extubation is shorter with the newer inhalational agents desflurane and sevoflurane. While no single anesthetic regimen has been shown to be superior in obese patients, newer agents may lessen residual postoperative anesthetic affects.

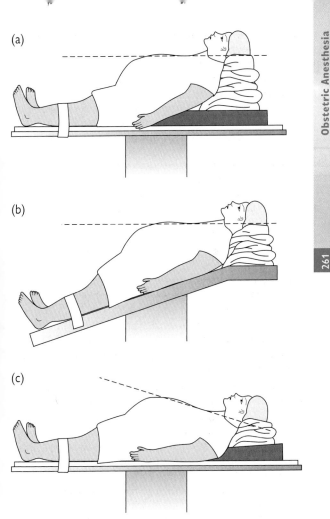

Figure 9.4 Proper positioning of the obese patient prior to induction of general anesthesia. Utilization of shoulder and head rolls alone (9.4a) or with reverse Trendelenburg positioning (9.4b), so that an imaginary line drawn between the external auditory meatus and the sternal notch is parallel to the floor, facilitates visualization of the vocal cords and tracheal intubation. The parallel alignment may be impossible to achieve using only a single pillow under the head (9.4c).

Intraoperatively, initiate ventilation with tidal volumes of 10–12 ml/kg ideal body weight and adjust as necessary.

- PEEP is rarely indicated and can worsen hypoxemia in obese patients. Large tidal volumes coupled with low chest wall compliance can produce high peak inspiratory pressures.
- High-inspired oxygen fractions may be required, thus limiting the use of nitrous oxide and possibly increasing the risk of intraoperative awareness.
- End-tidal capnography may be a poor guide to the adequacy of ventilation due to a large alveolar-to-arterial difference in carbon dioxide.
- During pregnancy, it is important to maintain $PaCO_2$ levels in the low to mid 30s, and arterial blood gas analysis may be required.

Following surgery and prior to extubation, gastric contents should be suctioned. Residual anesthetic effects, increased sensitivity to opioid analgesics, and neuromuscular blocking agents may postpone tracheal extubation.

- Airway obstruction must be avoided if at all possible in obese patients, since it can lead to cardiovascular decompensation.

Postpartum Care

Postoperatively, the morbidly obese patient remains at increased risk of respiratory insufficiency, and supplemental oxygen may be required for several days. The obese patient should be closely monitored for cardiopulmonary complications during the postoperative period.

Postoperative Pain Control

Opioids can depress respiration and should be used carefully in the morbidly obese. Following vaginal delivery omit use if possible.

In patients requiring operative delivery, pain control is important to encourage deep breathing and decrease the risk of atelectasis. Adequate pain control reduces side effects, improves respiratory function, and leads to early mobilization.

- Although the ideal method of pain control in obese patients remains unknown, a combination of opioid and nonsteroidal anti-inflammatory agent (NSAID) is recommended whenever possible, to produce superior pain relief while minimizing opioid-induced side effects.

- Subcutaneous and intramuscular injection routes should be avoided, since absorption may be less reliable in obese patients.
- Intravenous morphine, administered by either intermittent bolus, patient-controlled analgesia or neuraxial administration, can produce adequate pain relief.

Opioids administered by any route can result in respiratory depression, especially in obese patients with undiagnosed obstructive sleep apnea (OSA).

- Obese patients should be carefully screened for symptoms consistent with OSA. Consider continuous pulse oximetry in obese patients with suspected or documented OSA that receive opioids by any route (Table 9.9).
- Obese patients receiving opioids without OSA-related symptoms are candidates for standard postoperative monitoring, which usually consists of intermittent respiratory or sedation checks, or both.

Table 9.9 Recommendations for Patients with Documented or Suspected Obstructive Sleep Apnea (OSA)

- Preoperative
  - Assess patients for symptoms of OSA
  - Sleep study if suspected OSA and time allows
  - CPAP should be considered
  - Patient should be considered at high risk of difficult intubation
- Intraoperative
  - Regional anesthesia whenever possible
  - Avoid opioids whenever possible
  - Extubate awake in a lateral or semi-upright position and after full recovery of neuromuscular blockade
- Postoperative
  - NSAIDs whenever possible
  - Supplemental oxygen until baseline oxygenation is adequate
  - Continuous pulse oximetry
  - Utilization of CPAP when possible

Summary

Obesity during pregnancy increases the risk of maternal and fetal morbidity and mortality, and poses significant anesthetic challenges. Anesthetic risks may be reduced by early aggressive intervention.

Early epidural catheter insertion and testing, as early in labor as possible, is recommended to increase the likelihood of a successful regional anesthetic should an emergent cesarean section be required. General anesthesia should be utilized in obese parturients only when regional anesthesia is contraindicated.

Further Reading

1. Catalano PM. Management of obesity during pregnancy. *Obstet Gynecol.* 2007;109:419-433.
2. D'Angelo R, Dewan DD. Chapter 50: Obesity. In Chestnut DH, Polley LS, Tsen LC, Wong CA, eds. *Chestnut's Obstetric Anesthesia Principles and Practice 4th Ed.* Philadelphia, PA: Mosby Elsevier 2009:1079-1094.
3. Hamilton CL, Riley ET, Cohen SE. Changes in the position of epidural catheters associated with patient movement. *Anesthesiology.* 1997;86:778-784.
4. Hogan QH, Prost R, Kulier A, *et al.* Magnetic resonance imaging of cerebrospinal fluid volume and the influence of body habitus and abdominal pressure. *Anesthesiology.* 1996;84:1341-1349.
5. Hood DD, Dewan DM. Anesthetic and obstetrical outcome in morbidly obese parturients. *Anesthesiology.* 1993;79:1210-1218.
6. Perlow JH, Morgan MM. Massive maternal obesity and perioperative cesarean morbidity. *Am J Obstet Gynecol.* 1994;170:560-565.
7. Weiss JL, Malone FD, Emig D, *et al.* Obesity, obstetric complications and cesarean delivery rate - a population-based screening study. *Am J Obstet Gynecol.* 2004;190:1091-1097.
8. ASA Practice Guidelines for the Perioperative Management of Patients with Obstructive Sleep Apnea. *Anesthesiology.* 2006;104:1081-1093.
9. US Obesity Trends 1984-2008. From the CDC's Behavioral Risk Factor Surveillance System. Accessed at: http://www.cdc.gov/obesity/data/trends.html.

Chapter 10

Coexisting Disease and Other Issues

Michael J. Paech, FANZCA

Introduction

Almost any disease or malady may coexist with pregnancy, and many have a significant impact on the course of pregnancy, labor, and delivery. While comprehensive information about many diseases is beyond the scope of this chapter, key issues relevant to the most common or important conditions will be discussed briefly. An emphasis is placed on cardiac disease, which is the leading cause of indirect maternal death in most developed countries.

Cardiac Disease

Cardiac disease is present in 1%–3% of pregnancies. It is disproportionately responsible for maternal mortality and in developed countries it is the most common cause of indirect maternal death (10%–25% of all maternal deaths). There are a number of reasons why cardiac disease has become a leading cause of maternal death.

- As pregnancy becomes safer, more women with severe cardiac disease appear willing to accept the risk of becoming pregnant.
- More women with adult congenital heart disease or respiratory disease reach reproductive age.
- Rheumatic heart disease remains prevalent under poor socioeconomic conditions.
- Most deaths occur in women with undiagnosed disease.

Ischemic heart disease is now more prevalent among women of childbearing age, and the incidence increases with advancing maternal age. The extension of the reproductive age by assisted reproductive technologies and social change have been, in part, responsible for higher pregnancy rates among older women. The rising prevalence of diabetes and hypertension, particularly among the obese population, and increased recreational use of illicit drugs (e.g., cocaine, methamphetamine) also contribute to ischemic disease.

Most cardiac deaths in developed countries are now due to adult congenital heart disease, but the risk of death or serious morbidity from various conditions varies (Table 10.1).

Relevant Physiological Changes in Pregnancy

Physiologic adaptation to pregnancy (Chapter 2) often has an adverse impact on women with cardiac disease, who are likely to deteriorate symptomatically as gestation increases. The New York Heart Association Classification, based on exercise tolerance (Table 10.2), typically deteriorates at least one class, and Class III and IV are associated with higher maternal mortality.

The main physiologic changes contributing to worse outcomes are an increase in blood volume, oxygen demand, and cardiac output.

- Increased cardiac work may cause decompensation, with the prepartum increase in cardiac output frequently associated with symptomatic deterioration by late in the second trimester.

Table 10.1 Risk of Death or Severe Morbidity Based on Type of Cardiac Condition

High risk (mortality 5%–30%)
Pulmonary hypertension
Severe aortic stenosis
Marfan's syndrome with aortic valve or root involvement
Coarctation of the aorta with valvular involvement
Severe ventricular failure
NYHA classification 3 or 4
Moderate risk (mortality 1%–5%)
Single ventricle
Prosthetic heart valve
Systemic right ventricle / switch procedure
Unrepaired cyanotic congenital heart disease
Severe mitral or pulmonary stenosis
Moderate / mild aortic stenosis
Myocardial ischemia
Uncomplicated aortic coarctation
Low-risk (mortality 0.1%–1%)
Repaired congenital heart disease
Uncomplicated left-to-right shunts
Mitral valve prolapse; aortic, mitral or pulmonary regurgitation; moderate / mild mitral or pulmonary stenosis
Cardiac arrhythmia

Table 10.2 New York Heart Association (NYHA) Classification of Cardiac Disease

Class I: no undue symptoms associated with ordinary activity and no limitation of physical activity.
Class II: slight limitation of physical activity, patient comfortable at rest. Ordinary physical activity results in fatigue, palpitation, dyspnea or angina.
Class III: marked limitation of physical activity, patient comfortable at rest. Less than ordinary activity causes fatigue, palpitation, dyspnea, angina.
Class IV: inability to carry on any physical activity without discomfort. Symptoms of cardiac insufficiency or angina possible, even at rest.

Source: American Heart Association, Inc. *The Criteria Committee of the New York Heart Association. Nomenclature and Criteria for Diagnosis of Diseases of the Heart and Great Vessels. 9th ed.* Boston, MA: Little, Brown & Co; 1994:253–256.

- Maximum cardiac stress occurs early postdelivery, due to labor-induced sympathetic stimulation, autotransfusion of blood from the contracted uterus, and the relief of aortocaval compression.

General Considerations

Anesthesiologists must be part of the antenatal multidisciplinary assessment and planning team for women with more severe disease. Important care considerations are indicated in Table 10.3, and there are a number of questions and issues to consider (Table 10.4).

Table 10.3 Principles of Care for Patients with Cardiac Disease

Pre-conception counseling

Early antenatal assessment to determine the best location for delivery

Team management of those with significant disease by cardiologists, obstetricians and midwives, obstetric physicians, anesthesiologists and intensivists, neonatologists, psychologists, and community health care workers

Investigation to clarify diagnosis and severity of the pathophysiology
- electrocardiography
- echocardiography
- other specific investigations

Regular review of the impact of the physiological changes of pregnancy on the disease

Fetal surveillance

Correction of anemia and infection

Consideration of thromboprophylaxis

Stabilization of the disease and optimization of physical condition
- e.g., beta-blockers, pulmonary vasodilators, digoxin

Preparation for both elective and non-elective timing of delivery

Intrapartum management
- medical therapy (e.g., oxygen, oxytocics given slowly, avoid ergometrine and injected prostaglandins)
- antibiotic prophylaxis according to guidelines
- monitoring
- epidural analgesia
- fluid and drug therapies
- decision whether pushing can be allowed for vaginal delivery

Careful regional or general anesthesia for operative delivery and postpartum procedures

Postdelivery management
- high-dependency or coronary care unit observation
- medical management, watch for cardiac failure

Discuss contraception

Table 10.4 Anesthetic Questions Related to the Pregnant Woman with Cardiac Disease

What are the anatomical changes and pathophysiology of this cardiac disease?
What was the status before pregnancy and what is the current maternal and fetal condition?
What investigations have been and need to be performed?
What antenatal treatment must be instituted now?
Where is the parturient best delivered?
What is the plan for delivery, management of delivery and the puerperium?
Where is the best location for postpartum care?
What method of labor analgesia is advisable?
What method of anesthesia for cesarean delivery should be recommended?
What are the special considerations for the above?
What monitoring should be used?
How should hemodynamic or other emergencies be managed?

- While symptoms of breathlessness, fatigue, decreased exercise tolerance, and edema may be normal for pregnancy, they must not be dismissed, as they may be pathological.
- Flow murmurs are common, but atypical features mandate referral and investigation. Less severe congenital lesions may present for the first time in teenage or young adult pregnancy.
- Antibiotic prophylaxis against bacterial endocarditis is now considered to have a poor benefit-risk ratio but is occasionally warranted (Table 10.5).

Anticoagulant therapy with warfarin, while indicated in nonpregnant patients for atrial fibrillation, mechanical prosthetic heart valves, pulmonary hypertension, or a previous thromboembolic event, is usually avoided in pregnancy due to teratogenicity and other fetal effects. Substitution with unfractionated heparin or the longer-acting low-molecular-weight heparins has implications for regional block and labor or delivery (Chapter 3).

Rarely, cardiac surgery is required because of severe deterioration and failure of medical management (for example, mitral valvotomy for severe mitral stenosis).

- Cardiac surgical morbidity and mortality are higher in pregnant patients than nonpregnant.
- When necessary, surgery is normally performed during the late second trimester, when organogenesis is complete and the fetus is viable, or after delivery.

Table 10.5 **Antibiotic Prophylaxis against Endocarditis**[*]
When planning care, specific instructions should be recorded regarding intrapartum antibiotic prophylaxis
Required only for high-risk women having certain dental procedures or with infection that could cause significant or recurrent bacteremia (e.g., chorioamnionitis)
Consider the diagnosis of endocarditis in any woman with a cardiac defect who has positive blood cultures
Not required for vaginal or cesarean delivery in most cases, including mitral valve prolapse
Conditions where prophylaxis is recommended in the presence of infection or for certain dental procedures
Prosthetic heart valves or repair materials
Previous bacterial endocarditis
Complex cyanotic congenital disease • unrepaired cyanotic disease • repaired disease with residual defects
Suggested intravenous regimen 30–60 min before the procedure
Ampicillin 2 g or
Cefazolin or ceftriaxone 1 g
Vancomycin if enterococcus is a concern
Regimen for penicillin allergy
Cefazolin or ceftriaxone 1 g or clindamycin 600 mg
Oral: Amoxycillin 2 g

[*] Based on recommendations of the American Heart Association and endorsed by the American College of Obstetricians and Gynecologists 2008.

- During cardiopulmonary bypass, high rates of fetal mortality (10%–30%) can be reduced by: normothermic perfusion, pulsatile flow, maintaining hematocrit >28%, perfusion pressure >70 mmHg, normocarbia and pump flows > 2.5 L/min/m^2.

Cesarean delivery is usually performed for obstetric indications, and either regional or general anesthesia can be used safely (Tables 10.6 and 10.7) by an experienced anesthesiologist, paying attention to detail and maintenance of hemodynamic stability.

Specific Cardiac Conditions

Mitral Stenosis

Mitral stenosis may be isolated or part of mixed valvular disease, and is the most common valvular lesion (aortic stenosis is rare). Mortality is low (1%) unless associated with NYHA Class III or IV,

Table 10.6 Principles of Regional Analgesia and Anesthesia in Cardiac Disease

For labor and childbirth, regional analgesia is beneficial

Spinal or epidural opioid (with or without local anesthetic as an adjunct) initially followed by maintenance with low-dose plain local anesthetic and opioid by infusion or patient-controlled infusion plus small volume boluses

Careful fluid and hemodynamic monitoring
- avoid intravenous preloading or excessive administration
- continuous blood pressure monitoring in more serious cases
- avoid boluses of oxytocin and ergometrine

For regional anesthesia for operative delivery

Maintain hemodynamic stability
- continuous blood pressure monitoring in more serious cases
- prophylactic and therapeutic vasopressor
  - titrated phenylephrine or similar to avoid tachycardia, especially with stenotic valvular disease, hypertrophic cardiomyopathy or ischemic heart disease
  - titrated ephedrine to avoid bradycardia, especially regurgitant valvular disease or cardiomyopathy
- avoid sudden changes in pulmonary or systemic vascular resistance, especially with shunts, severe stenosis and cardiomyopathies
- avoid boluses of oxytocin and ergometrine

Establish the block slowly
- avoid single-shot spinal anesthesia (use sequential combined-spinal epidural or slow incremental epidural or spinal anesthesia)
- control maternal position (avoid aortocaval compression, nurse semi-upright if heart failure)

Provide good postoperative analgesia
- minimize tachycardia due to pain and consider mild peripheral vasodilation with epidural analgesia

or atrial fibrillation. Severe mitral stenosis (valve area < 1 cm^2) is most likely to be associated with large left atrial size and secondary pulmonary hypertension, leading to right ventricular failure (Figure 10.1).

Management involves control of arrhythmias and heart rate.

- Atrial fibrillation reduces preload from loss of atrial contraction.
- Rapid heart rates reduce diastolic filling time and increase left atrial pressure. Digoxin or β-blockers may be necessary.
- In the presence of atrial fibrillation, anticoagulation with heparin is indicated to prevent thrombus formation in the dilated left atrium.
- Other anti-arrhythmic drugs or cardioversion may also be indicated.

Although the cardiovascular stress of labor is usually well tolerated, epidural analgesia is indicated to reduce stress-induced tachycardia.

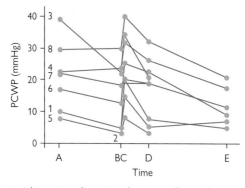

Figure 10.1 Intrapartum changes in pulmonary capillary wedge pressure (PCWP) in eight parturients with mitral stenosis. (A) First stage of labor; (B) second stage of labor, 15–30 min before delivery; (C) 5–15 min postpartum; (D) 4–6 hours postpartum; (E) 18–25 hours postpartum. Reprinted with permission from Clark SL et al. Labor and delivery in the presence of mitral stenosis: central hemodynamic observations. *Am J Obstet Gynecol*. 1985; 152(8):986.

Patients are at high risk of developing pulmonary edema at delivery, especially if preeclampsia is also present. For this reason intravenous fluid volumes should be minimized.

For cesarean delivery, either epidural or combined spinal-epidural anesthesia can be used, with care to minimize the impact of sympathectomy (Table 10.6).

Aortic Stenosis

This lesion is rare but serious. Pain and labor-induced tachycardia predispose to myocardial ischemia or heart failure due to inadequate coronary diastolic filling, and inadequate oxygen supply to the thickened left ventricle.

- Bradycardia may reduce cardiac output and cause heart failure.
- With severe stenotic lesions, balloon valvuloplasty is an option during the second trimester if medical therapy has failed.
- Valve replacement is associated with high fetal loss.

Valvular Incompetence

In contrast to stenotic valvular disease, regurgitant cardiac lesions such as mitral and aortic incompetence often improve during pregnancy as a result of the mild afterload reduction and increased blood volume.

- Mitral valve prolapse is common, and regurgitation usually trivial.
- With severe regurgitation, hypovolemia or tachycardia may decrease left ventricular volume, increase regurgitation, and cause a serious reduction in cardiac output.
- Atrial fibrillation is common with severe mitral regurgitation, and a plan for anticoagulation is important.

Labor and Anesthetic Management in Valvular Disease

In rheumatic valvular disease, good pain relief with epidural or spinal analgesia during labor (using opioids or low concentration local anesthetic/opioid combinations delivered slowly by infusion) is ideal.

- This minimizes the consequences of a sudden reduction in peripheral vascular resistance, maintains normal maternal heart rate, and allows controlled delivery without repeated Valsalva maneuvers.
- If epidural analgesia is contraindicated, parenteral meperidine (pethidine) is unsatisfactory and may cause tachycardia. Intravenous (IV) fentanyl or patient-controlled intravenous analgesia with remifentanil or fentanyl, plus control of heart rate with a β-blocker if required, is advisable for NYHA Class III or IV patients.

Monitoring of fluid balance to maintain normovolemia, judicious intravenous fluid, and vasoactive drug administration with α-agonists (e.g., phenylephrine) rather than ephedrine for vasoconstriction (to avoid its undesirable chronotropic effects) are recommended.

- Oxytocin should be delivered slowly by infusion, to avoid peripheral vasodilatation and tachycardia.
- Ergot uterotonics and injected prostaglandins are best avoided.
- Furosemide may be necessary to reduce the risk of postpartum pulmonary edema in the presence of severe mitral stenosis.

Regional or General Anesthesia in Valvular Disease?

In the absence of high levels of evidence regarding outcome, the merits of regional versus general anesthesia can be debated. Sudden increases in heart rate and afterload may precipitate pulmonary edema in mitral stenosis, or myocardial ischemia in aortic stenosis. Both single-shot spinal anesthesia (SA) and rapid establishment of epidural anesthesia (EA) may lead to sudden cardiovascular collapse, so if regional block is chosen it should be established slowly and in a controlled fashion, avoiding volume overload and bradycardia.

A suggested approach is:

- a sequential low spinal-epidural or slow EA approach
- optimization of maternal oxygenation

- direct arterial blood pressure monitoring and regular blood gas analysis
- cardiac output monitoring should be considered.

If using general anesthesia for severe aortic stenosis or cardiomyopathy, responses to anesthetic agents must be considered.

- Nitrous oxide increases pulmonary vascular resistance and should be avoided.
- Volatile anesthetics reduce systemic vascular resistance.
- The response to intubation should be attenuated (with opioids, magnesium, and/or vasodilators), and myocardial depression minimized (have inotropic drugs available).

Severe Congenital Heart Disease and Pulmonary Hypertension

In developed countries, maternal cardiac deaths from adult congenital heart disease exceed those from ischemic heart disease, aortic dissection, and valvular disease.

There are a large number of congenital disorders of varying complexity. Some are cyanotic (e.g., Tetralogy of Fallot) and others involve left-to-right shunts (such as patent ductus arteriosis, ostium secundum atrial septal defect, and ventricular septal defects). These vary in significance and require individual assessment.

- Some disorders may require only antibiotic prophylaxis, while others require aggressive control of physiological variables and management of hyperviscosity.

Acyanotic and Cyanotic Congenital Heart Disease

The acyanotic group includes a variety of cardiac structural and developmental abnormalities with good prognosis, especially if complex disease is satisfactorily corrected surgically in early childhood. If physical status is stable during pregnancy, regional analgesia and anesthesia are suitable and can be managed more or less routinely. Blood loss may cause an abrupt fall in cardiac output.

- Ebstein's anomaly is the downward displacement of the triscuspid valve with atrialized proximal portion of the right ventricle. This lesion may not present until late childhood, but has a good prognosis in pregnancy, despite paroxysmal arrhythmias and possible right-to-left shunting.
- The secundum atrial septal defect is one of the most common defects first diagnosed in pregnancy.
- Supraventricular arrhythmias are poorly tolerated as shunt is increased.

- Corrected ventricular septal defect, patent ductus arteriosus and aortic coarctation are other examples of acyanotic congenital lesions.

Pre-pregnancy polycythemia or oxygen saturation < 85% on air are poor prognostic indicators for the fetus in maternal cyanotic heart disease without Eisenmenger's syndrome.

Pulmonary Hypertension

This disease is of special concern, and is defined as pulmonary artery pressure greater than 30/15 mmHg and right ventricular hypertrophy, with or without cardiac failure. Electrocardiogram (ECG), such as right bundle branch block, may reflect this (Figure 10.2). Hypoxia, hypercarbia, and acidosis increase pulmonary artery pressure and resistance, so potential hazards include pain during prolonged labor, the respiratory depressant effects of systemic opioids, and inadequate hydration.

Pulmonary hypertension may be:

- Secondary—due to reversal of left-to-right shunts (Eisenmenger's syndrome; see Figure 10.3), prolonged severe mitral stenosis, or severe hypoxemia from respiratory disease (e.g., cystic fibrosis)
- Primary—a rare disorder that presents in women of reproductive age
  - Increases in pulmonary, and reduction in systemic, vascular resistance (e.g., hypovolemia or hypoxemia) are generally very poorly tolerated
  - Mortality is very high (30%–50%).

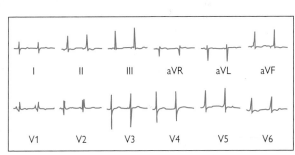

Figure 10.2 Electrocardiograph of a parturient with pulmonary hypertension, showing sinus rhythm with right atrial P waves (V1), an inferior axis, and evidence of right ventricular pressure overload (V1–2).

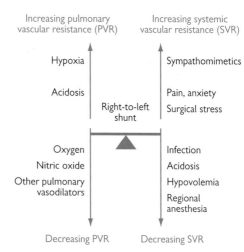

Figure 10.3 Factors affecting cardiac shunt.

Anesthetic management (whether regional or general) requires a thorough understanding of the original disease, the corrective surgery if relevant, and the current condition of the heart.

- In the presence of a shunt, loss-of-resistance to air for epidural placement is hazardous and air in intravenous infusion lines must be avoided, because of the possibility of IV air injection with subsequent paradoxical embolism.
- The implications of anticoagulation must be considered (Chapter 13).
- Prophylaxis against bacterial endocarditis may or may not be indicated (Table 10.5).
- Labor epidural analgesia is usually recommended and hemodynamic stability can be achieved using epidural or spinal opioids; maintenance may be with local anesthetic-opioid infusion or patient-controlled epidural analgesia.

General anesthesia for cesarean delivery (Table 10.7) may allow for cardiovascular stability, but has disadvantages such as morbidity from hemorrhage, infection, and thromboembolism. Regional analgesia and anesthesia require slow titration and intense monitoring to balancing factors affecting pulmonary and systemic resistance (Figure 10.4).

Table 10.7 Principles of General Anesthesia in Cardiac Disease

Perform an individual risk-benefit assessment, but consider general anesthesia rather than regional anesthesia for severe aortic stenosis, hypertrophic cardiomyopathy, and poorly controlled cardiac failure.

Be vigilant for hemodynamic changes, especially at intubation and extubation.

Obtund the sympatho-adrenal "stress response" to laryngoscopy and intubation
- appropriate doses of opioid eg. remifentanil 1 mcg/kg over 60 s; fentanyl 5–10 mcg/kg; alfentanil 10–20 mcg/kg
- magnesium 40–60 mg/kg post-induction
- vasodilators, e.g., glyceryl trinitrate (nitroglycerin) 250–500 mcg

Consider whether nitrous oxide is suitable (increases pulmonary vascular resistance)

Choose the most appropriate inhalational anesthetic with the least adverse cardiac and vascular effects

Maximize oxygenation

Choose the most appropriate neuromuscular blocking drug

Stabilize hemodynamics at extubation
- esmolol 0.5 mg/kg
- fentanyl 2 mcg/kg

Provide good postoperative analgesia
- patient-controlled intravenous analgesia with morphine
- adjuncts such as acetaminophen (paracetamol) and/or nonsteroidal anti-inflammatory drugs if no renal impairment or cardiac failure
- abdominal wall regional analgesia e.g., transversus abdominis plane (TAP) block

- Arterial oxyhemoglobin saturation is a valuable noninvasive tool for the detection of hypoxemia from shunt reversal or increased pulmonary pressures.
- Thermodilution pulmonary artery catheters and transesophageal echocardiography may be helpful in specific situations.
- Pulmonary vasodilators such as nitric oxide, 100% oxygen, aerosolized and intravenous prostaglandins (epoprostenol, iloprost or PGI2) or sildenafil may be tested to determine patient response, bearing in mind that platelet dysfunction may be induced, with implications for central neuraxial block. Bosentan may be introduced for pulmonary vasodilation after delivery.
- Intensive postpartum care is warranted, as death may still occur after an apparently uncomplicated intra- and early postpartum course.

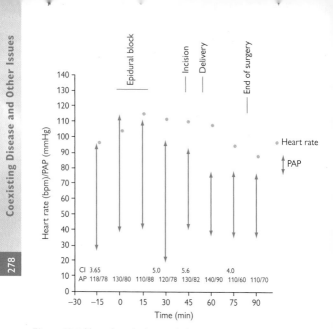

Figure 10.4 Hemodynamic changes during cesarean section in a parturient with primary pulmonary hypertension. CI, cardiac index (l/min); AP, arterial pressure (mmHg); PAP, pulmonary artery pressure (mmHg); bpm, beats per minute. Reprinted from the *International Journal of Obstetric Anesthesia, Vol. 5*, Khan MJ, Anesthetic considerations for parturients with primary pulmonary hypertension: review of the literature and clinical presentation, p. 38, Copyright (1996), with permission from Elsevier.

Myocardial Ischemia and Acute Coronary Dissection

Most cases of acute myocardial infarction occur in the third trimester in women > 35 years of age who have typical risk factors (obesity, smoking, hypertension, diabetes). Mortality is high (30%, rising the closer the infarct occurs to term gestation). During pregnancy and under regional anesthesia for cesarean delivery, changes in the ECG such as sinus tachycardia, left axis deviation and ST-T changes may make interpretation more difficult. However, unlike the muscle-brain isoenzyme of creatinine kinase (CK-MB), maternal troponin I levels are unchanged during pregnancy, and so a rise within 4 hours, lasting several days is specific for myocardial injury.

Medical therapies include:

- Nitrates, β-blockers and calcium-channel antagonists
- Heparin anticoagulation
- Aspirin and/or clopidogrel for unstable angina or acute infarction
  - clopidogrel precludes regional techniques for a week
- Percutaneous coronary intervention (the preferred management of acute syndromes)
- Thrombolysis (retaplase, alteplase) is associated with a very high risk of maternal hemorrhage

Vaginal delivery appears safer than cesarean after myocardial infarction during pregnancy. Regional analgesia is recommended for labor and delivery, and supplemental oxygen is recommended.

- Increases in oxygen demand due to shivering should be avoided (warm intravenous fluids, surface warm, use neuraxial opioid with local anesthetic, and intravenous clonidine 30 mcg to treat shaking).
- Monitoring of temperature, oxygenation, blood pressure and ECG are prudent and esophageal/transthoracic echocardiography may be helpful.
- Regional anesthesia (incremental epidural, sequential spinal-epidural or continuous spinal anesthesia) is suitable for operative delivery.
  - Spinal anesthesia or rapid epidural anesthesia are not ideal, due to the cardiovascular consequences of rapid uncompensated sympathectomy.
  - High thoracic epidural analgesia for postoperative analgesia favorably influences the endocardial to epicardial blood flow ratio.
- α1-agonist vasocontrictors (e.g., phenylephrine, metaraminol) are preferable to ephedrine.
- For general anesthesia, a modified technique should be used (Table 10.7).

Arrhythmias

During pregnancy, benign arrhythmias are common and serious arrhythmias (Figure 10.5) are rare.

- Some anti-arrhythmics such as phenytoin and amiodarone are associated with fetal effects (lidocaine may be preferable for ventricular tachycardia). β-blockers are preferred for acute rate control of atrial fibrillation or flutter.
- New onset atrial fibrillation is worrying; mitral valvular disease, thyrotoxicosis and other heart disease must be excluded. Manage by rate control with digoxin, and use anticoagulation if necessary.

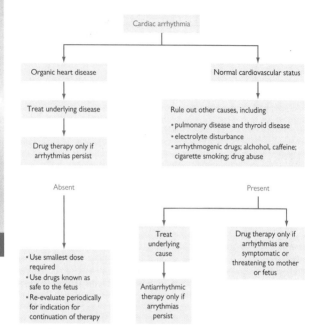

Figure 10.5 Management of cardiac arrhythmias during pregnancy.
Reprinted with permission from Rotmensch HH, *et al.* Management of cardiac arrhythmias during pregnancy. *Drugs.* 1987;33:628.

- Treat paroxysmal supraventricular tachycardias with vagal maneuvers and adenosine.
- Hemodynamic compromise from the sudden onset of any supraventricular arrhythmia can be treated with direct current cardioversion (starting at 50–100 joules under appropriate general anesthesia) because fetal heart rate changes are transient and benign.

Aortic Dissection

Most cases are due to Marfan's syndrome.

- This disease is an autosomal dominant disease of connective tissue (fibrillin gene mutations), and is associated with mitral valve prolapse or regurgitation, aortic root dilatation and regurgitation, and aortic dissection, especially in late pregnancy.

In addition to prepregnancy counseling, patients with an aortic diameter greater than 4 cm or progressive dilatation during pregnancy warrant:

- Aggressive control of hypertension
- Treatment with β-blockers
- Frequent transthoracic echocardiography to estimate aortic root size
- Epidural techniques for labor or operative delivery.

Hypertrophic Obstructive Cardiomyopathy

This disorder (commonly termed HOCM or idiopathic hypertrophic subaortic stenosis) is autosomal dominant with variable penetrance, involving a mutation at the myosin heavy chain gene. It usually presents in young adulthood.

- HOCM shares similarities with aortic stenosis, in that an asymmetric hypertrophy of the interventricular septum produces left ventricular outflow obstruction that is worsened by low ventricular volume, increased ventricular ejection velocity, or low arterial pressure.
- HOCM usually has a good outcome in pregnancy, but sudden death may occur due to ventricular arrhythmias and pulmonary edema.

Management is directed toward avoidance of hypovolemia and arrhythmias (especially the loss of atrial "kick" with atrial fibrillation or tachycardia).

- β-blockers are useful to reduce tachycardia (thus increasing end-diastolic ventricular filling and reducing myocardial oxygen demand and ventricular velocity).
- Implanted automated defibrillators may prevent sudden death from episodic ventricular tachycardia/fibrillation and require perioperative management.

Epidural or combined spinal-epidural analgesia during labor and delivery is valuable to reduce catecholamine release in response to pain. Direct arterial blood pressure monitoring is helpful. An individual risk-benefit assessment is necessary for operative delivery. Both careful slowly titrated epidural and general anesthesia have been used successfully, and direct-acting vasoconstrictors should be used so that ephedrine can be avoided.

Peripartum Cardiomyopathy and Heart-Lung Transplantation

Cardiomyopathy has various etiologies (e.g., viral myocarditis, drug-induced) but low-output cardiac failure without apparent cause ("peripartum cardiomyopathy") occurs in 1 in 2,000–4,000 pregnancies, often presenting during the third trimester or, most commonly (60%), postpartum.

In peripartum cardiomyopathy, women present with the rapid onset of global heart failure. Other dramatic symptoms include mural thromboembolism, severe hypotension, bradycardia and cardiac arrest at induction of general anesthesia.

The principal treatment is that of cardiac failure and anticoagulation.

- Mild reduction of afterload using appropriate regional analgesia is of benefit during labor, and well-managed regional block for cesarean delivery (avoiding single-shot spinal anesthesia) appears safe.
- Severely dyspneic patients who cannot tolerate a supine or semi-recumbent position may require general anesthesia, using a moderate to high dose opioid methods (Table 10.7).
- Invasive monitoring is indicated, with vasodilators and inotropes available. Intensive care or coronary care support must be available.

The prognosis is variable, and approximately 50% recover fully. Cardiac transplantation offers an alternative for those with persistent dysfunction.

In the rare case of successful pregnancy after cardiac transplantation, high rates of hypertension, preeclampsia and premature labor increase the likelihood of anesthetic involvement, although obstetric and maternal outcome is generally good. A balance must be struck between graft rejection and infection risk, and immunosuppressive therapy may need adjustment (for example, an increased dose of cyclosporine, which appears safe during pregnancy, due to the pharmacokinetic changes).

The denervated heart has higher resting heart rate due to loss of vagal tone, and is unaffected by indirect-acting drugs like atropine and ephedrine. The effects of direct-acting drugs may be exaggerated by β-adrenoreceptor upregulation, and the myocardial depressant effects of anesthetic agents predominate. Preload must be maintained, and local anesthetic containing epinephrine (adrenaline) avoided.

Diabetes

Diabetes is the most common metabolic disorder in pregnancy (incidence about 6% in the United States) and is increasing in prevalence. It may be present prior to pregnancy (usually insulin-dependent type 1) or arise during pregnancy due to physiological hormonal changes (gestational or Class A diabetes). Gestational diabetes is often managed with diet control, but some women require insulin.

In general, maternal risks are few, although obesity is common and preeclampsia also more common, especially among those with baseline proteinuria. In contrast, fetal morbidity is very common.

- There are higher rates of congenital abnormality.
- Intrauterine growth retardation and preterm delivery (and delayed lung maturation) are more common.
- Neonatal hypoglycemia is very common.
- Macrosomia is more common with poor maternal control because of hyperglycemia, hyperlipidemia and elevated amino acids. Consequences include shoulder dystocia at delivery, and obesity and diabetes in childhood or adolescence.

Management

The usual preoperative evaluation of the diabetic should include a careful evaluation of the airway, due to the increased risk of urgent delivery; gestational diabetics are often obese, which can also complicate anesthetic management.

- Diabetics should also be assessed for autonomic neuropathy because of its implications for regional anesthesia, hemodynamic instability, and delayed gastric emptying.

During labor, continuous maternal blood glucose control is important. Elevated intrapartum maternal glucose levels result in fetal hyperglycemia and hyperinsulinemia, which can in turn lead to fetal hypercarbia and acidemia.

- In Class A1 parturients, blood glucose should be checked every 2 to 4 hours during labor.
- In insulin-dependent diabetics, an intravenous insulin drip and dextrose infusion should be started (Table 10.8). Blood glucose should be checked via fingerstick hourly, and the rate of the infusions adjusted to maintain maternal glucose between 90 and 110 mg/dl. After delivery, insulin requirements fall quickly, so continued monitoring is necessary.

In the diabetic parturient, insulin requirements are increased but fall rapidly immediately after delivery due to the fall in human placental lactogen. Among gestational diabetics who have been managed with

Table 10.8 **Suggested Insulin and Glucose Infusion Rates Based on Finger Stick Glucose Measurements during Labor**

Glucose (mg/100 ml)	Insulin dose (units.hr)	Intravenous fluids 125 ml.hr
<100	0	D5 LR
100–140	1.0	D5 LR
141–180	1.5	Normal saline
181–220	2.0	Normal saline
>220	2.5	Normal saline

insulin, this is usually no longer required. In type 1 diabetics, insulin requirements usually rapidly return to prepregnancy levels.

Diabetes in the parturient is a relative indication for regional analgesia/anesthesia during labor.

- Epidural analgesia has been shown to decrease circulating catecholamines, which can decrease uteroplacental perfusion and increase insulin requirements.
- A functioning epidural catheter provides a route for rapid induction of surgical anesthesia if necessary urgently.

If a fluid load is considered before institution of regional anesthesia, only nonglucose-containing fluids should be used.

For scheduled (elective) cesarean deliveries, an early morning start time is best, as this minimizes the fasting period and makes insulin management easier.

- Blood glucose should be checked preoperatively and upon patient arrival, and insulin and dextrose infusions begun if necessary.
- Either spinal or epidural anesthesia is suitable.
- After delivery, the infant must be observed and monitored for hypoglycemia.

Pulmonary Disease

The significant changes that occur in pulmonary physiology and anatomy during pregnancy (Chapter 3) can alter the presentation and severity of pulmonary disease. Dyspnea is a common symptom during pregnancy, but occasionally is a result of undetected pulmonary and cardiac pathologies, so worsening symptoms must be investigated.

In part because of the impaired cellular immune response during pregnancy, both viral (influenza, mycoplasma and legionella) and bacterial pneumonia (streptococcus pneumoniae, pseudomonas aeroginosa and tuberculus pneumonia in those with human immunodeficiency virus) are serious diseases that lead to preterm delivery or pregnancy loss. The H1N1 influenza pandemic of 2009 illustrated the markedly increased mortality from adult respiratory distress syndrome associated with the pregnant condition.

It is recommended that smoking be avoided during pregnancy (Table 10.9).

Asthma

Asthma is the most common pulmonary disease of reproductive age, complicating up to 6% of pregnancies in the United States.

- It remains unchanged, improves or worsens during pregnancy in approximately equal proportions. It is unpredictable in the individual case, but may follow a recurrent pattern.

Table 10.9 Adverse Effects of Smoking During Pregnancy
Obstetric
Early pregnancy loss
Preterm delivery
Intrauterine growth retardation / low birth weight
Increased incidence of placental abruption
Neonatal
Impaired suckling
Sleep disturbance
Sudden infant death syndrome
Learning disorders
Childhood cancers
Physiologic
Increased mucus and decreased mucus clearance
Hyperactive airways
Small airway narrowing and closure
Increased carboxyhemoglobin concentration and lower oxygen affinity
Impaired immune response
Hepatic enzyme induction

- Approximately 10% of women with severe disease will require hospitalization.
- Severe asthmatics with increased airway hyperactivity during pregnancy may develop hypoxia that contributes to fetal morbidity or preterm delivery, or have acute exacerbations of bronchospasm and air-trapping.

Cesarean delivery rates are higher in women with moderate to severe disease, and undertreatment is an issue. If anesthesia is required in a severe asthmatic, or during an acute exacerbation, regional anesthesia is usually preferable to avoid airway manipulation.

- Avoid drugs that are bronchoconstrictors (e.g., ergot uterotonics, prostaglandin-$F_{2\alpha}$, morphine).
- Avoid triggers such as aspirin and nonsteroidal anti-inflammatory drugs.
- Bronchodilate with preoperative inhaled or nebulized β-sympathomimetics, inhaled steroids and other drugs.
- In the presence of acute intraoperative bronchospasm and hypoxemia, treat with short-acting inhaled β_2-sympathomimetics; if using general anesthesia, an increased concentration of volatile anesthetic during maintenance and induction with ketamine may be indicated.

Inhaled β_2-agonists, inhaled and oral steroids, anticholinergic drugs, methylxanthines, chromoglycates and possibly leukotriene-receptor antagonists appear safe during pregnancy. Breast-feeding may reduce the risk of childhood atopy.

Pulmonary Edema and /or Adult Respiratory Distress Syndrome

These conditions are uncommon to rare during pregnancy (adult respiratory distress syndrome 1 in 3,000–6,000; mortality 40%) and have multiple etiologies (Table 10.10). Management is similar to that during nonpregnancy, being treatment of the disorder, supportive respiratory care, fluid restriction and diuresis.

- Oxygen requirements are increased in pregnant patients compared to nonpregnant patients.
- The patient should be nursed upright with left tilt if possible.
- The lower colloid osmotic pressure of pregnancy makes cautious restricted fluid management vital.
- Regular fetal monitoring should be implemented.

Table 10.10 Etiology of Pulmonary Edema in the Pregnant Woman
Aspiration of gastric contents
Infection
Systemic sepsis
Influenza and other viral disease
Preeclampsia
Cardiac disease
Heart failure
Severe mitral stenosis
Fluid administration
Over-correction of hypovolemia
Associated with tocolytic drug infusion
Associated with oxytocic drug infusion
Transfusion-related acute lung injury (TRALI)

Neurosurgery and Neurological Disease

Neuroanesthesia

Neuroanesthesia is rarely required during pregnancy but may be necessary for:

- diagnostic or therapeutic interventions

- spinal surgery

- craniotomy for space-occupying masses or head injury

- trauma (which complicates 6%–7% of pregnancies and is a leading cause of incidental maternal death and morbidity)

In the absence of evidence-based guidance, the principles of neuroanesthesia and obstetric anesthesia must be reconciled and applied.

- Anticonvulsant therapy should be maintained through the perioperative phase (pregnancy changes the clearance, unbound fractions, and half-lives of some anticonvulsant drugs).

- Maintain effective pelvic tilt after 20 weeks gestation (if surgically acceptable, place the woman in the lateral position for long intracranial procedures).

- Have a low threshold for intraarterial blood pressure monitoring (aiming to preserve cerebral and uteroplacental perfusion), and maintain high normal blood pressure if the intracranial pressure (ICP) is raised.
- Use central venous access for inotropes or aspiration of air emboli.
- Maintain maternal arterial carbon dioxide tension in the low normal range ($PaCO_2$ 25–32 mmHg) to reduce ICP, while avoiding hyperventilation-induced uterine artery vasoconstriction and left-shift of the maternal oxyhemoglobin dissociation curve.
- Monitor and preserve body temperature (avoid induced hypothermia).
- Intracranial pressure can be controlled with a slight head-up position, low tidal volumes, and furosemide or mannitol 0.25–0.5 mg/kg (fetal hyperosmolality can reduce fetal lung fluid production, reduce urinary blood flow, and increase plasma sodium concentration).
- Isonatremic, isotonic and glucose-free intravenous fluids should be used.
- Safe, nonsedating antiemetic drugs include metoclopramide, antihistamines, droperidol and serotonin$_3$ receptor (5-HT3) antagonists.

With respect to anesthetic technique:

- In the operating room, the response to laryngoscopy should be attenuated; remifentanil is popular as it is very effective and also enhances rapid wakening.
- A propofol infusion, when used for many hours, is associated with mild metabolic acidosis.
- Volatile anesthetics such as isoflurane or sevoflurane reduce cerebral oxygen metabolic rate.
- Postoperative prophylactic tocolysis (nifedipine or nonsteroidal anti-inflammatory drugs) is generally only used to prevent premature labor if the risk of fetal loss is high.
- Intravenous heparin may have been used, especially for interventional radiology, and requires reversal in the event of emergency cesarean delivery or obstetric hemorrhage.
- Fetal monitoring may be appropriate, and the onset of labor postoperatively should be suspected if abdominal pain occurs.

Anesthetic Techniques

An approach to general anesthesia for cesarean delivery (to modify and minimize increases in cerebral blood flow and ICP) in a woman with raised intracranial pressure is shown in Table 10.11.

Table 10.11 Suggested General Anesthetic Technique for Cesarean Delivery for a Patient with Raised ICP

Pre-induction opioid
- e.g., intravenous (IV) remifentanil 1 mcg/kg over 60 seconds then titrated infusion, with or without post-induction IV magnesium 60 mg/kg

Total intravenous anesthesia with propofol (inhalational anesthetics suitable if normal ICP)

Avoid nitrous oxide
- elevates ICP, increases cerebral blood flow and cerebral oxygen metabolic rate, impairs autoregulation
- expands air bubbles

Oxytocin by infusion only
- to minimize bolus-induced cardiovascular effects such as transient hypotension, tachycardia and increase in cardiac output

Avoid venoconstrictors
- e.g., ergot uterotonics or prostaglandin $F_{2\alpha}$

Prophylactic antiemetics

Postoperative analgesia
- multimodal analgesia (local anesthetic infiltration or scalp blocks, opioids and acetaminophen)
- avoid tramadol
- cyclooxygenase$_2$ (COX-2) inhibitors do not increase bleeding but may be contraindicated for fetal reasons
- neuraxial opioids suitable after spinal surgery

Antithromboembolic stockings and calf compression perioperatively
- discuss heparin thromboprophylaxis with the neurosurgeon because of the potential hemorrhagic complications

Admission to a neurosurgical high-dependency unit or intensive care unit for observation or continued ventilation may be appropriate

If cesarean delivery is scheduled prior to a neurosurgical intervention, regional anesthesia can be recommended provided the patient is alert, cooperative, and has normal intracranial pressure. However, if ICP is high, dural puncture is dangerous because it may precipitate brain herniation or intracranial hemorrhage.

- Epidural injection will increase ICP, at least transiently.
- Epidural and spinal techniques have high failure rates after some types of spinal surgery and in the presence of ventriculoperitoneal shunt.

Cerebral vasospasm can complicate subarachnoid hemorrhage 3–6 days after the initial bleeding, and the recommended principles of "hypertension, hypervolemia and hemodilution" may require reassessment during pregnancy. The increased plasma volume and, to a lesser extent, red cell mass, are beneficial—but in preeclamptic patients, the mean arterial blood pressure should not be increased given the risk of eclampsia and other cerebral complications. Magnesium sulfate is safe and suitable for use, and nimodipine to control intracranial vasospasm appears safe, but may cause maternal hypotension.

Neurological Disease and Anesthesia

Many neurological disorders impact on either the efficacy or risks of neuraxial regional analgesia and anesthesia. Problems include:

- Technical difficulties (e.g., scoliosis)
- Potential trauma to lesions (e.g., vascular malformations, neurofibroma)
- Increased risk of inadvertent dural puncture or cord injury (e.g., spinal bifida)
- Increased risk of neurological deficits (e.g., spinal canal stenosis)
- Exaggerated or abnormal responses to drugs (e.g., multiple sclerosis, amyotrophic lateral sclerosis, polio, hereditary motor and sensory neuropathies such as Charcot-Marie Tooth disease or peroneal muscular atrophy)
- Abnormal autonomic responses (e.g., spinal cord injury)

Data are limited, but the largest series suggest that most women with preexisting neurological diseases usually experience uneventful epidural and spinal analgesia or anesthesia, and that these techniques are not contraindicated.

Multiple Sclerosis

This demyelinating disease of the central nervous system is characterized by episodic symptoms, then fixed deficits and increasing disability over time. It is not uncommon in women of reproductive age, and less severely affected individuals frequently conceive. During pregnancy, multiple sclerosis is largely unaltered, but the first 3 postpartum months are associated with higher rates of relapse (approximately 30%).

It is thus very important to engage the patient in the decision-making process.

The three major concerns about regional anesthesia are:

- Unmasking of silent demyelinated plaques by local anesthetic
- Exaggerated block responses (especially prolonged duration)
- Higher rates of disease relapse

Ideally, these women should be seen at an antenatal clinic. In obtaining consent for regional techniques during pregnancy, the anesthesiologist should take a number of steps.

- Document the current neurological condition of the patient.
- Inform the patient that there is no evidence of higher relapse rates associated with neuraxial local anesthetic administration.
- Take into consideration sporadic reports of more intense or prolonged block, especially in those with significant demyelination.
- Discuss the possibility of unmasking new deficits.

Experimental but not clinical evidence indicates that there is less risk of exacerbation with epidural techniques compared to spinal techniques (lower CSF local anesthetic concentration).

When general anesthesia is necessary, the anesthesiologist should be aware that multiple sclerosis and other similar diseases increase sensitivity to succinylcholine (with possible hyperkalemia) due to upregulation of nicotinic acetylcholine receptors.

Spinal Cord Injury

Pregnancy in women with spinal cord injury is no longer rare. As well as poor respiratory function and infection issues, especially in high quadriplegics, the major concern in patients who are paraplegic or quadriplegic is autonomic hyperreflexia, induced by labor or surgery-related nociception.

Autonomic hyperreflexia primarily affects those with injuries above T_8, and especially T_5. It results from sympathetic outflow in response to visceral stimulus (especially labor and perineal distension) in the absence of supraspinal inhibition (Figure 10.6). Neuronal and endocrine responses result in features such as:

- Severe vasoconstriction leading to hypertension, headache, sweating, flushing, and reflex bradycardia (vasodilator therapy with nifedipine or glyceryl trinitrate may be required)
- Potentially fatal maternal complications including cerebral hemorrhage or cerebral edema
- Fetal bradycardia or placental abruption

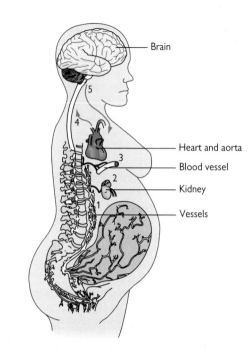

Figure 10.6 Mechanism of cardiovascular response to labor in autonomic hyperreflexia. Sensory afferents enter the cord below the level of the spinal cord lesion (1), eliciting reflex sympathetic outflow to (2) the adrenal medulla (T_5–T_9) and (3) the peripheral vasculature (T_1–L_1). These two responses provoke severe hypertension. Carotid and aortic baroreceptors (4) respond to the hypertension with afferent outflow to the brainstem, which in turn stimulates parasympathetic efferents to the sinus node via the vagus nerve (5), resulting in bradycardia.

If anesthetizing a patient with spinal cord injury, regional analgesia for labor and delivery should be instituted as soon as possible (detection of contractions indicating onset of labor may be difficult if the lesion is above T_{10}) as this is the best method of obtunding the abnormal autonomic response.

- A dense local anesthetic block is recommended, because motor block is not an issue.
- Reposition the patient regularly to prevent pressure sores.
- If an epidural is difficult to insert, consider continuous spinal analgesia.

- Monitor blood pressure and heart rate regularly, and assume hypertension reflects inadequate block. Have a low threshold for using continuous arterial blood pressure monitoring in the labile patient. If general anesthesia is required:
- Succinylcholine must be avoided in the first 6 or more months postinjury to minimize risk of hyperkalemic arrest (use rocuronium for rapid sequence induction).
- Maintain good analgesic depth and monitor postdelivery for up to 48 hours for signs of autonomic hyperreflexia.

Renal Disease

A number of changes in renal anatomy and function occur during pregnancy (Chapter 2), and maternal and fetal outcome in women with preexisting renal disease depends on the degree of renal dysfunction at conception, the underlying disease process, and the degree of hypertension. Diseases causing renal pathology during pregnancy include:

- Renal-specific diseases (e.g., focal segmental glomerulosclerosis, IgA nephropathy, reflux uropathy, polycystic kidney disease).
- Systemic diseases (e.g., diabetic nephropathy, hypertensive nephropathy, systemic lupus erythematosus, connective tissue disorders, vasculitides, Goodpasture's syndrome).
- Obstetric disorders (e.g., severe preeclampsia, obstetric hemorrhage).

Women with moderate or severe renal disease have a higher than normal rate of early pregnancy loss and stillbirth.

- Patients with severe renal disease have a variable course during pregnancy, but two-thirds experience deterioration and one in three develop end-stage renal failure.
- Those with mild renal dysfunction prior to pregnancy (serum creatinine 0.8–1.4 mg/dl or 80 to 124 micromol/l), or no established hypertension, have better outcomes.

Until recently, successful pregnancy among patients with severe renal disease was unusual, but with better medical monitoring and therapy it has become more common, even for those on dialysis. Of women of childbearing age receiving dialysis, approximately 10% will become pregnant and more than 50% achieve a live birth, although preeclampsia, preterm delivery and low birth weight are more common. All women with severe renal disease are at increased risk of pregnancy-related complications, and appropriate management plans must be established in liaison with obstetricians and nephrologists.

Renal Failure

Acute renal failure in pregnancy is rare (rate 1 in 10,000) and associated with:

- Severe preeclampsia (incidence 1%–2%)
- Hemorrhage (e.g., from abruption, amniotic fluid embolism)
- Acute fatty liver of pregnancy
- Obstructive uropathy

Chronic renal failure is defined as a progressive decrease in glomerular filtration rate (end-stage < 5 ml/min); diabetes mellitus and hypertension account for more than 50% of cases. Management problems include:

- Hypertension, hyperkalemia (ventricular dysfunction and acute arrhythmias), and hypocalcemia (QT interval prolongation)
- Sodium and water retention and hypoalbuminemia (pulmonary edema or hypovolemia)
- Gastric irritation or hemorrhage
- Normochromic normocytic anemia (fatigue, dyspnea) and uremia (nausea and vomiting)

In the perioperative period, postoperative atelectasis (decreased surfactant) and pneumonia (impaired response to infection) are more common.

Additional concerns for anesthetic management include:

- Peripheral neuropathies (document prior to regional block)
- Increased bleeding risk (defective von Willebrand factor)
- Changes in drug kinetics (low serum albumin, metabolic acidosis and reduced renal elimination)

Anesthesia for Patients with Renal Disease

The usual principles of anesthesia for patients with renal impairment or failure apply during pregnancy.

- Intravascular volume must be carefully assessed with a view to maintaining blood pressure, renal and placental perfusion (dialyse preoperatively if necessary); large fluid or blood losses are poorly tolerated.
- Anemia may require correction (preferably early, with erythropoietin, although this takes a week or more to increase hemoglobin concentration).

- Drugs that are primarily excreted by the kidneys should be avoided, as should nephrotoxic drugs, including nonsteroidal anti-inflammatory drugs.
- When general anesthesia is necessary, full precautions against gastric aspiration are indicated.
- Hypercarbia should be avoided (extracellular acidosis causes intracellular potassium to move into the extracellular compartment, exacerbating hyperkalemia).
- Succinylcholine-induced serum potassium rise (approximately 0.5 mmol/L) may prevent the use of succinylcholine for rapid-sequence induction.
- Exaggerated responses to anesthetic drugs occur (uremia may disrupt the blood brain barrier).
- Other general considerations include the use of heparin thromboprophylaxis, and an appropriate choice for postoperative care after delivery.
- When present, special care of arteriovenous fistula should be taken (bandage and pad and place intravenous cannula well away). The decision to insert an arterial cannula should also be made only after careful consideration and discussion with the nephrologists.

With respect to regional techniques, individual risk-benefit decisions are required.

- An attempt to assess the bleeding risk should be made (the platelet count and standard laboratory coagulation tests may be normal), preferably by means of specific tests in early consultation with a hematologist.
- Epidural and spinal anesthesia and analgesia are generally considered safe, with the usual provisos in relation to severe renal disease and anticoagulant drugs.

Hepatic Disease

A number of congenital or acquired liver diseases may be encountered during pregnancy. These include:

- preeclampsia
- viral hepatitis (A, B, C, D, E, and G viruses)
- hyperbilirubinemias (relatively benign disorders characterized by elevations of unconjugated bilirubin (e.g., Gilbert's disease) or conjugated bilirubin (e.g., Dubin-Johnson and Rotor syndromes)

- intrahepatic cholestasis of pregnancy
- acute fatty liver of pregnancy
- systemic diseases (e.g., lupus erythematosus and hemachromatosis)
- Wilson's disease, hydatid disease or cystic ecchinoccosis, cirrhosis, portal hypertension, acute liver failure or hepatic rupture

The most common (e.g., severe preeclampsia, Chapter 7) pose serious challenges, warrant multidisciplinary care led by physicians, and mandate a sound understanding of the anatomic, physiologic and functional changes in the liver induced by increased serum estrogen and progesterone during pregnancy.

Principles of Anesthesia

The choice of anesthetic technique is frequently determined by the degree of coagulopathy or rarely, in very severe disease, the state of obtundation. Regional techniques are preferable but may be contraindicated because of the risk of vertebral canal hematoma.

When general anesthesia is used, liver and renal blood flow should be maintained, and drugs which may be hepatotoxic avoided.

- Propofol exhibits normal pharmacokinetics in cirrhosis and causes no alteration of hepatic blood flow.
- Among inhalational agents, desflurane has negligible hepatic metabolism.
- Atracurium and cisatracurium show the least variability among the nondepolarizing relaxants.
- Beware exaggerated responses to anesthetics and analgesics in fulminant hepatic failure (poor metabolism and central depression associated with encephalopathy).

Viral Hepatitis

Through blood contact, health care workers are at risk of contracting hepatitis, especially HBV (the risk of seroconversion after exposure to a HBsAg+ woman is 1%–6% and HBeAg+ woman is 22%–31%), HCV and HDV. The application of universal precautions is essential. Women in the acute phase, or who have developed chronic hepatitis and cirrhosis, liver failure, or hepatocellular carcinoma, need special attention.

Intrahepatic Cholestasis of Pregnancy

The prevalence of this genetic disorder is < 1 in 1,000, but may be as high as 2%–15% in some countries. The disease is often subclinical and recurs in subsequent pregnancies. It usually presents after mid-pregnancy with:

- Pruritus in the extremities (palms and soles), then trunk and face (from reduced bile flow, bile and bile salt excretion).
- Mild jaundice (in 50% of cases, usually after 1–2 weeks).
- Malaise, nausea, abdominal discomfort and subclinical steatorrhea.
- A 10–100 times increase in serum bile acids and mildly elevated serum aminotransferases, resolving within 24 hours of delivery.

The fetus is at risk due to the direct effects of bile salts or preterm labor, and the neonate needs vitamin K to prevent intracranial bleeding. Once cholelithiasis has been excluded, supportive treatment is commenced with ursodeoxycholic acid, a hydrophilic bile acid that displaces toxic bile acids from hepatic membranes and relieves pruritus.

The anesthesiologist should assess the severity of liver dysfunction and coagulation disturbance, since vitamin K therapy and fresh frozen plasma may be required.

- Cesarean delivery may be necessary.
- Patients are at increased risk of postpartum hemorrhage.

Acute Fatty Liver of Pregnancy

Acute fatty liver is a rare and potentially fatal disorder (rate 1 in 20,000) of long-chain fatty acid metabolism that is specific to pregnancy. It typically presents close to term, and is difficult to diagnose because of similarity to severe preeclampsia with hepatic involvement.

A confirmed diagnosis requires prompt delivery of the fetus. Clinical presentation includes:

- Malaise, nausea and vomiting, abdominal pain, fever and jaundice
- Severe hypoglycemia
- Marked neutrophil leucocytosis, microangiopathic hemolytic anemia with thrombocytopenia, and disseminated intravascular coagulation
- Oliguria with serum electrolyte abnormalities, including high serum creatinine and ammonia
- Mildly elevated aminotransferases and bilirubin
- Metabolic acidosis from high serum lactate levels
- Renal failure, acute respiratory distress, and diabetes insipidus
- Pancreatitis, pseudocyst formation, and retroperitoneal bleeding

Other than delivery, therapy is mainly supportive. Initial therapy involves resuscitation and stabilization. Invasive monitoring is often necessary, and regular assessment of blood pressure, blood glucose, fluid and electrolyte, coagulation and acid-base status is essential.

- Hypoglycemia should be corrected.
- Coagulopathy usually requires correction (vitamin K and blood products), and prophylaxis against gastrointestinal hemorrhage with H2-receptor antagonists should be instituted.

Disease of the Biliary Tract

Late pregnancy and early postpartum increases in serum lipid concentrations, slowing of bile acid excretion and decreased small intestinal motility predispose women to cholelithiasis and cholecystitis. Acute cholecystitis is uncommon, and presents with:

- Right upper quadrant pain and tenderness
- Fever and leucocytosis
- Back pain and raised serum amylase (the latter indicating pancreatitis, which is also associated with alcohol or viral illness).

Most women with acute cholecystitis are suitable for conservative management, but the relapse rate is over a third and surgery may be preferable. Complications of gallstones represent the second most common nongynecologic condition requiring surgery during pregnancy.

Cholecystectomy is necessary in 1–8 per 10,000 pregnancies, but is associated with good maternal and fetal outcome, even when disease is severe.

- It can be performed with lead shielding of the uterus to minimize fetal exposure to radiation when cholangiography is necessary.
- Anesthetic management follows the usual principles, with attention to placental perfusion and gas exchange during laparoscopic surgery with pneumoperitoneum (Chapter 6).

Muscle, Neuromuscular and Musculoskeletal Disease

These diseases (e.g., myasthenia gravis, the muscular dystrophies, the myopathies such as mitochondrial myopathy, myotonic dystrophy, myotonia congenita, paramyotonia congenita, hyperkalemic periodic paralysis), whether myopathic or myotonic, have important implications for anesthesia and require close liaison with appropriate physicians. Regional anesthesia is usually well tolerated, but general anesthesia often requires modification.

Myotonic Disorders

Pregnancy is less likely in these diseases because of ovarian failure, but when it occurs, it may exacerbate all manifestations of the disease. Prolonged labor and uterine atony are more common, increasing the risk of postpartum hemorrhage.

Anesthesiologists must be familiar with these myotonic diseases because anesthesia and surgery may induce myotonia (muscle spasm and rigidity), which is difficult to abolish.

- Treatment options for a myotonic crisis are:
  - procainamide 1000 mg at 100 mg/min, watching for slowing of conduction
  - dantrolene, phenytoin, or direct injection of local anesthetic into the muscle
- Patients may display extreme sensitivity to some drugs and abnormal reaction to others.
- Muscle weakness and extramuscular features may be relevant.
- Susceptibility to malignant hyperthermia may be increased in some patients (e.g., myotonia congenita).

  The diseases may affect a number of systems:

- In myotonic dystrophy, cardiac conduction abnormalities are common (heart block, long QT), as are septal defects, and mitral valve prolapse can occur.
- Ventilation may be impaired, with restrictive defects and poor cough, or sleep apnea may be present.
- Pharyngeal weakness or delayed gastric emptying and other gastrointestinal problems contribute to an increased risk of aspiration.

General anesthesia in these patients is challenging.

- Doses of many medications should be modified and short-acting drugs used whenever possible.
- Undue sensitivity may be present to sedative and anesthetic drugs, and opioids.
- Prolonged responses (2–3 fold) occur with nondepolarizing neuromuscular blocking drugs (if muscle weakness is a feature).
- Succinylcholine causes dose-dependent myotonia of the jaw and chest that may prevent intubation and ventilation for up to 5 minutes.
- Anticholinesterases may precipitate myotonia.

Cold or shivering may precipitate myotonia, so temperature maintenance and monitoring are important. Neuraxial block induced shivering should be prevented (with warm solutions and neuraxial opioids) and treated promptly (e.g., IV clonidine, tramadol or meperidine).

Myasthenia Gravis

This chronic disease, characterized by weakness and fatigue of certain voluntary muscles, is most prevalent in females of childbearing age. IgG antibodies accelerate breakdown and partially block acetylcholine receptors. Treatment is with oral anticholinesterases, steroids, or thymectomy.

During pregnancy the course is unpredictable, with some women improving while others deteriorate. Premature labor is more common.

- Epidural analgesia during labor is usually suitable.
- During labor or the perioperative period, intravenous anticholinesterases are substituted for equivalent oral doses (e.g., IV neostigmine 0.7–1.5 mg for pyridostigmine 60 mg PO).
- Observation for bulbar weakness (such as difficulty swallowing, or with speech) and opthalmoplegia can guide therapy.
- Respiratory muscle weakness may be present.

For cesarean delivery, general anesthesia may be required to protect the airway, though regional anesthesia is suitable for well-controlled patients with minimal weakness.

- Neuromuscular blocking drugs should be used in very small doses or, preferably, be avoided (e.g., intubate using propofol and remifentanil).
- All drugs should be given in minimal effective doses.

Malignant Hyperthermia

Malignant hyperthermia (MH) occurs less often in pregnancy than in the rest of the population, making it extremely rare. The woman with MH susceptibility should be counseled in the antenatal period.

Early epidural analgesia during labor is advisable. Local anesthetics, adrenergic drugs, opioids, intravenous anesthetics, nitrous oxide, and aspiration prophylaxis drugs are safe.

- If possible avoid prostaglandins, which increase temperature, and drugs that cause tachycardia.
- Prophylactic dantrolene is not necessary.

If cesarean delivery is necessary, spinal anesthesia is the preferred option if no epidural catheter is present.

- Use a "clean" anesthetic machine (no vaporizers, flushed with oxygen, new circuitry, and carbon dioxide absorbent), even when a regional anesthetic is planned.
- Succinylcholine and volatile inhalational anesthetics are triggers and must be avoided if general anesthesia is required.
- A total intravenous anesthetic technique with propofol should be used for general anesthesia, with or without midazolam.
- Always monitor for an MH reaction (end-tidal PCO_2, temperature, etc.) and if necessary, treat an MH crisis as per recommended guidelines.

If the father is MH susceptible, the fetus has a 50% risk of MH, so all the preceding precautions are still necessary.

Musculoskeletal Disorders

Osteogenesis imperfecta, spinal muscle atrophic disease and dwarfism are rare in the pregnant population. A more common problem encountered is idiopathic scoliosis (incidence 1–4 per 1,000), which may have been arrested during adolescence by Harrington rod instrumentation of the spine. Scoliosis from any spinal muscular disorder is associated with a higher risk of cesarean delivery and poses problems with both regional and general anesthesia, so patients should be reviewed in the antenatal clinic.

Patients should be assessed for associated respiratory impairment or cardiac anomalies, and treated accordingly.

- Evaluate patients carefully for possible difficult intubation and plan accordingly.
- Regional techniques may need to be modified to maximize efficacy and safety. A careful assessment of spinal anatomy should be based on surgical history, examination of the spine, and anatomic imaging, including X-rays and ultrasound when available.
- Instrumented vertebral interspaces must be avoided when performing regional techniques.
- Subarachnoid techniques, including microspinal or macrospinal catheters in some cases, can be used to implement successful blocks, especially for cesarean delivery.

Despite careful planning, the patient should be warned about the need for multiple attempts, subsequent back pain, and other complications.

- The risk of unintentional dural puncture with an epidural needle is increased.

- Failure of regional block due to failure to locate the correct space, or subsequent drug maldistribution, is more likely.

Autoimmune or Connective Tissue Disease

In addition to Marfan's syndrome (see cardiac disease above), myasthenia gravis (see muscular disease above), idiopathic thrombocytopenic purpura and antiphospholid syndrome (see hematologic disease below), the most common diseases of relevance encountered are systemic lupus erythematosus, rheumatoid arthritis, and scleroderma.

Systemic Lupus Erythematosus

Systemic lupus erythematosus (SLE) is a chronic multisystem disease of young women. It is usually mild, and flares of disease respond well to treatment with steroids and antimalarial drugs (some anti-inflammatory or other immunosuppressive drugs are contraindicated during pregnancy).

- SLE has variable presentation, especially arthritis, cutaneous lesions, renal impairment, hypertension, cardiac disease (present in 50%), respiratory disease, mild thrombocytopenia, neurological and psychiatric abnormalities.
- A lupus anticoagulant antibody is present in 5%–10% of cases (see hematological disease). Thrombosis risk must be managed if the patient is lupus anticoagulant positive.

SLE follows an unpredictable course during pregnancy, but is associated with increased risk of preeclampsia.

Rheumatoid Arthritis

Most women with this chronic disease improve during pregnancy but deteriorate postpartum. Treatment must be managed appropriately, avoiding contraindicated drugs (anti-inflammatory drugs, penicillamine) and continuing those considered relatively safe (e.g., azathioprine).

The main anesthetic issue in rheumatoid arthritis is airway management.

- Look carefully for restriction of neck extension (atlanto-occipital and temporomandibular joint involvement, and cricoarytenoid dysfunction).
- Consider awake intubation if interincisor gap is <4–5 cm and the patient cannot protrude the mandibular incisors in front of maxillary incisors.

- Be very careful during intubation (atlanto-axial subluxation may cause acute cord injury).

Scleroderma

Scleroderma is a rare disease in pregnancy, sometimes treated with steroids and other immunosuppressive drugs. It is characterized by inflammation, vascular sclerosis (including Raynaud's phenomenon) and fibrosis of the skin and viscera, and runs an unpredictable course during pregnancy.

Anesthetic considerations include:

- Restrictive pulmonary disease is common.
- Check for gastroesophageal incompetence and reflux.
- Look for and treat hypertension and cardiac conduction abnormalities.
- Restricted mouth opening makes airway management difficult.
- Venous access may be difficult.
- Distal arterial cannulation is best avoided due to circulatory insufficiency.

Although individual decisions are based on consideration of all comorbidities and disease manifestations, regional analgesia and anesthesia is usually indicated (although blocks may be prolonged). Preparations should be made for potential difficult venous access or intubation, aspiration, and postoperative respiratory complications.

Hematologic Disease

Thrombophilias

The inherited thrombophilias encompass a variety of disorders—anticardiolipin antibody and lupus anticoagulant, heterozygosity or homozygosity for factor V Leiden mutation, heterozygosity for a prothrombin gene mutation variant, antithrombin deficiency, protein S and protein C deficiency, and hyperhomocysteinemia. These are associated with increased fetal loss, a modest increase in risk of preeclampsia, and a moderate to severe risk of thromboembolic events.

Based on risk assessment, women with these conditions are often receiving aspirin and unfractionated heparin (UFH); see "Management of the Anticoagulated Woman" below.

Antiphospholipid Syndrome

This syndrome is either primary or secondary (e.g., associated with systemic lupus erythematosus), and is one of the most common hypercoagulable states.

- Laboratory tests reveal Ig G and Ig M anti-cardiolipin antibodies and positivity to lupus anticoagulant, with *in vitro* prolongation of the activated partial thromboplastin time by lupus anticoagulant.
- Recurrent early pregnancy loss due to antibody activity at the placental trophoblast is common.
- Venous thrombosis occurs in up to 60%, but also arterial thrombosis in 10%; lower limbs are most commonly affected, but cerebral infarction can also occur.
- Thrombocytopenia, livedo reticularis (mottling of the skin), and hypertension (including pulmonary) are common.

Management during pregnancy involves aspirin and heparin to prevent pregnancy loss and thromboses, antithrombotic stockings, and prevention of hypothermia.

There is no contraindication to the use of regional anesthesia.

Postoperative anticoagulation is an important part of management. If there is no thrombosis history, prophylactic heparin plus warfarin is usually prescribed. If there is previous history of thrombosis, therapeutic doses of heparin are indicated with warfarin.

Von Willebrand's Disease

This is the commonest inherited (autosomal dominant) bleeding disorder, and affects 1%–2% of the population. It is most often due to abnormal production of von Willebrand factor (vWF), a protein produced by endothelial cells and platelets that carries factor VIII and aids adherence of platelets to vascular subendothelial layers. In addition to type I disease (70% of all cases and a quantitative defect) there are more severe variants (types II and III) which also have qualitative defects of function.

The disease is characterized by mucosal bleeding, easy bruising, and prolonged surgical bleeding.

- Laboratory tests show low concentrations of vWF antigen (15–60 units/dL) and factor VIIIc coagulation protein (40% of normal).
- Platelet function is abnormal in type II and III disease (binding of vWF to platelet glycoprotein, with ristocetin as a cofactor, is reduced by 40%).

During pregnancy, the levels of factor VIIIc and also vWF in type I disease rise substantially, usually exceeding 100% of the nonpregnant concentration.

- Treatment with 1-deamino-8-D-arginine vasopressin (DDAVP) to cause platelet release of vWF may be appropriate, especially if blood loss is expected.
- Regional anesthesia techniques are not contraindicated in type I disease.
- Factor concentrations fall rapidly postdelivery, so epidural catheters should not be retained.

Management includes consultation with a hematologist about the exact type of disease and previous response to management.

- Ideally, factor concentrations should be measured prior to delivery or undertaking neuraxial regional techniques.
- Intravenous DDAVP can be given 90 minutes prior to surgery (0.3 mcg/kg IV) to increase vWF concentrations by 2–4 fold to normal i.e., > 100 units/dL. Daily repeat doses of DDAVP show tachyphylaxis.
- Predelivery administration of factor VIII concentrates to those with qualitative defects of vWF antigen or severe autosomal recessive disease may be necessary.

Thrombocytopenia

There are a number of causes of low platelet count during pregnancy.

- Gestational thrombocytopenia
  - incidence 5%
  - counts often 120–150 $\times$ 10^9/L but rarely < 100 $\times$ 10^9/L
- Preeclampsia (Chapter 7)
- Idiopathic or autoimmune thrombocytopenic purpura (ITP)
  - incidence 2–6 per 100,000
  - associated with antiphospholipid syndrome
  - treatment with steroids, then high-dose IV immunoglobulin if unresponsive
  - aim for counts > 50 $\times$ 10^9/L to avoid primary bleeding risks and use platelet transfusion to achieve these levels immediately prior to surgery
  - observe the neonate, as platelet count nadir is 2–5 days postdelivery

- Thrombotic thrombocytopenia purpura or hemolytic uremic syndrome (both rare)
- Heparin-induced thrombocytopenia (rare to very rare with low-molecular-weight heparin)
  - platelet factor 4 antibodies
  - associated with serious thromboses
  - commences 5–10 days after exposure or on reexposure

In most bleeding disorders, including those involving platelets, there is no specific platelet count at which regional anesthesia can be defined as "safe" with respect to the risk of vertebral canal hematoma (see Chapters 3 and 7) . Such an event is exceptionally rare, and retrospective series indicate that neuraxial block may be uneventful even when platelet counts are extremely low.

Anemia

Pregnant women are predisposed to both iron deficiency and megaloblastic anemia, and require additional iron and folate during pregnancy. Inherited disorders of hemoglobin synthesis (thalassemias) or structure (hemoglobinopathies) may produce mild asymptomatic maternal anemia, through to severe disease with high perinatal morbidity. Most women with a thalassemia (quantitative defects in the production of globin chain subunits) are carriers with asymptomatic disease, who compensate well for their mild anemia. Homozygotes for hemoglobin C or E also usually have mild disease, with chronic hemolysis.

- Anesthetic considerations are based on assessment of the impact of chronic anemia on oxygen carriage and cardiac function (Table 10.12).

Table 10.12 **Anesthetic Management of the Anemic Pregnant Patient**
Check that a diagnosis has been made and appropriate therapy introduced (consult with hematologist or physician if required)
Consider the implications of the underlying disease
If well compensated chronic anemia, blood transfusion is usually unnecessary if hemoglobin concentration is above 7 g/dl
Only treat compensated anemia if there is ongoing bleeding
Give supplemental oxygen as required
Treat coexisting blood factor abnormalities (e.g., thrombocytopenia, leukocytosis)
Regional techniques may be contraindicated by thrombocytopenia (e.g., aplastic anemia) or platelet dysfunction (e.g., uremia)

Sickle cell trait is benign, but some sickling disorders (e.g., sickle cell disease due to HbSS and SC) have significant implications during pregnancy, such as:

- Severe anemia
- Vaso-occlusive crises
- Increased infection risk
- Fetal growth retardation and increased fetal loss

Psychiatric Disease

A number of mental health disorders peak in incidence during the reproductive period.

- There is a 5-fold increase in depression in the year after delivery, such that postnatal depression leading to suicide is now one of the most common causes of indirect maternal death in developed countries.

The obstetric anesthesiologist may have his or her technical and non-technical skills tested, especially by women with major personality disorders or schizophrenia.

Good antenatal management requires:

- Consideration of the implications and interactions of medications. (Table 10.13)

Table 10.13 Implications of Medications Prescribed for Psychiatric Patients

Major tranquilizers (e.g., haloperidol, thioridazine, fluphenazine)
- extrapyramidal side effects
- sedation
- orthostatic hypotension
- poor response to blood loss (α_1-adrenergic antagonism)
- cardiac conduction changes (heart block, prolonged QT interval)
- neuroleptic malignant syndrome (rare, potentially fatal drug-induced condition with similarities to malignant hyperthermia)

Antidepressants
- lowered seizure threshold from tricyclic antidepressants
- avoid meperidine (pethidine) in those on moclobemide (but no interaction with selective serotonin reuptake inhibitors [SSRIs])
- awareness of serotonin syndrome from the combination of SSRIs and tramadol

Anti-anxiety drugs
- use intravenous midazolam 1 mg repeated or clonidine 25 mcg repeated for panic attacks
- consider dexmedetomidine for procedural sedation

- Consultation with psychiatrists and physicians to develop management plans before the onset of labor or need for surgery.
- Seeking informed consent early.
- Facing challenges because of aggressive, paranoid or uncooperative behavior.
- The need to involve other parties with Power of Attorney or legal guardianship.
- Empathy and use of suitably quiet and private environs when consulting patients.

Depression

Depression, including manic-depressive illness, is associated with:

- Poor health and lack of antenatal care
- Nausea and vomiting
- Increased rates of cesarean delivery
- Poor compliance with medication because of (mainly unfounded) fears about fetal effects.

Anesthesia may be needed to support treatment of severe depression with electroconvulsive therapy (ECT). ECT is safe during pregnancy and anesthetic principles are shown in Table 10.14.

Management of the Drug-Dependent Pregnant Woman

Nearly 90% of women who abuse drugs are of childbearing age, and substance abuse during pregnancy is prevalent in many societies (30 per 1000 deliveries in Australia, with opioid dependence alone 11 per 1000). Polysubstance abuse is common, and frequently used drugs are alcohol, nicotine, marijuana, opioids, cocaine, amphetamines, benzodiazepines and toluene-based solvents. A combination of the clinical manifestations of drug abuse, the physiological changes of pregnancy, and the pathophysiology of pregnancy-related disease often leads to mental confusion, poor fetal outcomes, and serious or even life-threatening maternal complications. Acute admissions of women who have not accessed antenatal care should raise suspicion.

Women who are dependent on illicit drugs present challenges and place high demands on obstetric, anesthetic, and pain management services during pregnancy and childbirth. Up to 80% will require anesthetic services in the perinatal period.

Table 10.14 **Anesthesia for Electroconvulsive Therapy**
Continue usual antidepressant medication but consider drug interactions
Prevent aortocaval compression if > 20 weeks
Give aspiration prophylaxis
Use a rapid sequence induction if symptoms or gestation (> 20 weeks) warrant
• e.g., propofol 2 mg/kg and succinylcholine (suxamethonium) 0.5–1 mg/kg
Ventilate to normocapnia for pregnancy (30–32 mmHg) after the ECT and until extubation
Monitor the fetus after the ECT (> 24 weeks)
• transient severe fetal bradycardia occurs rarely
Monitor for uterine contractions or blood loss after the ECT

ECT = electroconvulsive therapy

- Early antenatal referral to an anesthesiology clinic is recommended.
- Care plans should be organized by teams including obstetricians, midwives, family practitioners, psychologists, community support groups, and medical services personnel.

The assessment of the acutely intoxicated parturient is difficult, as is obtaining consent for procedures. These women often suffer from poor diet and untreated coexisting disease.

- Co-morbidities include hepatitis, cellulitis, poor dentition, respiratory infections, untreated abscesses, and endocarditis.
- Peripheral venous access is often difficult or impossible.
- Specific pharmacological effects of the drugs used may be evident.
- Caution must be exercised when handling needles and body fluids that may be positive for hepatitis and other transmissible viruses.

Anesthesia and analgesia requirements may be altered due to opioid dependency, naltrexone use or abnormal opioid receptor density and function (opioid receptor "downregulation" from cocaine abuse). Regional analgesia for labor and postoperative regional analgesia have significant advantages.

- Despite very large doses of systemic opioids, analgesia is often unsatisfactory.
- Adverse drug reactions (or interactions) during anesthesia include sympathomimetic stimulation by cocaine or amphetamine, and a lack of effect of indirect-acting α_1-adrenergic agonists.
- Additional analgesic interventions during regional anesthesia for cesarean delivery are often required (consistent with the theory of

opioid-induced abnormal pain sensitivity or "opioid-induced hyper-algesia").

- Postoperative pain relief is often inadequate. A multimodal approach, which may include the use of gabapentinoids and keta-mine, is warranted.

Management of the Anticoagulated Pregnant Woman

The obstetric anesthesiologist is very likely to encounter women who are on antiplatelet or anticoagulant drugs. These drugs impact on peripartum and perioperative care, including anesthesia and the risk of obstetric or surgical bleeding. The normal pregnant state is prothrombotic, making thromboembolic events up to 5 times more likely during pregnancy (see Chapter 13). A number of prepregnancy and pregnancy-specific conditions merit prophylactic or therapeutic anticoagulation:

- High risk of thromboembolic disease
- Recent deep vein thrombosis and/or pulmonary embolism
- Inherited thrombophilias
- Prolonged bed rest
- Certain cardiac diseases
- Mechanical prosthetic heart valves
- Malignancy

Anticoagulant Therapy

Warfarin is often used in the postpartum period, but infrequently during pregnancy because it crosses the placenta and has adverse fetal effects. These are:

- Embryopathy (facial hypoplasia, scoliosis, short limbs and phalanges, chondral calcification) unless stopped within 6 weeks of conception (5% risk with exposure between 6–9 weeks gestation).
- Fetal hemorrhage (leading to acute or subacute central nervous system and opthalmological abnormalities) associated with expo-sure in the second or third trimesters.

Therapy with heparin is usually substituted prior to pregnancy in patients who require maintenance anticoagulation. Consequently, most pregnant women receive heparin during the antenatal and perinatal periods (Table 10.15). Management decisions should be

Table 10.15 Typical Doses of Heparin		
Drug	*Prophylaxis*	*Therapeutic*
Enoxaparin	40 mg SC daily	1 mg/ kg SC bd or 1.5 mg/kg SC daily
Dalteparin	5000 iu SC daily	100 iu/kg SC bd
Unfractionated heparin	7,500–10,000 iu SC bd	5,000–10,000 iu IV then IV infusion to maintain therapeutic range for aPTT

SC = subcutaneous. iu = international units. aPTT = activated partial thromboplastin time.

made in collaboration with obstetricians and hematologists, including regarding the optimum duration of therapy. Heparins do not cross the placenta due to their high molecular weight, and both unfractionated heparin (UFH) and low-molecular-weight heparin (LMWH) are used in different circumstances.

LMWH (e.g., enoxaparin, dalteparin) is often preferred because of greater efficacy for prophylaxis, more reliable pharmacokinetics, and reduced monitoring requirements.

- LMWH has a longer duration of action and higher patient acceptability than UFH.
- Dosing is more convenient when used for therapeutic anticoagulation; UFH must be administered intravenously, as opposed to subcutaneous administration of enoxaparin.
- LMWH is associated with a lower incidence of heparin-induced thrombocytopenia (<1%).

Unfractionated heparin (UFH) is administered IV for acute therapeutic anticoagulation (aiming for an activated partial thromboplastin time [aPTT] 2–3.5 times normal).

- To treat acute thrombus or thromboembolus, or prior to delivery in patients with a mechanical heart valve.
- Uptitration of doses may be necessary because of altered pharmacokinetics in pregnancy (placental heparinases, altered plasma protein binding, and increased renal clearance).
- Reversal of anticoagulation (with IV protamine) is easier than with LMWH.

Disadvantages of UFH include higher rates of maternal hemorrhage when used intravenously, and higher rates of heparin-induced thrombocytopenia and osteoporosis than LMWH.

Peripartum Management

Anticoagulation should be reversed fully or minimized at the time of labor and delivery to avoid severe obstetric or operative bleeding, which will also allow neuraxial block by decreasing the risk of vertebral canal hematoma.

- Warfarin needs to be stopped 4–5 days prior, until vitamin K-dependent coagulation factor concentrations are restored, and the international normalized ratio (INR) has returned to < 1.5.
- Prophylactic LMWH should be stopped at least 12 hours prior to planned regional block or anticipated labor and delivery.
- Therapeutic LMWH should be stopped at least 24 hours or more prior to planned regional block (to ensure low anti-Xa activity).
- Therapeutic anticoagulation with LMWH should be changed to shorter-acting and reversible IV UFH and this continued until approximately 4–6 hours before labor or surgery.
- Subcutaneous UFH may be stopped at least 4 hours prior to regional block or delivery (although epidural hematoma risk appears negligible with prophylactic subcutaneous UFH).

After surgical delivery or procedures, reintroduction of LMWH should be delayed for at least 4 hours and not restarted until at least 2 hours after epidural catheter removal (to avoid potential breakdown of clot and thus epidural bleeding).

- An epidural catheter should be removed if therapeutic anticoagulation is planned.
- An epidural catheter may be retained if thromboembolism prophylaxis is planned, but steps must be taken to ensure scheduled postpartum removal at a time of minimal anticoagulant activity—at least 12 hours after a prophylactic dose of LMWH.

A number of organizations such as the American College of Chest Physicians and the Obstetric Medicine Group of Australasia have produced practice guidelines for the management of venous thromboembolism, thrombophilia and antithrombotic therapy during pregnancy. The American Society of Regional Anesthesia and similar European societies have published guidelines about regional anesthesia and analgesia in patients on antiplatelet and anticoagulant drugs.

Medications other than the heparins may have significant effects on coagulation.

- Drugs with mild, reversible effects on platelet function (e.g., nonsteroidal anti-inflammatory drugs) or a mild to moderate irreversible effect (e.g., low-dose aspirin) do not alone contraindicate regional techniques or surgery.

- Herbal medications that alter platelet function (garlic, ginseng, ginkgo) also show no evidence of a significant increase in clinical bleeding risk.
- Drugs with profound effects on platelet function (e.g., clopidogrel) are rarely encountered in pregnant women but contraindicate neuraxial block for a week.
- Thrombin inhibitors and factor Xa inhibitors (e.g., fondaparinux) cross the placenta, confer an unknown risk of bleeding, and also contraindicate neuraxial techniques while active.

Further Reading

1. Burt CC, Durbridge J. Management of cardiac disease in pregnancy. *Continuing Education in Anaesthesia, Critical Care and Pain.* 2009;9:44-47.
2. Dob DP, Yentis SM. Practical management of the parturient with congenital heart disease. *Int J Obstet Anesth.* 2005;15:137-144.
3. Madden BP. Pulmonary hypertension and pregnancy. *Int J Obstet Anesth.* 2009;18:156-164.
4. Galvagno SM, Camann W. Sepsis and acute renal failure in pregnancy. *Anesth Analg.* 2009;108:572-575.
5. Wang LP, Paech MJ. Neuroanaesthesia for the pregnant woman. *Anesth Analg.* 2008;107;193-200.
6. Hebl JR, Horlocker TT, Schroeder DR. Neuraxial anesthesia and analgesia in patients with preexisting central nervous system disorders. *Anesth Analg.* 2006;103:223-228.
7. Madan R, Khoursheed M, Kukla R, et al. The anaesthetist and the antiphospholipid syndrome. *Anaesthesia.* 1997;52:72-76.
8. Choi S, Brull R. Neuraxial techniques in obstetric and non-obstetric patients with common bleeding diatheses. *Anesth Analg.* 2009;109: 648-660.
9. Ludlow J, Whybrow T, Paech MJ, et al. Drug abuse and dependency during pregnancy: anaesthetic issues. *Anaesth Intensive Care.* 2007; 35:881-893.
10. A Working Group on behalf of the Obstetric Medicine Group of Australasia. Anticoagulation in pregnancy and the puerperium *MJA.* 2001;75:258-263.
11. Horlocker TT, Wedel DJ, Rowlingson JC, et al. Regional anesthesia in the patient receiving antithrombotic or thrombolytic therapy: American Society of Regional Anesthesia and Pain Medicine evidence-based guidelines (3rd edition). *Reg Anesth Pain Med.* 2010;35:64-101.

Chapter 11

Complications of Labor and Delivery

Craig M. Palmer, MD

Introduction

Despite the best efforts and intentions of obstetricians and anesthesiologists in caring for the parturient, complications can arise which impact the management of labor and delivery, and have implications for anesthesia care. As with complications such as hemorrhage (Chapter 8), understanding the underlying pathophysiology improves our approach to anesthetic management.

Prematurity and Preterm Labor

Definitions

Preterm labor is defined as regular uterine contractions occurring at least once every 10 minutes and resulting in cervical change prior to 37 weeks gestation. A preterm infant is any infant delivered before 37 weeks of gestation.

- Any infant weighing less than 2500 grams at birth is a low birth weight (LBW) infant.
- Any infant below 1500 grams at birth is a very low birth weight (VLBW) infant, regardless of gestational age.

At 29 weeks gestation, over 90% of estimated fetal weights are below 1500 grams.

Incidence

Prematurity is the leading cause of perinatal morbidity and mortality in the United States. The high incidence of preterm delivery is one of the major reasons the U.S. ranks so low (28th in 1998) among developed nations in infant mortality.

- The overall incidence of preterm delivery in the United States was 12.7% in 2007, but there was a significant disparity between racial groups—the incidence was 11.6% in white parturients, and 18.3% in black parturients.

Neonatal Morbidity and Mortality

Perinatal mortality approaches 90% for infants born before 24 weeks gestation; by 30 weeks gestation, survival exceeds 90% (Figure 11.1). Within this 6-week time frame, even minimal delays in delivery can have a significant impact on neonatal survival.

- Between 25 and 26 weeks gestation, each day that delivery can be delayed improves survival rate by up to 5 percentage points.
- By 34 weeks gestation, neonatal survival should exceed 98%.
- Delay of delivery from a gestational age of 25 weeks to 31 weeks improves neonatal survival rate from just over 15% to almost 95%.

Neonatal mortality figures shed little light on the complications these infants suffer and subsequent impact on their lives. While advances in

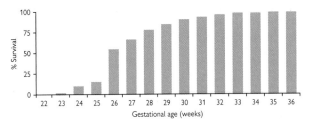

Figure 11.1 Predicted survival by gestational age derived from logistic regression equation.

neonatology have decreased mortality for very low birth weight infants, such neonates still usually encounter a stormy course following delivery (Figure 11.2).

- Very low birth weight (VLBW) infants are at risk of significant morbidity from a number of complications, including:
  - Respiratory distress syndrome (RDS). The incidence of RDS is near 90% in infants born before 27 weeks gestation, and declines almost linearly to near 0% by 36 weeks.
  - Necrotizing enterocolitis and sepsis. The incidence of both sepsis and necrotizing enterocolitis are gestational age related.
  - Intraventricular hemorrhage (IVH). The incidence of serious (Grade III and IV) IVH exceeds 30% at 26 weeks gestation, but declines rapidly to near 0% by 31 weeks.

Treatment of these problems is tremendously expensive, often requiring stays of several months in a neonatal intensive care unit setting.

- It has been estimated that for infants of 900 grams, about 26 weeks gestational age, the total cost per survivor exceeds the expected lifetime earnings per survivor.

Even beyond the immediate perinatal period, survivors are often left with neurologic abnormalities, chronic pulmonary problems, and visual disturbances (Figure 11.3). Because of this overwhelming impact on the infants, their families, and the health care system, it becomes imperative for all involved to do whatever is possible to avoid preterm delivery.

Obstetric Management

Current obstetrical practice focuses on delaying delivery in patients who develop preterm labor (PTL). The initial assessment of a patient with PTL consists of a thorough physical examination to eliminate treatable medical conditions that may have precipitated labor, and a pelvic exam to rule out premature rupture of membranes. Bed rest, intravenous hydration, continuous fetal heart rate monitoring, and tocography are almost universally indicated. Bed rest and hydration alone are effective in a substantial portion of patients. If these conservative measures are ineffective, ultrasonography is undertaken to establish gestational age; on occasion, amniocentesis will be used to assess fetal lung maturity and to rule out infection.

Once the diagnosis is established, the obstetrician must decide whether to institute pharmacologic tocolytic therapy.

- This decision is based on the estimated gestational age, fetal weight, and the presence or absence of fetal distress and infection.

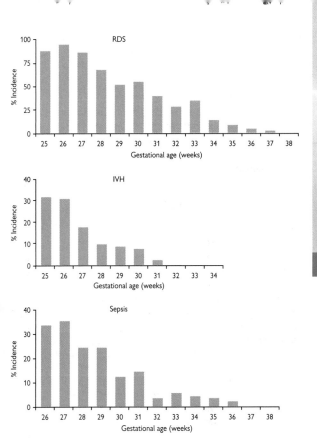

Figure 11.2 The incidence of respiratory distress syndrome (RDS), intraventricular hemorrhage (IVH), sepsis, and necrotizing enterocolitis (NEC) related to gestational age at birth. This article was published in the *American Journal of Obstetrics and Gynecology, Vol. 166*, Robertson PA et al. Neonatal morbidity according to gestational age and birth weight from five tertiary care centers in the United States, 1983–1986, pp. 1629–1645, Copyright Elsevier (1992).

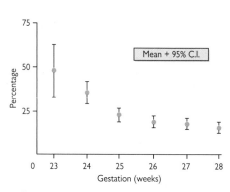

Figure 11.3 Estimated rates of major permanent disability versus gestational age at birth in preterm infants. Reprinted with permission from Wood N and Marlow N. The contribution of preterm birth to outcomes in children, pp. 1071–1086. In: Rodeck CH and Whittle MJ, *Fetal Medicine: Basic Science and Clinical Practice.* 1999, Elsevier.

- In general, a gestational age between 20 and 34 weeks, with a fetal weight less than 2500 gm and a reassuring fetal heart rate are indications for tocolytic therapy.

Physiology and Treatment of Preterm Labor

While the processes that initiate labor are incompletely understood, the physiology of uterine contraction is well understood. Like all smooth muscle, the myometrium contains myosin and actin filaments that generate the contractile force. Pacemaker cells within the myometrium are capable of initiating spontaneous contractile activity, which spreads throughout the myometrium via gap junctions between cells.

Calcium plays a critical role in uterine contractility. Prior to contraction, the intracellular calcium concentration increases, due to release of calcium from the sarcoplasmic reticulum and/or flux across the sarcolemma. Calcium interacts with calmodulin (a regulatory enzyme), which in turn activates myosin light-chain kinase (MLK). Activated MLK phosphorylates myosin, which then binds with actin. Adenosine triphosphate (ATP) is hydrolyzed by myosin ATPase, releasing the energy that causes movement of the actin-myosin elements and myometrial contraction. A reduction in intracellular calcium concentration, or dephosphorylation of myosin, inhibits the actin-myosin interaction, causing relaxation.

There are several pharmacologic avenues to inhibit preterm labor and uterine contractility (Table 11.1):

- **Adrenergic agents**. Activation of beta-2 adrenergic receptors within the myometrium activates adenyl cyclase, converting ATP to cyclic-AMP. Increased cyclic-AMP decreases intracellular calcium, inhibiting MLK and decreasing contractile activity.

- **Magnesium**. Magnesium sulfate decreases uterine activity, probably by decreasing intracellular free calcium concentration, and competitively inhibiting calcium through competition for binding sites. It may also activate adenyl cyclase, increasing synthesis of cyclic-AMP.

- **Calcium channel blockers**. By blocking voltage dependent calcium channels in the cell membrane (or altering intracellular uptake and release mechanisms), calcium channel blocking agents decrease the concentration of free calcium within the myometrium.

- **Prostaglandin synthetase inhibitors**. Prostaglandins $F_{2\alpha}$ and $E_{2\alpha}$ are potent stimulators of uterine activity. During labor, their concentration increases in maternal blood and amniotic fluid. The nonsteroidal anti-inflammatory agents that inhibit prostaglandin synthetase can inhibit the production of these prostaglandins.

Table 11.1 Pharmacological Agents for Control of Preterm Labor

Agent	Site of action	Mechanism
Magnesium sulfate	Intracellular Ca^{2+} binding sites Possibly Adenylate cyclase	Direct competition for binding sites Increases cAMP systhesis
β-agonist agents Terbutaline Ritodrine	β_2-Adrenergic receptors	Activates adenylate cyclase, increases cAMP
Calcium channel blockers	Voltage-dependent calcium channels	Decrease intracellular Ca^{2+} concentration
Nonsteroidal anti-inflammatory agents (NSAIDs)	Prostaglandin synthetase	Inhibit production of prostaglandins $F_{2\alpha}$ and $E_{2\alpha}$

Anesthetic Implications

No single agent is uniformly successful as tocolytic therapy for all patients, and each agent possesses side effects that can limit its usefulness.

- Each of the tocolytic agents currently in use has the potential for significant interactions with commonly used anesthetic agents.

- Because of the high stakes and long-term consequences involved in the care of the preterm infant, it has proven difficult to compare the efficacy of agents in randomized clinical trials.
- The degree of prematurity of the infant itself may have implications for the route of delivery (i.e., vaginal or abdominal).

Magnesium Sulfate

Magnesium is the intravenous tocolytic agent of choice in many centers, probably because of a relatively low incidence of serious side effects.

- The normal serum magnesium level ranges from 1.4 to 2.2 meq/l.
- Therapy for termination of preterm labor is initiated with an intravenous bolus of 4–6 gm, followed by a continuous infusion.
- The infusion is titrated to maintain a serum concentration of 5–8 mg/dL; while often sufficient to inhibit uterine activity, even at this concentration, magnesium is not always successful.
- Increasing the serum concentration is not usually more effective, and increases side effects.

Physiologic Effects

Magnesium causes peripheral vasodilation, and parturients often experience warmth, flushing, and nausea. Maternal tachycardia and hypotension may result, but are transient.

At higher serum concentrations, other effects are seen (Table 11.2):

- <10 meq/l: Widening of the QRS complex and prolongation of the PR interval are uncommon, but can be seen at therapeutic levels.
- 10–12 meq/l: Deep tendon reflexes are lost (deep tendon reflexes can be followed as a rough clinical measure of serum concentration).
- 15–18 meq/l: Respiratory arrest can occur.
- 25 meq/l: Cardiac arrest may occur.

Fetal effects are infrequent; decreased fetal heart rate variability has been reported, as has a reduced biophysical profile score (see Chapter 12). Respiratory depression, hyporeflexia, and decreased tone have been reported in neonates following prolonged maternal magnesium therapy.

Management of Regional Anesthesia

Due to vasodilation, hypotension tends to occur more often in these patients during regional anesthetics.

- Careful attention to maternal blood pressure allows the use of either epidural or spinal anesthesia.

Table 11.2 Clinical Effects of Magnesium Sulfate Therapy	
Serum concentration (mEq/l)	Clinical effects
1.4–2.2	Normal serum concentrations
5–8	Therapeutic concentration for inhibition of preterm labor
6–10	Widening of QRS complex and PR interval on ECG
10–12	Loss of deep tendon reflexes
15–18	Respiratory arrest; S-A and A-V block on ECG
25	Cardiac arrest

- The slower onset of epidural techniques may make them preferable to spinal anesthetics, as intravenous fluids can be titrated to maintain maternal blood pressure.

Management of General Anesthesia

Parturients receiving magnesium are more susceptible to muscle relaxants. At the neuromuscular junction, magnesium inhibits release of acetylcholine and decreases sensitivity of the postsynaptic endplate to acetylcholine. When general anesthesia is necessary in a parturient receiving magnesium, the response to any relaxant must be carefully monitored.

- Following the use of succinylcholine, the train-of-four response must be closely followed with a peripheral nerve stimulator to guide further use of relaxants.
- When necessary, further relaxants should be administered in very small doses because of their exaggerated effect.

While magnesium has been shown to decrease the MAC of halothane at therapeutic levels, this is not a clinically significant effect.

β-2 Adrenergic Agents

Both ritodrine and terbutaline (by virtue of their β-2 receptor activity) are tocolytic, but only ritodrine is FDA approved for tocolysis.

- Both are usually administered by continuous intravenous infusion, titrated in response to the uterine contraction pattern.
- Terbutaline is sometimes administered as a single intravenous or subcutaneous dose for prompt but temporary inhibition of uterine activity.

Physiologic Effects

Both ritodrine and terbutaline have significant β-1 receptor effects, accounting for the majority of their side effects.

- β-1 activity can cause vasodilation (resulting in hypotension).
- Hyperglycemia (often requiring insulin therapy) and hypokalemia are frequently seen in these patients, as is tremulousness (Table 11.3).

Direct β-1 activity increases myocardial contractility and heart rate, leading to increased cardiac output. The most significant side effects of β-agonist therapy are due to these cardiac effects.

- Pulmonary edema occurs in up to 1% of patients, and may be either cardiogenic or noncardiogenic in nature. It requires discontinuation of therapy but, fortunately, discontinuation usually leads to resolution of the pulmonary edema.
- Myocardial ischemia has also been reported, manifesting as chest pain and ECG change; this also resolves with discontinuation of therapy.

Management of Anesthesia

When anesthesia is required, a period of 60–90 minutes between discontinuation of therapy and the anesthetic is ideal; because of the short half-life of these agents, this allows their acute effects to subside. Unfortunately, a delay of this magnitude may jeopardize the fetus.

- The vasodilation accompanying β-agonist therapy can aggravate hypotension when regional techniques are used.
- Epidural anesthesia, with its slower onset, is probably preferable to spinal anesthesia.
- Intravenous fluids can be used to support maternal blood pressure, but aggressive hydration may precipitate or exacerbate pulmonary edema.

Table 11.3 Side Effects of β-agonist Therapy	
Side effect	Reported incidence (approx.)
Hypokalemia[a]	50
Hyperglycemia[a]	30
Shortness of breath or chest pain	10
"Ischemic" ECG change	5
Cardiac arrhythmias	3
Hypotension	3
Pulmonary edema	<2

[a]Transient (less than 24 hours).

- Vasopressor therapy may need to be used more aggressively to maintain maternal blood pressure; due to the likelihood of an already elevated maternal heart rate, phenylephrine is the vasopressor of choice for most patients; the fetal heart rate should be continuously monitored.

Prostaglandin Synthetase Inhibitors

Prostaglandins $E_{2\alpha}$ and $F_{2\alpha}$ are potent stimulators of uterine activity, and also cause softening of the cervix near term. Prostaglandin synthetase inhibitors (PSIs) prevent the conversion of arachidonic acid into the active prostaglandins.

- While all drugs in this class possess this capacity, only indomethacin is widely used in the treatment of preterm labor. It can be administered both orally and rectally, but fetal side effects (below) usually limit the duration of therapy. Therapy can be continued for several weeks.

Physiologic Effects

In contrast to magnesium and beta-agonists, indomethacin has few maternal side effects.

- It may affect maternal coagulation, but despite widespread use in parturients, this does not seem to be of major clinical importance. In an otherwise healthy parturient without clinical evidence of impaired hemostasis, further evaluation of maternal coagulation status is generally not indicated.

These agents may have significant fetal effects, however.

- PSIs may result in premature closure of the fetal ductus arteriosus *in utero*; this effect appears related to gestational age, and is less of a problem prior to 32 weeks' gestation.
- Indomethacin may cause decreased fetal urine excretion, leading to oligohydramnios and, rarely, neonatal renal failure.
- An increased incidence of necrotizing enterocolitis, intracranial hemorrhage, and bronchopulmonary dysplasia has been noted in neonates following *in utero* indomethacin therapy (Table 11.4).

Because of these side effects, the total recommended dose of indomethicin is 400 mg; this limitation means indomethicin therapy is usually limited to 48 hours or less.

Calcium Channel Blockers

By inhibiting transmembrane calcium flux, the calcium channel blockers reduce myometrial contractility. Nifedipine is most widely used

Table 11.4 **Reported Fetal Effects of Indomethacin Therapy for Preterm Labor**
Premature closure of fetal ductus arterious
Pulmonary hypertension
Oligohydramnios
Neonatal renal failure
Increased neonatal incidence of: • necrotizing enterocolitis • intracranial hemorrhage • bronchopulmonary dysplasia

for tocolysis. The drug has a rapid onset following sublingual administration, and therapy is maintained via the oral route.

Physiologic Effects

Maternal side effects of nifedipine therapy are generally mild.

- Nifedipine has few cardiac effects, but vasodilation and decreased blood pressure may be seen. This may be associated with a reflex tachycardia, headache, and nausea.
- It has few clinically significant fetal effects.

Management of Delivery

It is important to remember that the uterine relaxant properties of all these agents do not stop with delivery.

- Depending on the duration of therapy and the half-life of the agent, all may contribute to uterine hypotonia.
- Vigorous pharmacologic therapy may be necessary to restore uterine tone and prevent significant maternal blood loss (see Chapter 8).

Despite aggressive therapy, tocolysis often fails and labor progresses. When delivery becomes inevitable, a choice as to the best route of delivery must be made. Currently, the lower limit of viability hovers around 24 weeks gestational age.

Some obstetricians have advocated routine cesarean delivery for all infants with an estimated gestational weight below 1500 g, to reduce head trauma and subsequent intracranial hemorrhage, but there is little evidence to support this position.

- No difference has been shown in the incidence of intracranial hemorrhage in infants under 1500 g with vertex presentation and vaginal delivery, compared with cesarean delivery.

- There is no evidence to suggest that the routine use of outlet forceps provides protection against head trauma.
- In the preterm infant with breech presentation, however, there is evidence to indicate that a cesarean delivery is safer than a vaginal delivery; the advantages of surgical delivery for the infant must be weighed against the increased maternal morbidity of cesarean delivery.

When the vaginal delivery of a preterm infant is planned, epidural anesthesia has several theoretical advantages.

- It can help avoid a precipitous delivery that may increase the risk of intracranial hemorrhage.
- "Pushing" efforts by the mother before full cervical dilation must be avoided.
- A well-relaxed perineum allows for controlled delivery of the infant's head.

Each of these goals can be achieved with solid epidural blockade. Likewise, if delivery is known to be imminent, spinal anesthesia can be used to the same ends.

> It is probably most important, when planning for the delivery of a very premature infant, to ensure the presence of trained neonatal personnel for resuscitation, and ready access to a neonatal intensive care unit for subsequent care. Such neonatal expertise and facilities are responsible for lowering the gestational age of viability to the point where it stands today.

Multiple Gestation

Incidence

The incidence of multiple gestation has been increasing over the last 15 years due primarily to the proliferation of assisted reproduction technology and increased use of ovulation-inducing drugs. Currently in the United States, 3% of all pregnancies are multiple.

- Naturally, about 1 in 90 pregnancies is a twin gestation, about 1 in 9800 is triplet, and only about 1 in 70,000 are higher order gestations.
- Considerable geographic and ethnic variation exists—the rate of twin pregnancies is 50 per 1000 pregnancies in Nigeria, while only 4 per 1000 in Japan.

- Multiple gestation is more common in older parturients and those of higher parity.

Physiologic Effects

A number of physiologic changes are associated with multiple gestation, which can increase maternal risk (Table 11.5).

- Cardiac output increases more in multiple gestation than singleton pregnancies, and the increase occurs earlier in gestation.
- There is an increased incidence in anemia, due to a greater increase in blood volume but a relatively smaller increase in red cell volume.
- The size of the uterus is larger, and the increase in size occurs earlier in gestation, placing the parturient at greater risk of supine-hypotension syndrome and aortocaval compression.
- The larger size of the uterus contributes to a lower total lung capacity (TLC), a decreased functional residual capacity (FRC), and an elevated closing volume. Together with an increased metabolic rate and greater oxygen consumption, these factors contribute to an increased risk of hypoxemia during apnea (as occurs during induction of general anesthesia).
- The larger size of the uterus increases cephalad pressure on the stomach, placing parturients at greater risk of aspiration.

Table 11.5 **Maternal Consequences of Multiple Gestation (Compared with Singleton Pregnancies)**		
System	*Consequence*	*Comments*
Cardiovasular	Increased cardiac output	Occurs earlier in gestation
Hemotologic	Increased incidence of anemia	Increase in blood volume relatively greater than increase in RBC mass
Respiratory	↓ Total lung capacity ↓ Functional residual capacity ↑ Closing Volume	All increase risk of hypoxemia on induction of general anesthesia
Metabolic	↑ O_2 consumption ↑ Metabolic rate	Also increases risk of hypoxemia
Reproductive	Larger uterus	Increased incidence of aorta compression when supine Contributes to lower total lung capacity and FRC Greater risk of aspiration

Obstetric Implications

Apart from the physiologic changes, multiple gestation entails other pregnancy-related risks.

- Preterm labor complicates 40%–50% of multiple gestations. The requirement for tocolytic therapy is likewise increased, increasing the risk of tocolytic interactions with anesthetic agents noted above. The inherent risks of tocolytic therapy for the parturient, such as pulmonary edema, are also likely increased in this population. The risk of uterine atony and postpartum hemorrhage after delivery are increased by both the use of tocolytic agents and the increased distention of the uterus at term.
- Pregnancy-induced hypertension is as much as 5 times more common in multiple gestation than single gestation.
- The risk of placental abruption, placenta previa, and malpresentation are all increased with multiple gestation.

Fetal mortality is increased in multiple gestation; the risk of fetal mortality is 5–6 times higher in twin pregnancies than singleton pregnancies.

- Most of this risk is due to a greater incidence of prematurity.
- Mortality of the second twin is also increased over that of the first twin, due to intrapartum events including placental abruption, cord prolapse or entrapment, and malpresentation.

Obstetric Management

The course of obstetric management depends upon the intrauterine presentation of the fetuses. Ultrasonography is used to determine as precisely as possible their orientation.

- The route and method of delivery are also highly dependent on the expertise of the individual obstetrician attending the delivery. With triplet or higher gestations, delivery will almost always be *via* cesarean section.

Vaginal delivery is possible for most twin gestations. Several combinations of presentation are possible with twins:

- Twin A vertex/Twin B vertex (occurring in about 42% of cases)
- Twin A vertex/Twin B non-vertex (about 38%)
  - The second twin (Twin B) must be smaller than Twin A, but over 1500 g estimated fetal weight. Twin B may be delivered from either a vertex or breech presentation. Maneuvers including external cephalic version or internal podalic version may be used to turn Twin B after delivery of Twin A; delivery of Twin B may be accomplished with either partial or complete breech extraction.

- Twin A non-vertex (about 19%).
  - In the former two cases, vaginal delivery is usually feasible, while in this case, cesarean delivery is usually performed.

The time interval between deliveries is not critical, though continuous fetal heart rate monitoring of Twin B is necessary until delivery is accomplished. On occasion, surgical delivery (i.e., cesarean section) is necessary for delivery of the second twin.

Anesthetic Considerations

The anticipated vaginal delivery of a parturient with a twin gestation is a very strong indication for epidural anesthesia. Effective epidural anesthesia will facilitate any manipulations necessary, as well as provide a method of inducing surgical anesthesia if cesarean delivery becomes necessary.

- The epidural catheter should be placed as early in labor as practical, and its function assured; if any doubt as to the reliability of the catheter exists, it should be replaced.
- Due to the increased risk of postpartum hemorrhage, large bore (16-g or larger) intravenous access should be established, and blood sent for type and crossmatch.
- Because of the relatively greater size of the uterus, aortocaval compression must be carefully avoided.

Delivery should take place in an operating room where everything necessary for surgical intervention (both from an obstetric and anesthetic standpoint) is readily available. Routine monitors should be applied to the parturient. Oxygen via simple face mask may improve fetal oxygenation.

- Communication with the obstetrician is of vital importance: the obstetric plan can change quickly and dramatically depending on the course of the delivery, and anticipating obstetric interventions can save valuable moments.

During labor and through the delivery of Twin A, the nature of the epidural block should not differ greatly from epidural analgesia supplied to any other routine vaginal delivery. After delivery of Twin A however, it may be necessary to rapidly densen the block to allow obstetric manipulations as noted above. 2-chloroprocaine, 3%, is the local anesthetic of choice when rapid establishment of a surgical block is necessary. It can be used for perineal anesthesia for episiotomy or application of forceps, for internal version of Twin B, or for cesarean delivery. In cases of dire fetal distress, it may be necessary to induce general anesthesia.

For internal manipulations, uterine relaxation may be necessary.

- Intravenous nitroglycerin is an effective agent for this purpose; an initial dose of 100 ug should be used, and can be increased as necessary, up to 500 ug.
- It should rarely be necessary to use inhalational agents solely for uterine relaxation, though they are effective at high concentrations.

Following delivery, be alert for excessive bleeding due to uterine atony; aggressive therapy including methergine and prostaglandin $F_{2\alpha}$ may be necessary.

For elective cesarean delivery of multiple gestations, regional anesthesia, either epidural or spinal, is preferable to general anesthesia, in part to decrease the risk of neonatal depression. From a maternal perspective, greater weight gain associated with multiple gestation can contribute to a higher incidence of difficult intubation in these patients and, together with the propensity to rapid desaturation and increased aspiration risk, makes avoidance of general anesthesia preferable.

Abnormal Presentation

Definitions

The "presentation" of the infant refers to the most dependent (or "presenting") part of the infant. The "lie" refers to the long axis of the infant; longitudinal lies are by far the most common, but they may be either vertex (cephalic) or breech (caudal).

- Vertex presentation, with infant's head delivering first, is the most common presentation—but, depending on the flexion, extension, and rotation of the fetal head, may still constitute a malpresentation.

In normal labor, the fetal head presents with a flexed cervical spine (the fetal chin on its chest) and the fetal face turned posteriorly ("occiput anterior" or "OA"). This presentation gives the greatest chance of a successful spontaneous vaginal delivery.

Breech Presentation

Breech presentation is the most common malpresentation. It may be further classified as complete, frank, or incomplete (footling), depending on the position of the lower extremities (Figure 11.4).

At term, about 3% of singleton fetuses are in breech presentation. It has long been known that the fetus is at increased risk when vaginal delivery is attempted with breech presentation:

- The risk of fetal death is 16 times greater than vertex presentation.

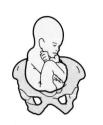 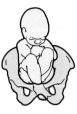 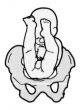

Complete breech   Incomplete breech   Frank breech

Figure 11.4 Classification of breech presentation. Reprinted with permission from Seeds JW. In: Gabbe SG, Niebyl JR, and Simpson JL, *Normal and Problem Pregnancies*. 1986, Elsevier.

- The risk of asphyxia is over 3 times greater.
- Birth trauma is 13 times more common.
- The risk of cord prolapse is increased 15 times with incomplete breech presentation, and 5 times with complete breech presentation.

Maternal risk is also increased:

- The likelihood of perineal trauma is increased.
- The risk of uterine atony and postpartum bleeding resulting from use of tocolytic agents.
- Infectious risk increases due the intrauterine manipulations that often are necessary with vaginal delivery.

This increased risk has led some to advocate cesarean delivery for all cases of breech presentation, but this does not completely eliminate fetal risk; delivery of the fetus can be difficult even at surgery. This stance also does not take into account the increased maternal morbidity of a surgical delivery.

- Regardless, at present over 90% of breech presentations in the United States are delivered by cesarean section.

Anesthetic Considerations

There are three main methods to accomplish a vaginal breech delivery.

- **Spontaneous delivery**. With a spontaneous delivery, there is no obstetric intervention or manipulation involved.
- **Partial breech extraction**. With partial breech extraction, the infant is allowed to deliver to the level of the umbilicus, and then the obstetrician assists with the delivery of the thorax and head, either manually or with Piper forceps.

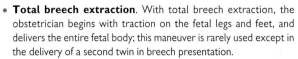

- **Total breech extraction**. With total breech extraction, the obstetrician begins with traction on the fetal legs and feet, and delivers the entire fetal body; this maneuver is rarely used except in the delivery of a second twin in breech presentation.

The attempted vaginal delivery of a breech presentation is a very strong indication for epidural anesthesia. Epidural anesthesia has several advantages:

- It provides excellent maternal pain control.
- It can inhibit the maternal urge to push until full cervical dilation is achieved.
- It provides excellent perineal relaxation to facilitate a controlled delivery.
- An in-situ epidural catheter provides a quick and effective route to rapidly increase the density of blockade to facilitate the obstetric maneuvers noted above, or to convert to anesthesia for cesarean delivery if necessary.

During labor (until full cervical dilation), standard regimens of epidural analgesia should prove adequate, unless a deeper block is necessary to inhibit maternal pushing urges.

During the actual delivery, a deeper block, such as obtained with bupivacaine 0.25%, is usually helpful.

A surgical block (as obtained with 2-chloroprocaine 3% or lidocaine 2%) is helpful for forceps-assisted deliveries, though the level of the block should not need to exceed T_8.

> As with twin deliveries, clear communication with the obstetrician is essential! Ideally, the obstetrical plan of management should be discussed beforehand.
>
> - A means of rapidly providing uterine relaxation, such as intravenous nitroglycerin, should be readily at hand.

For an elective cesarean delivery, regional techniques (either spinal or epidural) are equally efficacious.

Other Abnormal Presentations

Vertex malpresentations include **face and brow presentations**, and persistent **occiput posterior** ("OP") presentation.

Face and brow presentations result when the fetal cervical spine fails to flex with descent to the pelvic brim; in a face presentation, the cervical spine is in an extended position, and in brow presentation, it is neutral. Either of these presentations poses problems because a larger diameter is presented to the pelvic inlet.

- With a face presentation, a successful vaginal delivery is most likely if the fetus is in a mentum anterior (chin anterior) position.
- Brow presentations usually convert spontaneously during the course of labor to either a face or occiput anterior presentation.

Vaginal delivery with a persistent occiput posterior presentation can usually be expected, though the parturient may experience more discomfort than usual and have a longer labor.

Generally speaking, management of labor analgesia in these situations will be the same as for a routine occiput anterior presentation and labor.

A **transverse lie or shoulder presentation** usually mandate a cesarean delivery.

External Cephalic Version

External cephalic version (ECV) is the rotation of the fetus from breech to vertex presentation by manipulation of the uterus through the abdominal wall. When performed close to term, the maneuver is successful in 50%–80% of cases. The maneuver is attempted after 36 weeks gestation for several reasons:

- If spontaneous version to a cephalic presentation was to occur, it would likely have happened by 36 weeks.
- Risk of reversion of a successful version is lower after 36 weeks (reversion rate is as low as 2%).
- If complications arise, the infant is close enough to term to be delivered.

Complications

Complications are rare, but include placental abruption, hemorrhage, preterm labor, and even fetal demise.

Anesthetic Considerations

A tocolytic is often administered to facilitate the procedure. The use of regional anesthesia for ECV is somewhat controversial, but appears to be increasing. Epidural or spinal anesthesia certainly increases maternal comfort during the procedure, and several recent series have shown an increased success rate with no increase in morbidity when regional anesthesia is used.

- Use of anesthesia is resisted by some obstetricians who feel that maternal discomfort is an important gauge of the amount force which can be applied during the procedure.
- Reports of the successful use of epidural anesthesia for ECV have utilized extensive blockade, to the T_6 level, and the use of surgical concentrations of local anesthetics (i.e., 2% lidocaine).
- Spinal anesthesia with less extensive block (i.e., sufentanil 10 ug or bupivacaine 2.5 mg with an opioid) has also been associated with high success rates, comparable to those obtained with extensive epidural blockade. The use of a combined spinal-epidural technique for providing anesthesia probably provides the greatest flexibility, allowing epidural extension of the block if the intrathecal injection proves inadequate.
- The American College of Obstetricians and Gynecologists does not make any recommendations for or against the use of anesthesia for version.

Shoulder Dystocia

Definition

Shoulder dystocia is defined as a delivery that requires additional maneuvers beyond modest downward traction on the fetal head to effect delivery of the shoulders. In most cases, after delivery of the fetal head, the anterior shoulder becomes lodged behind the pubic symphysis.

Implications

Shoulder dystocia can result in significant morbidity and even mortality for the infant.

- If delivery is not accomplished promptly, umbilical cord compression may result in asphyxia.
- Traction on the fetal head may cause damage to the fetal brachial plexus ("Erb's palsy"); this damage can be permanent.
- Maneuvers to effect delivery may result in fractures, most often the fetal humerus.

Parturients developing shoulder dystocia are at increased risk of postpartum hemorrhage and fourth degree lacerations of the perineum.

Risk Factors

Among identified risks for shoulder dystocia are:

- macrosomia

- history of a previous macrosomic infant
- maternal obesity
- maternal diabetes
- history of a prior delivery with shoulder dystocia.

Anesthetic Management

The majority of management options for shoulder dystocia are obstetric, though prompt anesthetic involvement can be helpful. Among obstetric options are:

- Extension of episiotomy
- Suprapubic pressure to dislodge the impacted anterior shoulder
- Hyperflexion of the maternal thighs in an attempt to elevate to pubic symphysis ("McRoberts maneuver")
- Rotation of the shoulders to an oblique presentation within the maternal pelvis
- Attempted delivery of the posterior shoulder
- Replacing the fetal head in the vagina and pelvis and rescue of the infant with an abdominal cesarean delivery ("Zavanelli maneuver").

If an epidural catheter is in place, good perineal anesthesia will facilitate each of these options. Surgical anesthesia, as can be achieved with lidocaine 2% or chloroprocaine 3%, is indicated. Should it become necessary to attempt a cesarean delivery, rapid induction of anesthesia is essential. Conceivably this can be done with rapid dosing of a functional epidural catheter, but more likely induction of general anesthesia will be necessary. Attempting to position the patient for a spinal anesthetic would likely slow delivery; positioning usually proves difficult, and the fetal heart rate should be continuously monitored throughout induction.

Vaginal Birth After Cesarean Delivery (VBAC)

As the rate of cesarean delivery has climbed steadily in the last 50 years, the number of women presenting for delivery who have had a previous cesarean delivery has steadily risen also. Many of these parturients will opt for an elective repeat cesarean delivery, but a substantial number will attempt to delivery vaginally, opting for a trial of labor after cesarean delivery, or "TOLAC." Labor in these patients poses 2 distinct problems:

- The same circumstance which prevented their vaginal delivery with the previous pregnancy may reoccur.

- The uterine scar may rupture, significantly increasing maternal and fetal mortality (see also Chapter 8).

The practice of offering a "trial of labor" to parturients who have had a previous cesarean delivery (TOLAC) has been controversial over the past decade. In the mid 1980s, the American College of Obstetricians and Gynecologists (ACOG) determined that almost all parturients with a prior low-uterine-segment cesarean delivery could safely undergo a trial of labor and vaginal delivery. Subsequent reviews have indicated that even in these patients, attempting TOLAC entails a small, but significant and serious increase in morbidity and mortality for both mother and infant due to uterine rupture. This risk led ACOG to adopt the position that the procedure should be attempted only in facilities which have obstetrical, anesthesia, and nursing services "immediately available" to perform operative delivery if indicated. This resulted in TOLAC generally being offered only in larger facilities with such round-the-clock staffing. In 2010, the National Institutes of Health in the U.S. convened a consensus conference on TOLAC and VBAC rates, which urged ACOG to revisit their position, as ACOG's position has limited access to the procedure for many women who appeared at "low risk." Partially in response to this pressure, ACOG has reaffirmed its position that the "immediate availability" represents optimal practice, but if a patient is fully informed of, and accepts, the risks of a TOLAC, she should be allowed to proceed in facilities with lower staffing levels.

Anesthetic Considerations

When trial of labor after cesarean delivery procedures first began to be widely employed in the 1980s, some obstetricians believed regional anesthesia was contraindicated, fearing that epidural block would mask the pain associated with uterine rupture and delay diagnosis. However, experience has shown that pain is not the only, or even most prominent, symptom of intrapartum rupture in TOLAC patients; further, when present, the pain associated with rupture is atypical of labor and usually readily distinguished.

Several large series have indicated that not only can regional anesthesia be safely employed, it can actually increase the chance of successful vaginal delivery by allaying maternal pain and anxiety.

- In many large practices where VBAC deliveries are commonly attempted, a TOLAC is considered a strong indication *for* epidural regional analgesia.
- Prudence still dictates that the lowest concentration of local anesthetic that provides adequate analgesia should be used in these patients; combination techniques using opioids and epinephrine can allow very low concentrations (bupivacaine 0.0625% or lower, or ropivacaine 0.5%) to be used.

Amniotic Fluid Embolism

Definition

Amniotic fluid embolism (AFE) is one of the most catastrophic complications of pregnancy, labor, and delivery. The cause of AFE was originally thought to be an embolic event, the passage of amniotic fluid into the maternal circulation. For many years, the diagnosis could only be definitively made by identifying fetal squamous cells in the maternal pulmonary circulation. More recent investigations have proposed an immunologic basis for the syndrome, and at present the diagnosis is made based on presenting symptoms and clinical course, rather than specific laboratory or pathologic findings.

Risk Factors

The true incidence of AFE is unknown, but based on one of the largest reviews to date is likely between 1 in 13,000 to 20,000 pregnancies. No specific risk factors have been identified, making prediction impossible.

- It may occur intrapartum or in the immediate postpartum period.
- Maternal mortality has been reported as high as 80% in some series, but more recent reports indicate it is between 20%–30%.
- Survivors may be left with severe and permanent disability.
- Neonatal mortality is probably about 25%, with 50% of survivors suffering significant neurologic deficit.

> Reports over the last several decades appear to indicate a decrease in maternal mortality associated with AFE. It is not clear whether this change in maternal mortality represents improvement in the resuscitation and critical care of these patients or recognition that *less* catastrophic cases can occur; the decrease may also be an artifact of changing diagnostic criteria and reporting methods.

Symptoms and Presentation

Typically, the onset of symptoms is abrupt and includes a sudden dramatic drop in blood pressure and circulatory collapse, respiratory arrest, and rapid onset of hypoxia. Awake patients become unresponsive and may exhibit seizure activity. Eventually, coagulopathy is present in all cases. The diagnostic criteria for AFE are listed in Table 11.6.

Anesthetic Management

Without aggressive resuscitation, a patient suffering AFE will likely die, and even heroic efforts may be unsuccessful or have a poor outcome.

In general, management is straightforward but challenging:

- Maintain maternal blood pressure with fluids, vasopressors and inotropes if necessary.
- Maintain maternal arterial oxygen saturation. Intubation is usually necessary, especially in light of altered mental status.
- Aggressively treat alterations in coagulation.
  - All cases of AFE exhibit coagulation abnormalities, with over half developing clinical disseminated intravascular coagulation (DIC).

While randomized clinical trials have not been published (and for obvious reasons will not likely ever be performed), a number of interventions associated with successful resuscitation of AFE have been described in case reports.

- Cardiopulmonary bypass
- Extracorporeal membrane oxygenation
- Intra-aortic balloon counterpulsation
- Hemofiltration
- Plasma exchange
- Inhaled nitric oxide

Table 11.6 Diagnostic Criteria for Amniotic Fluid Embolism (AFE) (All must be present for diagnosis.)
Acute hypotension or cardiac arrest
Acute hypoxia
Coagulopathy
Onset during labor, cesarean delivery or dilation and evacuation - or - Onset within 30 min of evacuation of the uterus

Heart failure, particularly right heart failure, appears to be a common symptom in these patients, and temporary mechanical support may allow time for the myocardium to recover.

> An attribute of parturients who suffer AFE which should not be underestimated is that prior to the insult, they were young and healthy with excellent physiologic reserve. This justifies continuation of resuscitative efforts and use of extraordinary interventions when they might otherwise be abandoned as hopeless in other patient populations. Case reports have shown that good outcomes have been achieved despite otherwise dismal prognostic indicators, when extraordinary efforts have been applied.

The Febrile Parturient

Fever is not uncommon laboring or pregnant women, and can pose challenges for anesthetic management. While fever can result from a wide variety of causes, from an anesthetic standpoint infectious causes usually give rise to concern when a regional technique is planned. The reason is the theoretical risk of spreading the infection to the neuraxis, the spinal cord and meninges, during a bacteremic or viremic episode. When a general anesthetic is planned in an acutely ill, febrile patient, anesthetic concerns are the same as they would be in a nonpregnant patient.

Fever in the parturient may be viral or bacterial in origin.

Viral Causes

Among common viruses encountered during labor are:

- Herpes simplex types 1 and 2
- Hepatitis
- HIV

Herpes Simplex

- HSV1 is associated with oral lesions (cold sores) and transmission occurs through oral secretions.
- HSV2 is associated with lesions on mucous membranes or skin of the genital tract, and is spread through sexual contact.
- Generally speaking, viremia is uncommon during *recurrent* outbreaks of either type, so regional anesthesia can be safely employed.

- Primary infection is associated with a transient viremia, but such outbreaks should be uncommon during labor. The safety of regional anesthetics during primary infections has not been confirmed.

Hepatitis

- At least 5 varieties of hepatitis (A, B, C, D, E) have been identified.
- Parturients with chronic hepatitis B and C are most frequently encountered, though only acute infections will typically be febrile.
- As hepatic function may impact maternal coagulation, a platelet count and clotting studies should be checked before regional anesthesia in patients with chronic disease.
- If a parturient with acute hepatitis requires anesthesia, concerns are the same as those in a nonpregnant patient.

Human Immunodeficiency Virus (HIV)

- HIV seropositivity alone has little anesthetic implication.
- CNS infection occurs early in the infection process with HIV, so there is no validity to the concern that a neuraxial anesthetic may spread HIV to the CNS.
- If necessary, epidural blood patch can be safely performed in HIV (+) parturients.

Bacterial Causes

Fever of infectious origin in the laboring parturient is usually bacterial in origin. Common bacterial sources of fever in parturients include:

- Urinary tract infection (UTI)
- Chorioamnionitis

Urinary Tract Infection

- UTI is probably the most common bacterial infection in parturients, and asymptomatic bacteruria may occur in 10% of pregnant patients.
- Pyelonephritis is the most severe form of UTI, and requires prompt treatment with antibiotics.
- Induction of regional anesthesia in patients with UTI must take into account potential hemodynamic instability secondary to dehydration and vomiting.
- Intravenous antibiotics should be administered before regional anesthesia is induced; a single dose of antibiotics is sufficient for this purpose.

Chorioamnionitis

- Intra-amnionotic bacterial infection has been associated with post-partum uterine atony and hemorrhage.
- Neonatal complications of chorioamnionitis include neonatal sepsis, respiratory tract infections, and an increased incidence of cerebral palsy.
- Once the diagnosis is suspected, antibiotics should be administered promptly.
- As with UTI, regional anesthesia can be induced after antibiotic therapy is begun.

Summary

When abnormalities occur in the process of labor and delivery, a more aggressive anesthetic approach is necessary to ensure an optimal outcome. Familiarity with the medications associated with preterm labor is essential, as most have the potential for interaction with common anesthetic agents and techniques; the anesthesiologist must be aware of the medications the parturient may be taking, must understand these interactions, and prepare or alter the anesthetic plan accordingly. Finally, during delivery of the patient with a multiple gestation or abnormal presentation, communication with the obstetrician can be the key to ensuring a successful outcome. Anticipating what the obstetrician need to do, and knowing what is necessary in terms of anesthesia to accomplish it, can save valuable time in an urgent situation. Communication, anticipation, and understanding separate the average obstetric anesthesiologist from the excellent one.

Further Reading

1. Bottoms SF, Paul RH, Mercer BM, *et al.* Obstetric determinants of neonatal survival: antenatal predictors of neonatal survival and morbidity in extremely low birth weight infants. *Am J Obstet Gynecol.* 1999;180:665-669.
2. Childress CH, Katz VL. Nifedipine and its indications in obstetrics and gynecology. *Obstet Gynecol.* 1994;83:616-624.
3. Katz VL, Farmer RM. Controversies in tocolytic therapy. *Clin Obstet Gynecol.* 1999;42:802-819.
4. Hill WC. Risks and complications of tocolysis. *Clin Obstet Gynecol.* 1995;38:725-745.

5. Lanni SM, Seeds JW. Malpresentations. In Gabbe SG, Niebyl JR, Simpson JL, eds. *Obstetrics: Normal and Problem Pregnancies*. New York: Churchill Livingstone, 2002:473-501.

6. McIntire DD, Bloom SL, Casey BM, *et al*. Birth weight in relation to morbidity and mortality among newborn infants. *New Engl J Med*. 1999; 340:1234-1238.

7. Palmer CM. Preterm labor. In: Atlee JL (ed.): *Complications in Anesthesia*. Philadelphia, PA: W.B. Saunders, 2006:763-765.

8. Preterm birth. In Cunningham FG, Gant NF, Leveno KJ, *et al*. (eds.) *Williams Obstetrics, 21st Edition*. New York: McGraw-Hill, 2001:689-727.

9. Vaginal Birth after previous cesarean delivery. Practice Bulletin No.115. American College of Obstetricians and Gynecologists. *Obstet Gynecol*. 2010;116:450-63.

10. Van Zundert, A, Vaes, L, Soetens, M, *et al*. Are breech deliveries an indication for epidural analgesia? *Anesth Analg*. 1991;72:399-403.

11. Wilkins IA, *et al*. Efficacy and side effects of magnesium sulfate and ritodrine as tocolytic agents. *Am J Obstet Gynecol*. 1988;159:685-689.

12. Wood N, Marlow N. The contribution of preterm birth to outcomes in children. In: Rodeck CH, Whittle MJ, eds. *Fetal Medicine: Basic Science and Clinical Practice*. London: Churchill Livingstone, 1999:1071-1086.

Chapter 12

Fetal Assessment and Care

Laura S. Dean, MD
Robert D'Angelo, MD
Craig M. Palmer, MD

Introduction

Obstetric anesthesia is unique among anesthetic subspecialties in its responsibility to not one, but two patients: the parturient and the fetus. Not only must anesthetic interventions be in the best interests of the mother but they must also, as far as possible, be in the best interests of the unborn infant. Often, the "best" interests of these two patients are at odds with each other, and there is no single "best" course of action. The appropriate anesthetic interventions will depend upon the clinical circumstances, and the judgment and experience of the individual anesthesiologist.

Obstetric anesthesiologists need to be familiar with available means of fetal assessment for two reasons.

- All maternal anesthetic interventions have at least the potential to impact fetal well-being.

- In most emergent situations, anesthetic interventions are undertaken on the mother because of the fetus: understanding the role and limitations of fetal assessment is the knowledge that allows the anesthesiologist to exercise appropriate judgment.

Normal Fetal Growth and Development

- Estimated gestational age (EGA) is defined by obstetricians as the time from the first day of the last menstrual period. The actual time of fertilization is about two weeks later.
- On average, delivery occurs about 280 days from the first day of the last menstrual period, amounting to 40 weeks, or roughly 9 months. This 9-month gestation period is often divided into trimesters of 3 months each, corresponding to various obstetrical milestones.
- About one week after ovulation and fertilization (which are closely related temporally) the blastocyst implants in the uterine lining. Development of the placenta and chorionic villi begin almost immediately; once this development begins, the products of conception are termed an "embryo."

During gestation and trophoblastic invasion, the spiral arteries that supply the endometrium lose smooth muscle and the ability to constrict. Abnormal trophoblastation is integral to the pathophysiology of preeclampsia.

- By three weeks after fertilization, a true intervillous space has developed, and maternal blood supply to the placenta is established.
- Most major structures of the embryo have been formed by 8 weeks after fertilization.
- By 12 weeks EGA (10 weeks after fertilization), the uterus has enlarged enough to be palpable above the pubic symphysis.
- At midpoint of the pregnancy, 20 weeks EGA, the fetus weighs roughly 300 g.
- Over the next four weeks, weight more than doubles to over 600 g, and passes 1000 g (2.2 lbs.) by an EGA of 28 weeks. While the fetus is small, survival after delivery at this gestational age is almost 100% with skilled neonatal care. At term, 40 weeks EGA, average fetal weight is about 3400 g (Table 12.1).

Table 12.1 Fetal Developmental Milestones		
Average Fetal Weight (grams)	Estimated Gestational Age (weeks)	Characteristics
—	2	Fertilization
<1	3	Implantation
14	12	Intestines in abdomen. Eyes closed
45	14	Identifiable external genitalia
200	18	Prominent ears. Lower limbs well-developed
460	22	Lanugo (hair) visible. Vernix present
820	26	Fingernails present. Little adipose tissue
1000	28	Eyelashes present
1700	32	Toenails present. Testes descending
3400	40	Fingernails beyond fingertips. Testes in scrotum

Reprinted with permission from Cunningham FG, Macdonald PC, Gant NF, et al. The morphological and functional development of the fetus, pp. 165–207. In: *Williams Obstetrics, 19th ed.* 1993, McGraw-Hill.

Uteroplacental Physiology

The placenta is the organ of interface and communication between the mother and the fetus; through the placenta, oxygen and nutrients pass from the maternal circulation to the fetus, and carbon dioxide and waste products pass from the fetal circulation to the mother. There is no direct communication between maternal and fetal circulations. Fetal blood stays within the fetal capillaries of the chorionic villi, and maternal blood stays within the intervillous space of the placenta.

In order for a substance to pass from the maternal to the fetal circulation, it must traverse the trophoblast (cells that form the boundary between the intervillous space and the chorionic villi), the stroma of the intravillous space, and the fetal capillary wall, or endothelium. Transfer across this barrier is not strictly passive; the trophoblast can actively speed or slow the transfer of many substances, particularly those of high molecular weight.

Other important factors that impact placental transport include:

- concentration gradients
- the degree of protein binding
- the rate of both maternal and fetal blood flow
- total surface area of the placenta

Molecules with a molecular weight under 500 d move primarily by simple diffusion; this is the mechanism for transport of oxygen, carbon dioxide, water, and electrolytes. Anesthetic gases, being relatively small molecules, also traverse the placenta via passive diffusion. The rate of oxygen transfer across the placenta is limited by maternal and fetal blood flow. The placenta supplies approximately 8 ml/min/kg fetal body weight of oxygen to the developing fetus. Because of mixing of blood within the intervillous space, oxygen saturation of maternal blood in the intervillous space is lower than maternal arterial oxygen saturation (about 70%) with a PO_2 of 30 to 35 mmHg. Oxygen saturation of fetal blood in the umbilical vein is about the same, but the PO_2 is lower (Table 12.2).

Despite this low PO_2, the fetus has several adaptations allowing it to grow and thrive *in utero*. These factors increase oxygen delivery at the tissue level:

- Higher cardiac output per body weight than adults
- Increased oxygen affinity of fetal hemoglobin
- Higher hemoglobin concentration than adults

Table 12.2 Oxygen, Carbon Dioxide, and pH Values in Maternal and Fetal Blood

Variable	Uterine		Umbilical	
	Artery	Vein	Artery	Vein
PO_2 (mmHg)	95	40	15	27
SaO_2 (% Saturation)	98	76	30	68
O_2 Content (ml/dl)	15.8	12.2	6.4	14.5
Hemoglobin (g/dl)	12.0	12.0	16.0	16.0
O_2 Capacity (ml O_2/dl)	16.1	16.1	21.4	21.4
PCO_2 (mmHg)	32	40	48	43
CO_2 Content (mM/L)	19.6	21.8	26.3	25.2
HCO_3 (mM/L)	18.8	20.7	25.0	24.0
pH	7.40	7.34	7.35	7.38

Based on Cunningham FG, MacDonald PC, Gant NF, et al. (eds.) The morphological and functional development of the fetus. In: *Williams Obstetrics, 19th ed.*, Norwalk,CT: Appleton & Lange, 1993:165–207.

Carbon dioxide transfer is by simple passive diffusion. Carbon dioxide crosses the placenta faster and more readily than oxygen. The pCO_2 in fetal blood returning to the placenta via the umbilical arteries is slightly higher than maternal venous pCO_2, which facilitates diffusion, as does the mild maternal hyperventilation and resulting respiratory alkalosis in the third trimester.

Fetal Circulation

The fetal circulation is highly adapted to this metabolic environment (Figure 12.1). Oxygenated fetal blood returns from the placenta via the umbilical vein; the umbilical vein enters the abdomen and follows the abdominal wall to the liver, where it divides. The smaller division carries blood to the portal sinus and hepatic veins, while the major division joins the inferior vena cava (IVC). In the inferior vena cava, the oxygenated placental blood mixes with deoxygenated blood returning to the heart from the lower half of the fetal body. While mixing results in a lower PO_2, the oxygen content of blood returning to the fetal heart from the IVC is still considerably higher than that returning from the superior vena cava (SVC).

Upon entering the heart, blood from the IVC is shunted primarily through the foramen ovale; this has the effect of delivering the better-oxygenated blood to the left ventricle, and thence to the heart and brain. Blood from the SVC enters the right ventricle and pulmonary artery, before being shunted via the ductus arteriosus to the descending aorta. A portion of this blood flows through the umbilical arteries to return to the placenta.

This pattern of shunts allows the fetal ventricles to pump in series while *in utero*, rather than in parallel as in adults. This series arrangement contributes to a higher cardiac output per weight (as much as 3 times that of an adult at rest), and helps compensate for the lower O_2 content of fetal blood.

Prepartum Fetal Assessment

The primary goal of intrauterine fetal surveillance is to prevent fetal demise, or stillbirth, and to decrease neonatal morbidity. An ideal prepartum test would be:
- quick and simple to perform
- inexpensive

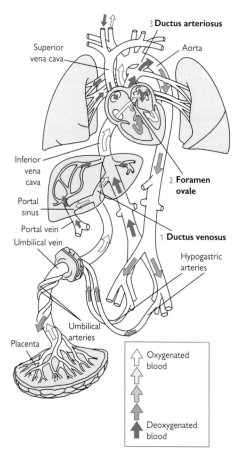

Figure 12.1 Fetal circulation. See text for complete explanation. Well-oxygenated blood returning from the placenta is selectively shunted to the heart and brain via the ascending aorta. The three major shunts of the fetal circulation are the ductus venosus (1), the foramen ovale (2) and the ductus arteriosus (3). After: The morphological and functional development of the fetus. Reprinted with permission from Cunningham FG, Macdonald PC, Gant NF, et al. *Williams Obstetrics,* 19th ed, pp. 165–207. 1993, McGraw-Hill.

- accurate
- able to produce objective results

There is no single test that meets these criteria. However, a number of prepartum tests are used by obstetricians, often in selected populations, to improve the outcome of pregnancy. The results of these tests may have implications for the anesthesiologist in the timing and urgency of delivery, and are reviewed below.

Fetal Movement

Quantification of fetal activity perceived by the mother was one of the earliest prepartum fetal assessment tests devised. It has the advantage of being simple and cheap to perform, and can therefore be applied to large numbers of patients. The underlying premise is that fetal movement is decreased by hypoxia. Fetal movements decrease significantly during uterine contractions that are associated with decreases in fetal heart rate. In contrast, fetal activity remains normal if not associated with significant fetal heart rate changes during uterine contractions.

- In the simplest form of fetal activity monitoring, the mother is instructed to count the number of times she feels the fetus kick, turn, or otherwise move during a set time period.
- The average time it takes to feel 10 fetal movements in the third trimester is about 18 minutes; a one-hour time period for 10 movements is greater than 3 standard deviations beyond the mean.
- To perform the test, the mother records the amount of time it takes for her to feel 10 movements; if she fails to feel 10 movements within one hour, further fetal evaluation is indicated.

Contraction Stress Test

Contraction stress testing combines the use of continuous fetal heart rate and uterine contraction monitoring; it was a direct outgrowth of the use of intrapartum fetal heart monitoring, which linked fetal hypoxia and asphyxia with certain fetal heart rate patterns, particularly late decelerations.

- Uterine contractions can be induced in the nonlaboring patient during the third trimester by either nipple stimulation or intravenous oxytocin administration.
- A satisfactory test requires three contractions within 10 minutes while the fetal heart rate is continuously recorded.
- In a confusing twist of terminology, a negative test is reassuring, with no decelerations associated with contractions; a positive test

indicates the presence of decelerations and the need for further evaluation.

- Disadvantages of the test include the time, effort, and equipment necessary; further, it is contraindicated in conditions such as placenta previa and premature rupture of membranes, where labor must be avoided.

Nonstress Test

The nonstress test was derived from the contraction stress test when it was observed that contraction stress tests were rarely abnormal as long as fetal heart rate accelerations were associated with fetal movement.

- This simplifies the test and eliminates the need for uterine contractions.
- The fetal heart rate (and usually uterine activity) is monitored for 20 to 40 minutes, while the mother simultaneously notes fetal movement.
- A normal, or reactive, test exhibits a normal baseline fetal heart rate, adequate variability, and at least two fetal heart rate accelerations of 15 beats per minute or more, lasting 15 seconds and associated with fetal movement.

Due to its simplicity, the nonstress test is currently the mainstay of prepartum fetal surveillance and is typically performed twice weekly when indicated for ongoing evaluation.

Maternal and fetal indications for nonstress testing include:

- Diabetes mellitus
- Collagen vascular disorders
- Chronic disease
- Intrauterine growth retardation
- Multiple gestation
- Decreased fetal movement

Ultrasonography

The widespread availability and accuracy of ultrasonography has made it an essential tool in the prepartum and intrapartum evaluation of fetal well-being.

- Among the most valuable information which ultrasonography can provide is an estimate of gestational age.
- Particularly in the late first and early second trimesters, fetal measurements obtained with ultrasound are the most accurate means available of determining gestational age.

- Accurate dating is especially useful for determining options when pregnancy is threatened before fetal viability, or when viability is marginal.
- Ultrasonography is also highly useful in identifying fetal anomalies. As with accurate dating, identification of lethal fetal anomalies permits rational choices to be made regarding route of delivery. Identification of serious but nonlethal anomalies prior to delivery allows planning for appropriate postpartum care of the neonate, to optimize outcome; on occasion, such anomalies may be amenable to improvement with *in utero* therapy.

Biophysical Profile

The biophysical profile utilizes ultrasonography to measure several parameters, in conjunction with a nonstress test, to provide an assessment of the fetus's overall development and well-being. Five elements are assessed for the biophysical profile (Table 12.3); each is assigned a score of either 0 or 2.

- A score of 8 to 10 is generally associated with a favorable outcome (Table 12.4)
- A score of 0 to 6 indicates a high perinatal mortality rate that usually requires intervention.

The amniotic fluid volume tends to receive greater weight in determining a course of action with intermediate values (Table 12.4). Testing is usually performed at 34 to 36 weeks gestation, but may be performed as early as 28 weeks.

Table 12.3 Elements of Biophysical Profile

Variable	Description	Score*
Nonstress Test	Reactive test	2
Fetal Breathing Movements	At least one episode of breathing of 60 s duration	2
Gross Fetal Body Movements	At least three episodes	2
Fetal Tone	At least one episode of extension and return to flexion of extremities or spine	2
Amniotic Fluid Volume	At least one fluid pocket of at least 1cm in depth	2

*10 total points available.

Table 12.4 Interpretation and Management of Biophysical Profile Score

BPP Score	Perinatal Mortality*	Management
10	<1/1000	Routine
8: Normal Amniotic Fluid	1/1000	Routine
8: Low Amniotic Fluid	89/1000	If functioning renal tissue and intact membranes, deliver for fetal indications
6: Normal Amniotic Fluid	Variable	Deliver mature fetus, repeat test in 24 hrs for immaturity
6: Low Amniotic Fluid	89/1000	Deliver for fetal indications
4	91/1000	Deliver for fetal indications
2	125/1000	Deliver for fetal indications
0	600/1000	Deliver for fetal indications

*Perinatal mortality within 1week without intervention.

This article was published in the *American Journal of Obstetrics and Gynecology*, Vol. 157, Manning FA, Morrison I, Harman CR, *et al.* Fetal Assessment based on fetal biophysical profile scoring: Experience in 19,221 referred high-risk pregnancies, p. 880, Copyright Elsevier (1987).

Intrapartum Fetal Heart Monitoring

To understand the fetal response to labor, it is necessary to understand the hemodynamics of uteroplacental blood flow. Uterine perfusion pressure (UPP) is approximated as mean maternal uterine arterial pressure minus mean uterine venous pressure; the maternal mean arterial pressure minus the maternal central venous pressure is a slightly higher approximation. In a healthy parturient, UPP is approximately 60 mmHg, which is slightly lower than predicted due to the vascular resistance of intraplacental vessels (Figure 12.2). During a normal uterine contraction, intrauterine pressure can easily exceed 60 mmHg. As the pressure increases during a contraction, first the uterine venous pressure will be exceeded, which constricts uterine outflow, and eventually uterine arterial pressure will be exceeded, preventing perfusion.

The fetal circulation through the placenta continues throughout the contraction; therefore, at the peak of most contractions, there is a period where uterine blood flow is essentially cut off, and no

$$UPP = (M.M.U.A.P - M.M.U.V.P.)$$
$$\approx 70 \text{ mmHg} - 10 \text{ mmHg}$$
$$\approx 60 \text{ mmHg}$$

UPP – Uterine Perfusion Pressure
MMUAP – Mean Maternal Uterine Arterial Pressure
MMUVP – Mean Maternal Uterine Venous Pressure

Figure 12.2 Calculation of Uterine Perfusion Pressure.

exchange occurs. The analogy can be made that the fetus is required to "hold its breath" for a few moments every few minutes during labor. A healthy term fetus has sufficient metabolic reserve to tolerate this stress without problems.

Monitoring the fetal heart rate (FHR) is the primary means of assessing fetal status during labor, specifically the response of the fetus to the added stress of uterine contractions. While ultimately interpretation of the fetal heart trace is the responsibility of the obstetrician, it is important that the anesthesiologist be familiar with the basics of FHR monitoring, as he or she is often the first physician in the position to identify potentially ominous signs and take corrective action.

Elements of the FHR to be considered in interpretation include:

• baseline fetal heart rate
• variability of the FHR
• presence or absence of decelerations and accelerations

Baseline FHR

The normal baseline FHR is between 110 and 160 beats per minute (bpm). Fetal tachycardia is a persistent FHR above 160 bpm and does not usually require urgent intervention, as long as variability is maintained.

Fetal tachycardia can be the result of:

• Maternal fever or infection (particularly chorioamnionitis).
• Medications administered to the mother can also cause fetal tachycardia—atropine and beta-sympathomimetics (terbutaline or ritodrine, often used for tocolysis).

Fetal bradycardia is defined as a FHR below 110 bpm. In contrast to adults, cardiac output of the fetus is highly rate dependent; the fetus has a very limited ability to compensate for decreased heart rates by increasing stroke volume.

- At a FHR below 90 bpm, cardiac output falls, resulting in the shunting of blood to the brain, heart, and vital organs; other tissue will become progressively anaerobic, and PO_2 and pH will decrease.
- While a healthy fetus can probably tolerate a heart rate of 90 to 100 bpm for a prolonged period due to metabolic reserve, a stressed infant will experience progressive hypoxemia unless the heart rate is increased.
- Due to the episodic interruptions of uterine blood flow during labor described above, even a healthy infant cannot tolerate such a low heart rate during active labor.

Bradycardia may be associated with:

- Some congenital heart lesions.
- Maternal medications (beta-blockers and high levels of local anesthetics).
- More significantly, fetal bradycardia is often a response to a hypoxic insult.

Variability

Variability in the FHR refers to the minute fluctuations between the R-waves of the fetal ECG. The SA node sets the intrinsic FHR; in the absence of any other influences, the R–R interval would be constant, and the FHR trace would appear as a straight, flat line. A constantly changing balance of autonomic influences affect the SA node, however, with the result that that the R–R interval is constantly changing slightly. This results in the jagged, "sawtooth" pattern seen in normal FHR monitor strips (Figure 12.3). Normal variability is defined as fluctuation of 6–10 bpm. The presence of variability in the FHR is taken as evidence of an intact, functional neuraxis: appropriate CNS traffic between aortic arch and carotid chemoreceptors and baroreceptors, through the cerebral cortex and brainstem, and out through the vagus nerve and cardiac sympathetics. Diminished or absent variability is taken as a sign of CNS hypoxia.

Decelerations

Decelerations are periodic FHR changes that occur in response to fetal insults, and may be related to the uterine contraction pattern. They are defined as *early, variable,* and *late.*

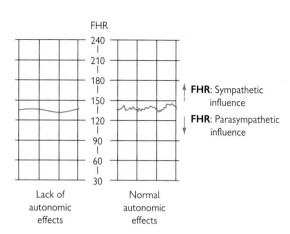

Figure 12.3 Autonomic influences and the fetal heart rate. Sympathetic influences tend to increase the baseline heart rate, while parasympathetic influences tend to decrease it. Reprinted with permission from Huddleston JF, Management of acute fetal distress in the intrapartum period. *Clin Obstet Gynecol.* 1984;27(1):84–94.

Early Decelerations

Early decelerations are considered to be a vagal response to fetal head compression during contractions. They begin with the onset of the contraction, with a gradual decrease in the FHR and a gradual return to baseline before the end of the contraction; they are sometimes said to "mirror" the contraction (Figure 12.4). They are generally considered benign.

Variable Decelerations

Variable decelerations are considered to be a vagal reflex to umbilical cord compression. Their temporal relation to uterine contractions is appropriately "variable." They are characterized by an abrupt onset and abrupt return to baseline, and are irregular in shape (Figure 12.5).

• They are considered "severe" when the FHR drops 60 or more bpm below baseline for 60 seconds or more.
• If repetitive and severe, variable decelerations may lead to progressive fetal acidosis, and efforts to eliminate them should be undertaken.

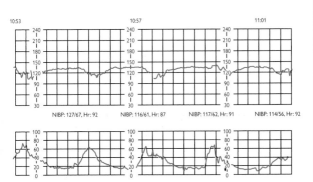

Figure 12.4 Early decelerations. Early decelerations in a 23-year-old parturient in early labor. The decelerations tend to "mirror" the uterine contraction pattern, and the FHR returns to baseline before the end on the contraction. (Note: The uterine contraction pressure scale is not accurate.)

Late Decelerations

Late decelerations are considered ominous, because they are assumed to indicate uteroplacental insufficiency. As noted above, uterine blood flow ceases at the peak of normal uterine contractions; this leads to a brief period during each contraction when oxygen exchange is markedly reduced and fetal PO_2 falls slightly (Figure 12.6). A healthy

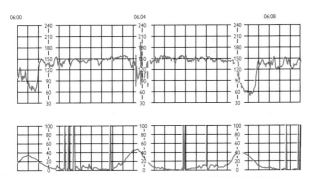

Figure 12.5 Variable decelerations. Severe variable decelerations in a 30 year old parturient in active labor. The decelerations begin after the start of the uterine contraction, and the fetal heart rate has returned to baseline before the end of the contraction. (Note that FHR variability is well maintained between the decelerations.)

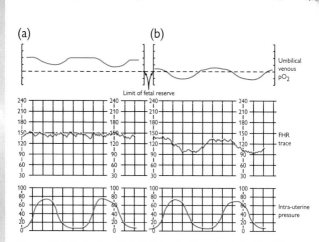

Figure 12.6 Mechanism of late FHR decelerations. As uterine blood flow decreases during a uterine contraction, placental oxygen exchange is briefly disrupted, resulting in a transient drop in fetal pO₂. A healthy fetus has sufficient reserve to tolerate this brief interruption, but in a stressed fetus, the fetal pO₂ drops below a critical level causing a vagally-mediated decrease in fetal heart rate. Reprinted with permission from Huddleston JF, Management of acute fetal distress in the intrapartum period. *Clin Obstet Gynecol.* 1984;27(1):84–94.

fetus has sufficient reserve to tolerate this brief interruption, but a stressed fetus may not be able to tolerate even these brief interruptions in oxygen supply. The result is that blood is shunted to the brain and heart, and away from peripheral tissues. This activates a vagal reflex due to transient fetal hypertension, activating baroreceptors of the aortic arch and carotids.

- Late decelerations are characterized by a smooth decrease in FHR from baseline after the start of the contraction, and a smooth return to baseline after the end of the contraction (Figure 12.7).
- If repetitive, late decelerations can lead to progressive fetal acidosis and deterioration. Aggressive efforts to eliminate the decelerations or to deliver the fetus should be made.
- Late decelerations with absent variability are a particularly ominous sign, indicating severe fetal hypoxemia; every effort should be made to deliver the infant as quickly as possible.

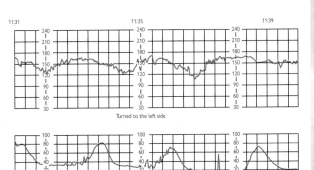

Figure 12.7 Late decelerations. Repetitive late decelerations in a 31-year-old parturient in active labor. The decelerations in the FHR lag behind the uterine contraction pattern: the drop in FHR begins after the start of the contraction, and persists after the contraction has resolved. (Note: The uterine contraction pressure scale is not accurate.)

In Utero Resuscitation

In utero resuscitation, or fetal resuscitation, is the first intervention that should be attempted when fetal compromise or distress is suspected. It may prevent the need for urgent intervention and delivery, or at least may improve fetal status during the period before delivery can be effected. *In utero* resuscitation consists of several distinct interventions that should all be applied at the same time, as it is rarely possible to determine exactly which step will alleviate the fetal insult.

Interventions

Position Change

The rationale for maternal position change is to eliminate aortocaval compression that may be impeding uterine blood flow.

- Avoidance of supine positioning, and use of the left uterine displacement position should be routine during all phases of labor, but the mass of the gravid uterus may still impinge on the abdominal aorta in certain situations in some patients. This can restrict uterine blood flow to the placenta.
- The "supine-hypotension syndrome" results from similar compression of the abdominal vena cava; in this instance, however, the

decrease in venous return because of caval compression results in maternal hypotension.

- With either situation, the mother should be turned to the full lateral position, either left or right; if one side does not relieve the problem, the other should be tried.

- In extreme situations, the mother should be placed in the "knee-chest" position, i.e., turned prone and positioned with her knees and upper chest or anterior shoulders on the bed. This tends to move the fetus's weight cephalad, and can decrease umbilical cord compression or fetal head compression at the pelvic brim.

Oxygen Administration

Despite large increases in maternal PO_2 with increasing FiO_2, maternal blood oxygen content does not increase significantly, because even on room air ($FiO_2 = 0.21$) maternal hemoglobin is nearly saturated with oxygen.

- Fetal hemoglobin has a different affinity for oxygen, however, and available evidence indicates that fetal PO_2 and oxygen saturation increase significantly with increases in maternal FiO_2.

- If fetal oxygen delivery decreases for any reason (decreased uterine blood flow, increased uterine tone, or umbilical cord compression), increasing fetal blood oxygen content may improve fetal status (Table 12.5).

- Unfortunately, it is not usually possible to increase maternal FiO_2 to 1.0 in the standard labor suite (though this can be accomplished with an anesthesia machine). Administering oxygen via simple face-mask at high flows (15 l/min or more) can significantly increase

Table 12.5 Relation between Maternal FiO$_2$ and Umbilical Artery and Vein Oxygen Gradient		
Maternal FiO$_2$	Umbilical venous blood oxygen content*	Umbilical arterial blood oxygen content*
0.21	13.2 +/− 0.5	5.3 +/− 0.6
0.47	15.9 +/− 0.8	7.9 +/− 0.4
1.0	17.7 +/− 0.1	11.8 +/− 0.8

*In: ml O$_2$/100 ml blood

Reprinted with permission from Ramanathan S, Gandhi S, Arismandy J, et al. Oxygen transfer from mother to fetus during cesarean section under epidural anesthesia. Anesth Analg. 1982;61:576–581.

maternal FiO_2, and it is reasonable to assume a corresponding improvement in fetal blood oxygen content.

Blood Pressure Support

Since decreases in maternal blood pressure can clearly result in decreases in uterine blood flow, increasing maternal blood pressure may improve uterine and placental perfusion.

- Except in those unusual circumstances where maternal blood pressure is known to be excessive (as in severe preeclampsia), empirically increasing maternal blood pressure in the face of fetal compromise is indicated.

- The most rapid means of elevating maternal blood pressure is with intravenous phenylephrine 40–80 mcg (alternatively, ephedrine 5–10 mg); this should be accompanied by vigorous intravenous fluid administration, with nonglucose containing fluids (normal saline, lactated Ringer's solution, or Plasmalyte®).

- Closely monitor blood pressure response during and following interventions.

Decreasing Uterine Tone

Since the cause of the decelerations is the uterine contractions, one of the first steps to take is to stop the contractions. If the contractions can be stopped, or at least slowed, the fetus may have a chance to recover and the urgency or need for delivery may be avoided. A very rapid contraction pattern may not allow a fetus sufficient time between contractions to recover from the episodic decrease in oxygen delivery.

- If contractions are augmented with the pitocin, the infusion should be reduced or stopped when there is evidence of fetal compromise.

- The most widely used method of decreasing uterine tone or stopping uterine contractions is probably terbutaline, either subcutaneous or intravenous, 0.25 mg.

- Nitroglycerin, either intravenous or sublingual, is another agent that has proven effective for rapidly producing uterine relaxation.

- Intravenous nitroglycerin should be administered beginning at a dose of 50 mcg: the dose can be escalated upwards to as high as 500 mcg until the desired relaxant effect is seen. Intravenous nitroglycerin has a rapid speed of onset (30–45 sec) and a short duration of action (1–2 min), so it should be viewed as a temporizing measure.

- Sublingual nitroglycerin, either tablets or spray, has also been shown to be effective. Careful maternal blood pressure monitoring is necessary, as both terbutaline and nitroglycerin can cause significant decreases in maternal blood pressure.

Further Reading

1. American College of Obstetricians and Gynecologists. Fetal heart rate patterns: monitoring, interpretation, and management. *ACOG Technical Bulletin No. 207*;1995.

2. Evertson LR, Gauthier RJ, Schifrin BS, et al. Antepartum fetal heart rate testing: I. Evolution of the nonstress test. *Am J Obstet Gynecol.* 1979; 133:29-33.

3. Longo LD. Respiration in the fetal-placental unit. In Cowett RM, ed. *Principles of Perinatal-Neonatal Metabolism*. New York: Springer-Verlag, 1991:304-315.

4. Manning FA, Morrison I, Harman CR, et al. Fetal assessment based on fetal biophysical profile scoring: experience in 19,221 referred high-risk pregnancies. *Am J Obstet Gynecol.* 1987;157:880-884.

5. Moore KL. *The Developing Human: Clinically Oriented Embryology, 4th Ed.* Philadelphia, PA: WB Saunders, 1988.

6. Moore TR, Piacquadio K. A prospective evaluation of fetal movement screening to reduce the incidence of antepartum fetal death. *Am J Obstet Gynecol.* 1990;162:1168-1173.

7. Parer JT. (1999) Fetal heart rate. In Creasy RK, Resnik R, eds. *Maternal-Fetal Medicine, 4th ed.* Philadelphia, PA: WB Saunders, 1999:270-299.

8. Platt LD, Paul RH, Phelan J, et al. Fifteen years experience with antepartum fetal testing. *Am J Obstet Gynecol.* 1987;156:1509-1515.

9. Ramanathan S, Gandhi S, Arismandy J, et al. Oxygen transfer from mother to fetus during cesarean section under epidural anesthesia. *Anesth Analg.* 1982;61:576-581.

10. Vintzileos AM, Dnuppel RA. Multiple parameter biophysical testing in the prediction of fetal acid-base status. *Clin Perinatol.* 1994;21:823-848.

Chapter 13

Management of Later Complications of Obstetric Anesthesia and Analgesia

Michael J. Paech, FANZCA

Post-Dural Puncture Headache

Incidence and Risks of Post-Dural Puncture Headache

Post-dural puncture headache (PDPH) (also termed post-spinal headache) is the most common major complication of neuraxial block in the obstetric population. It leads to substantial health care costs, mainly as a result of delayed hospital discharge. The incidence after spinal techniques, which are widely used for elective cesarean delivery and in many units also for labor analgesia, is largely determined by the selection of spinal needle. Meta-analysis shows that the incidence falls with the use of:

- Needles of smaller gauge.
- Needles of non-cutting bevel design (i.e., pencil point, Whitacre, Sprotte or other "atraumatic" needle tip; see Figure 3.5).

Choice of Spinal Needle and Insertion Technique

The incidence of PDPH associated with specific needles is shown in Table 13.1. In practice, a more rigid 24 or 25 gauge Sprotte needle or a long Gertie-Marx needle is useful and the author routinely uses a 27 gauge pencil-point style needle, which:

- Provides tactile sensation of dural puncture (the "dural pop" from tenting the posterior dural surface anteriorly) in approximately 80% of cases.
- Allows rapid efflux of cerebrospinal fluid (CSF) into the needle hub.
- Is associated with a PDPH rate of approximately 1 in 200.

The spinal needle is introduced through a short (approximately 3 cm) introducer needle placed into the interspinous ligament. When performing a combined spinal-epidural technique, or having difficulty, a spinal needle can be placed through a correctly located epidural needle.

Risks for Unintentional Dural Puncture

The incidence of unintentional dural puncture with an epidural needle (a "dural tap") depends on the experience of the operator (with fatigue a possible additional factor). In teaching units the incidence varies widely (<0.5%–4%) but headache follows in 40%–80% of cases, possibly varying with gauge and type of epidural needle. Patient factors determining PDPH are also undetermined.

- Morbidly obese women appear more likely to suffer "dural tap" but less likely to experience PDPH.
- Women with a history of headache may be at greater risk.

Diagnosis

The key diagnostic features of PDPH are described in Table 13.2, and the differential diagnosis in Table 13.3. Post-dural puncture headache

Table 13.1 The Incidence of Post-Dural Puncture Headache Associated with Specific Spinal Needles	
22 G Quincke	30%–40%
22 G Sprotte	10%
24 G Sprotte	2%
25 G Quincke	5%–10%
25 G Whitacre	3%–8%
27 G Quincke	2%–4%
27 G Whitacre	0.5%–1%
29/30 G Quincke	<0.5%

G = gauge.

is a clinical diagnosis, based on criteria such as those suggested by the International Headache Society, namely a headache that is:

- Postural in nature.
- Of onset within 5 days of a dural puncture (usually within 48 hours and often much earlier after a "dural tap").
- Associated with at least one other symptom, such as neck stiffness, tinnitus, hyperacusia, photophobia, or nausea.

Laboratory tests and conventional imaging are of little diagnostic value, although meningeal enhancement seen on computed tomography (CT) scan when investigating possible low CSF pressure headache is suggestive. In approximately 30% of apparent PDPH there has been no difficulty with epidural needle or catheter placement, or no CSF leak noted at the time of the procedure.

- The key diagnostic element is the postural nature of the headache or neck pain, with improvement or resolution when supine and onset or exacerbation when erect or ambulant, within hours to days of a spinal or epidural technique.

Table 13.2 Key Diagnostic Features of Post-Dural Puncture Headache

Postural influence – headache worse when erect and usually markedly or completely diminished when fully recumbent
Variable intensity and nature – depending on the type of needle used and the patient response
Often bi-temporal or occipital in location and sometimes confined completely to the posterior neck
Onset within 48 hours in 90% of cases
Without treatment, symptoms gradually improve – 70% resolve within one week and 95% within 6 weeks if PDPH is due to a spinal needle – 70% persist at one week and 10% at one month if PDPH is due to an epidural needle
Headache sometimes accompanied by other symptoms – nausea and vomiting, dizziness, photophobia or visual disturbance, tinnitus or auditory disturbance
Rarely associated with cranial nerve palsies – most commonly the abducens (6th cranial) nerve but also oculomotor, trochlear, facial and vestibulocochlear nerves
Very rarely associated with potentially life threatening complications – spinal abscess, meningitis, seizure, subdural hematoma, intracranial hemorrhage and cerebellar tonsillar herniation

PDPH = post-dural puncture headache.

Table 13.3 Differential Diagnosis of Post-Dural Puncture Headache
Preeclampsia
Tension or migraine headache
Cervicogenic and musculoskeletal neck and occipital pain
Sinus headache
Caffeine or amphetamine withdrawal
Intracranial tumor
Pituitary hemorrhage
Cerebral vein thrombosis
Cerebral or subarachnoid hemorrhage
Subdural hematoma
Meningitis

More common causes are listed first. The etiology of early postpartum headache, which has an incidence of 30%–40%, is frequently multifactorial.

Importantly, if atypical features are present, or a headache recurs after effective therapy, careful consideration of alternative diagnoses is essential, and thorough neurological assessment and imaging may be warranted.

Prevention of PDPH

PDPH Associated with Spinal Techniques

To prevent PDPH when using a spinal needle:

- Use the smallest practical spinal needle with an atraumatic tip.
- If the only available needle is a sharp-bevel/cutting-edge (Quincke) needle, the bevel should be directed parallel rather than perpendicular to the longitudinal (cephalad-caudad) orientation of the dura and arachnoid. The stylet should be replaced prior to withdrawing the spinal needle.

Avoiding "bearing down" or "pushing" at the time of delivery, bed rest and pharmacological therapies such as oral caffeine are not preventative.

PDPH Associated with Epidural Techniques

There is little evidence for strategies to avoid unintentional "dural tap" (and subsequent PDPH) when inserting an epidural needle. It appears that:

- Loss-of-resistance to saline is preferable to loss-of-resistance to air, as immediate or early onset headache occurs from subarachnoid air entering the cranium.

- Directing the epidural needle tip laterally rather than cephalad reduces the risk of dural puncture (but is associated with a higher failure rate, so is not recommended).
- The greater the depth to the epidural space the higher the risk (but underweight women are at risk because the epidural space may lie within 2.5–3 cm of the skin). Use of ultrasound may assist determination of the correct depth of needle insertion.
- Needle design and size (17 or 18 gauge versus 16 gauge) is probably relevant, with less severe headaches associated with smaller epidural needles.
- Rotation of the needle after identification of the epidural space should be avoided.

After "dural tap" suggested strategies to reduce either the incidence or severity of PDPH that have *not* been confirmed by large randomized trials, are:

- Intrathecal placement of the epidural catheter (PDPH onset is usually delayed until after removal of the catheter).
- Injection of subarachnoid saline 10 ml (immediately or later at the time of catheter removal).
- Injection or infusion of epidural saline through a re-inserted epidural catheter (30–60 ml intermittent boluses several hours apart, or an infusion at 30–60 ml/h).
- Repeated doses of epidural morphine 3 mg through a re-inserted epidural catheter.
- A prophylactic epidural blood patch (EBP) through a re-inserted epidural catheter. There may be a minor benefit but this does not reliably reduce the incidence of PDPH, the need for therapeutic EBP, or improve the mother's interaction with the infant and has infection risks.

Treatment of PDPH

Symptomatic, Expectant Treatment

Headache is common in the postpartum period. The diagnosis of PDPH is one of exclusion, so a multidisciplinary plan for evaluation and management is recommended. Refractory or recurrent and persistent headache requires further investigation, to avoid missing potentially life-threatening causes. There are no particularly effective pharmacological therapies for PDPH. Remaining recumbent while waiting for spontaneous resolution of headache will at least partially relieve symptoms, as intracranial CSF volume and pressure are restored to normal. However, prolonged periods lying flat prevent normal care of the infant and are poorly tolerated and this expectant management leads to longer hospital stay, more staff work and more post-discharge hospital visits. It is recommended that:

- The recumbent position should be encouraged whenever practical.
- Mild severity PDPH may respond to caffeine (500 mg IV or 300 mg tds oral) or sumatriptan (6 mg subcutaneous) but moderate to severe headache does not and both drugs have undesirable side effects (insomnia, agitation, seizures).
- Therapeutic EBP should be offered if headache is moderate or severe or persistent, after obtaining informed consent. EBP cures 90% of "post-spinal" PDPH, but less than 50% of "dural tap" PDPH It is more effective if delayed at least 24 hours after dural puncture with a spinal needle, and 48–72 hours after "dural tap."

Epidural Blood Patch: Application and Efficacy

Epidural blood patch is the only effective therapy for PDPH. It rapidly relieves vasodilatory headache symptoms by increasing neuraxial pressure, redistributing CSF upward to normalize intracranial volume and pressure, thus reducing cerebral blood flow by adenosine-mediated vasoconstriction. Blood also forms an adherent clot over the puncture site, preventing continued CSF loss and assisting the fibroblastic proliferative response and collagen repair of meningeal damage. Restoration of normal epidural anatomy usually occurs fully and rapidly, within 24 hours.

EBP is most appropriate when PDPH is severe, causing functional disability, or when headache fails to resolve despite a trial of expectant treatment. Contraindications are:

- Coagulopathy.
- Systemic sepsis, fever or local infection.
- Anatomical abnormality indicating a high risk of repeat dural puncture.

EBP results in complete or partial relief of PDPH after a "dural tap" (20 gauge needle or larger) in 80%–90%, but complete relief in only 30%–50%.

- Lack of success is most commonly due to headache recurrence after 12–36 hours, in which case a third of women request another EBP.
- EBP causes mild back pain in most women but serious complications are rare, although not well quantified (Table 13.4).

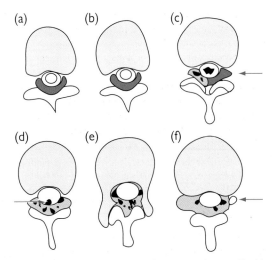

Figure 13.1 Six figures representing equidistant images between T_{10} (a) and L_3 (f), showing the distribution of blood 3 hours after an epidural blood patch. Blood is shown as black and darker areas. There is general compression and anterior displacement of the thecal sac. In (c) the arrow points to blood extending out of the neural foramen. In (d) the arrow points to clot adherent to dura and within the intrathecal sac. In (f) the arrow indicates the dorsal root ganglion, which is displaced down and anterior by blood clot. Reprinted with permission from Beards SC, *et al.* Magnetic resonance imaging of extradural blood patches: appearances from 30 min to 18 h. *Br J Anaesth.* 1993;71(2):183.

Table 13.4 **Complications of Epidural Blood Patch**
Back pain during injection
Transient bradycardia
Short-term post-procedural back pain (mild to moderate for 1–5 days)
Radicular pain or paresthesia in the buttocks or lower limbs
Neck or thoracic pain
Cranial nerve palsies
Cauda equina syndrome or arachnoiditis
Acute meningeal irritation, epidural abscess, pyrexia
Subdural hematoma
Deterioration of mental status, seizures, acute exacerbation of headache

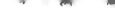

Epidural Blood Patch: Timing and Technique

The levels of evidence with regard to many procedural aspects of EBP are weak, so practices vary. Epidural blood patch appears less successful if performed too soon after dural puncture. Despite greater success if delayed, this approach also increases the duration of suffering. It is suggested that EBP:

- Is considered any time after 24 hours from onset of "post-spinal" PDPH.
- Is considered after 48 hours from "dural tap".
- The lateral position for insertion of the epidural needle is usually more comfortable for the patient, but may make identification of the epidural space more difficult and prolong the procedure.
- Be performed at the same or an adjacent lower intervertebral level to the puncture (no proven outcome benefit, but supported by imaging studies).
- Involve injection of 20 ml of sterile venous blood, although the volume of blood that can be injected may be limited by back pain during injection.
- Be followed by patient rest, lying supine for approximately 1–2 hours.

Other Therapies for Post-Dural Puncture Headache

A number of other treatments have been suggested or investigated, but have not been subjected to randomized evaluation, large clinical trials, or are limited in their clinical suitability. Some patients are unwilling to receive blood, or have contraindications to its injection. These alternatives are unproven so cannot be recommended currently.

- Epidural saline or Dextran injection (to briefly elevate epidural space pressure and give short-term relief of mild PDPH). Complications include retinal hemorrhage, orbital pain, interscapular pain, neuropraxia, dysesthesias and anaphylaxis.
- Surgical closure of the puncture site at laminectomy.
- Percutaneous injection of tissue adhesive (fibrin glue).

Back Pain

Back pain is very common before, during and after pregnancy, mainly due to muscular, vertebral and pelvic joint stress (as a result of gravitational changes and hormonal effects on joint laxity associated with pregnancy), and secondary to increased lumbar lordosis. Disc degeneration due to these stresses is also more common.

In the postpartum period, the physical demands of breastfeeding and childcare contribute to musculoskeletal pain and 25%–50% of women report lower back pain until 6–12 months. Epidural analgesia for labor and childbirth, and regional anesthesia for operative delivery, do NOT increase the risk of postpartum back pain.

Predictors of back pain within 48 hours of delivery are:

- Back pain before pregnancy (the only predictor of persistent pain).
- Maternal age less than 25 years.
- Labor duration of 12 hours or more.

Women of younger age in whom multiple needle passes are made are more likely to have localized tenderness at the insertion site over the first 48 hours postpartum. Very rarely, the needle insertion site alone remains tender, possibly due to neuroma formation in the skin.

Infection

Infection Control

Strict attention to infection control is an essential element of safe anesthesia care, especially when regional techniques are used. Although many suggestions for asepsis are not evidence-based, and are extrapolated from studies of intravascular catheter placement, consensus recommendations (the American Society of Anesthesiologists *Practice Advisory for the Prevention, Diagnosis, and Management of Infectious Complications Associated with Neuraxial Techniques*) are available (Table 13.5).

Most skin and soft tissue infections (up to 90%) involve staphylococcal species, especially skin commensals such as *S. aureus* and *S. epidermidis*. Very occasionally, a regional technique is contraindicated by extensive local folliculitis or furuncles, or by the presence of severe distant infection (e.g., an abscess), but more common risk factors are considered to be:

- Diabetes
- Intravenous drug use
- Immunocompromise or steroid therapy
- Prolonged epidural catheterization

Nevertheless, infections occur in otherwise healthy women, with sources of microorganisms including contaminated equipment or

Table 13.5 Infection Control Recommendations for Epidural and Spinal Techniques in Obstetrics

Wear a hat and face mask.
Wash your hands with an antiseptic solution after removing jewelry and watches.
Wear sterile gloves.
Consider wearing a sterile gown if a catheter technique is being employed.
Clean the skin site thoroughly with antiseptic (e.g., 0.5%–2% chlorhexidine in alcohol 70%–80%), moving away from the site to cover a large field. Repeat the application once the solution has dried.
Cover the field with a large sterile drape.
Use a "no touch" technique, avoiding handling of needles and the catheter that will enter the patient.
Use sterile-packed epidural and intrathecal solutions if available.   • Wipe the neck of nonsterile ampoules with antiseptic before breaking to allow drawing up.
Apply a sterile transparent dressing to the skin site (consider an antiseptic impregnated dressing at the puncture site if catheterization beyond 48 hours is planned).
Consider use of a 0.22 μm bacterial filter in the epidural catheter system.
In the event of accidental catheter disconnection, the safest policy is to remove the catheter.
The epidural insertion site should be checked daily for signs of infection, and the catheter removed as soon as clinically indicated.
Use an aseptic approach when accessing the epidural catheter system and minimize the number of times it is breached.
Do not give prophylactic antibiotics, but treat distant infection or bacteremia before the procedure.

dispersal from the operator, contaminated injectate, bloodstream bacteremia from distant sites and, most commonly, tracking inward from the skin. A 2010 report from the Centers for Disease Control in Atlanta documented 5 cases of meningitis associated with neuraxial labor analgesia, one fatal, in parturients. All were associated with preventable lapses in technique by the anesthesiologist.

Epidural Skin Site Infection

Despite usually short periods of epidural catheterization, bacterial colonization of the catheter increases significantly after 48 hours, suggesting that increased duration of catheterization is a major risk factor.

If an epidural catheter is retained after cesarean delivery, the incidence of skin inflammation is 2%–5% and minor infection at the insertion site 0.1%–0.5%. Appropriate management steps are to:

- Remove the epidural catheter if still in place, and culture the tip.
- Swab the skin and send the specimen for culture and sensitivity.
- If skin redness, tenderness, purulent discharge or subcutaneous fluctuation indicate that antibiotic therapy is necessary, appropriate IV antibiotics should be used until a clinical response occurs and microbiological diagnosis and sensitivities are available. Oral antibiotics should be continued for at least 7 days and sometimes much longer, based on specialist advice.
- Ensure follow-up examination of the patient and provide post-discharge information about progression and symptoms and signs that require reassessment.

Epidural Abscess

Deep vertebral soft tissue infections (bacterial epidural, paraspinous, pyriformis or sacroiliitis abscesses) appear very rare, and the incidence has been difficult to quantify. However, these infections are now more frequently reported and appear to be increasing in frequency. Some speculate that this relates to use of epidural opioids and low local anesthetic concentrations, which do not share the antibacterial properties of concentrated local anesthetic. Prolonged epidural catheterization is often noted, but some cases arise despite only a few hours of catheterization.

The exact incidence is unknown and varies across different sites.

- Large databases, including a U.K. audit of persisting neurological complications, suggest an incidence of < 1 in 100,000. This is likely to be a large underestimate, because in most cases diagnosis and treatment occurs prior to the onset of neurological complications, preventing persisting neurological injury.
- Prospective series indicate an incidence of 1 in 2,000–10,000.
- Retrospective or prospective data from individual maternity units have found an incidence of 1 in 800–3,000.

Clinical Features

The signs and symptoms of these serious infections are shown in Table 13.6. The presentation tends to be delayed (days rather than hours) and may be insidious. Thus, both a high index of suspicion and post-discharge recognition are needed to reduce diagnostic delay, which compromises the chance of early treatment and full recovery.

Table 13.6 Signs and Symptoms of Epidural Abscess or Deep Vertebral Canal Infection

Back pain
- often severe

Fever and malaise
- may precede pain

Clinical and laboratory signs of infection
- tachycardia
- neutrophilia with left shift
- raised C-reactive protein
- raised erythrocyte sedimentation rate

Tenderness to palpation at or near the site

Neurological deficit
- sphincter incontinence
- lower limb weakness
- lower limb or buttock paresthesia
- sensory changes
- radicular pain

Associated skin site infection
- erythema
- tenderness
- warmth
- fluctuation
- discharge

Signs of meningeal irritation or meningitis
- headache
- photophobia
- nuchal rigidity
- vomiting
- agitation
- change in conscious state

If infection is suspected, early consultation with other specialists is imperative.

- Consult with radiologists and organize magnetic resonance imaging (MRI), preferably with gadolinium (CT scan may be inconclusive; see Figure 13.2).
- Consult with infectious disease specialists about optimal antibiotic therapy (usually necessary for 6 weeks and longer for adjacent osteomyelitis).
- Consult with neurosurgeons as to whether surgical intervention with drainage is required.
- Do not perform lumbar puncture through an infected area (infection may spread).

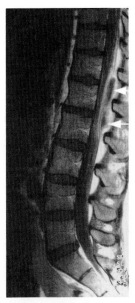

Figure 13.2 Sagittal T_1 weighted magnetic resonance image of a posterior epidural abscess (arrowed) in a parturient. The abscess was predominantly on the left and is shown compressing the spinal cord anteriorly. Reprinted with permission from Collier CB and Gatt SP. Epidural abscess in an obstetric patient. *Anaesthesia and Intensive Care.* 1999;27:663.

Management

Conservative (antibiotic) management alone is appropriate for selected patients with small, superficial infections and no neurological symptoms. Rapid surgical intervention (open laminectomy or, rarely, percutaneous drainage) may be required to define pathology, obtain tissue specimens and material for microbiological diagnosis, and to decompress and drain larger abscesses. When indicated by the onset of neurological signs and symptoms, immediate surgery (within hours) is associated with the best chance of a good outcome. Worse outcomes are associated with:

- Thoracic abscess (compared lumbar).
- Spinal canal stenosis (very rare in the obstetric population).
- Atypical microorganisms (bacteria or tuberculus, fungal or parasitic organisms).
- A longer duration of neurological signs and delay in decompression.

Meningitis

Meningitis is rare, though due to incomplete reporting the true incidence is unknown. The incidence has been estimated at 1–4 per 100,000, although clusters of cases occur. The presenting features are:

- Headache and neck stiffness.
- Drowsiness and lethargy.
- Fever.

These symptoms may be confused with PDPH or with headache associated with distant infection. A careful history is necessary because community-acquired viral or bacterial infection can present coincidentally. Causative organisms include streptococcus viridans, beta-hemolytic streptococcus and pseudomonas, but blood cultures are often negative. Lumbar puncture (revealing low glucose, increased protein and high leukocyte count in the CSF) can establish a microbiological diagnosis, with polymerase chain reaction to identify the causative organism, but is contraindicated if cellulitis, subcutaneous or deep tissue pus is present. Compared with community-acquired bacterial meningitis, the outlook is relatively good if appropriate antibiotic therapy is begun early.

Vertebral and Intracranial Hematoma and Vascular Events

These complications are exceptionally rare, with none reported among hundreds of thousands of neuraxial obstetric blocks performed in the U.K. registry of cases in 2006 and 2007. The presentation of these complications is not always clearly related to regional anesthesia or analgesia. The major complication categories are:

- Vertebral canal hematoma with signs of spinal cord compression or ischemia
- Intracranial subdural hematoma (usually following dural puncture, with or without epidural blood patch)
- Intracranial extradural, subarachnoid or intracerebral hemorrhage
- Posterior reversible encephalopathy syndrome from cerebral vasospasm
- Cortical vein thrombosis
  - Causes headache that can be confused with PDPH
  - Is probably underdiagnosed (incidence 1 in 10,000–25,000)
  - May not be causally related to regional techniques or dural puncture

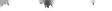

Vertebral Canal Hematoma (Spinal Epidural Hematoma)

Vertebral canal hematoma (spinal epidural hematoma) is exceptionally rare, despite an incidence of venous bleeding during epidural insertion of 5%–10%. Case reports of epidural hematoma have been reported in women with disordered coagulation and rarely, with severe preeclampsia (Table 13.7). Other rarities include hematoma from trauma, vascular malformations or tumors, and a cervical or thoracic location. The decision whether to perform a regional technique in the presence of an increased risk of vertebral canal bleeding must be individualized (also see Chapter 10) and care should be exercised in women at increased risk of bleeding. Potential risks include:

- Severe thrombocytopenia from preeclampsia or idiopathic thrombocytopenic purpura.
- Platelet disorders.
- Patients taking antiplatelet drugs other than low-dose aspirin (e.g., clopidogrel).
- Severe renal failure.
- Falling platelet number or declining platelet function (e.g., severe preeclampsia, von Willebrand's disease).
- Patients with an epidural catheter who receive postpartum heparin thromboprophylaxis.
- Anticoagulated patients.

Caution must be exercised at the time of epidural catheter removal, as well as at insertion.

Presentation and Management

The signs and symptoms of spinal or epidural hematoma are shown in Table 13.8. Most cases associated with regional block present within hours (sometimes days) of catheter insertion or removal. Signs progress

Table 13.7 Factors Associated with Spinal Hematoma
Traumatic insertion
Severe preeclampsia
Epidural techniques associated with higher risk than spinal techniques
Coagulation abnormalities
• Indwelling epidural catheter while on LMWH • Immediate or early postoperative (< 4 hours) LMWH dosing • Combination of LMWH with other drugs affecting platelet function (e.g., nonsteroidal anti-inflammatory drugs) or other anticoagulant drugs • Twice daily or therapeutic dose of LMWH

LMWH = low molecular weight heparin.

over hours, and leg weakness in the absence of recent epidural drug administration is very concerning. Routine measures to improve safety include:

- Regular postpartum surveillance of patients who have received regional blocks (sensory and motor assessment).
- Protocols for the investigation of abnormal or recurrent motor block.
- Access to magnetic resonance imaging (the diagnostic investigation of choice).
- Access to neurosurgical assessment and care (surgical decompression, preferably within 8 hours, provides the best chance of neurological recovery).
- Maintenance of normal to high blood pressure to maintain spinal cord blood supply until decompression.

Anterior spinal artery syndrome or rupture of a vertebral canal arteriovenous malformation may lead to a similar presentation. In about 15% of the population, the branches of the internal iliac artery provide the major blood supply to the conus medullaris, placing these people at greater risk of an ischemic spinal cord injury, although the event is exceptionally rare and unpredictable.

Intracranial Hematoma

Subdural and extradural hematoma can arise spontaneously, after no apparent or minor trauma, but the former are most often associated with dural puncture. Subdural hematoma is thought to develop because of stretching and tearing of dural veins, consequent to a fall in

Table 13.8 **Clinical Features of Subarachnoid or Epidural Hematoma**
Lower limb weakness • often bilateral and asymmetric
Absent or reduce lower limb reflexes
Bladder dysfunction
Anal dysfunction • absent sphincter tone or perineal sensory change
Numbness and sensory loss • variable
Local or radicular back pain • transient local pain occurs but possibly in a minority • many cases are silent, with no abnormal local findings on examination of the back

CSF pressure, whereas spontaneous hematoma are thought to be due to rupture of small epidural arteries, secondary to local anatomical aberrations and mechanical forces during spinal movement. It is unclear whether high pressures generated by epidural blood patch further contribute to the etiology.

Pathology may be either unilateral or bilateral. The presentation can be acute, subacute or chronic, but often occurs several days (and occasionally weeks) after delivery. Features include:

- Headache (usually nonpostural).
- Seizures (common, and in the early postpartum period often misdiagnosed as eclampsia).
- Change in conscious state (including confusion or prolonged postictal drowsiness).
- Focal neurological signs (e.g., hemiparesis).
- Signs of raised intracranial pressure (e.g., papilloedema, nausea and vomiting that is more prominent than that associated with PDPH).

Diagnostic imaging is with contrast CT scan or MRI of the head. In many cases, unless the blood collection is small and the neurological state is improving, neurosurgical decompression will be required.

Neurological Deficit

Background and Etiology

Nerve injuries result from mechanisms such as:

- Compression and stretching.
- Ischemia.
- Direct needle injury.
- Intraneural drug injection.

Neurological complications during pregnancy are common, and are contributed to by the increase in soft tissue pressure from fluid retention and fat deposition, by musculoskeletal changes, and by compression of nerves at the pelvic brim during delivery. Examples are:

- Conditions causing neuropathic pain (e.g., sciatic nerve entrapment or compression by disc prolapse or nerve root trauma).
- Nerve entrapment syndromes.
  - Carpal tunnel (incidence up to 20%).
  - Meralgia paresthetica (sensory loss and dysesthesia in the lateral anterior thigh due to compression of the lateral cutaneous nerve of the thigh from L_2–L_3 in the pelvis or under the inguinal ligament).

- Cranial nerve palsies (especially the sixth or abducens nerve). Mechanisms include previously silent pathology such as pituitary or other intracranial tumors or loss of CSF following dural puncture.
- Immediate postpartum transient sensory changes in the lower limbs (incidence 20%).
- Clinically significant deficits (incidence up to 1% of peripartum women).

Most neurological injuries do not arise from anesthetic procedures (see also below) but are due to:

- Obstetric events (e.g., femoral or obturator nerve palsies among nulliparous women having a prolonged second stage of labor).
- Positional compression (e.g., sciatic nerve compression in the buttock or posterior thigh, and compression of dorsal rami of the sacral nerves that supply skin over the lower sacrum and buttock during cesarean delivery).
- Other pathologies (e.g., prolapsed intervertebral disc, inherited neuropathy or ischemia due to spontaneous bleeding into the vertebral canal in patients with bleeding or clotting disorders or on anticoagulants).

Focal demyelination usually causes short-term deficits, whereas axonal loss is more likely to produce a prolonged deficit. Approximately one-third of obstetric nerve injuries are associated with a motor deficit.

Assessment and Management

An anesthesiologist is frequently the first physician consulted, so he or she must be able to perform a reasonably thorough neurological examination, and have good knowledge of the differential diagnoses. Anesthesiologists should show good judgment as to when neurologic referral is warranted, and be able to recognize the signs and symptoms of rare pathologies that mandate immediate intervention (e.g., vertebral canal hematoma or epidural abscess).

Management depends on the specific condition or lesion, but should be coordinated among health care disciplines. Except in cases of mild sensory dysfunction, and patients in whom symptoms and signs appear likely to resolve rapidly, management principles are:

- Consult a neurologist with an interest in this area of medicine.
- Perform magnetic resonance imaging to:
  - Exclude neuraxial mass lesions.
  - Identify spinal cord or nerve root syrinxes or hematoma or increased signals suggestive of trauma.

- Exclude preexisting pathology such as vertebral canal tumor, stenosis or arteriovenous malformation (if a space-occupying lesion is identified, neurosurgical consultation is required).
- Consider nerve conduction studies or electromyography for diagnostic and prognostic value.

Fortunately, full recovery from most neurological deficits is the norm, although in more severe cases this may take weeks to months.

Direct Complications of Neuraxial Block

Direct complications of neuraxial regional anesthesia are very rare.

- The estimated incidence is 1 in 5,000–10,000.
- Spinal techniques appear to have a higher rate of complications than epidural techniques.
- Permanent injury is exceptionally rare:
  - Comprehensive national audit data from the UK show a "worst case scenario" incidence of permanent injury (persisting more than 6 months) of 1 per 100,000, and of paraplegia or death rate of 0 (confidence interval 0–0.7) per 100,000.

Case reports have described a variety of injuries:

- Spinal cord conus medullaris injury from spinal techniques performed too high in the vertebral column (L_2–L_3 interspace or higher). Although the spinal cord usually terminates at L_1, in 20% of the population it terminates below this level, and rarely it is tethered to low lumbar vertebral levels. The most common problem is incorrect identification of the interspace, because 50% of anesthesiologists estimate the space to be lower than it is (Figure 13.3).
- Nerve root injury (Table 13.9) from needle trauma or injection of solution, despite most cases being associated with severe paresthesia or lancinating pain at the time of insertion or injection.
- Vertebral canal "mass" lesions (e.g., hematoma, abscess).
- Arachnoiditis (leading to pain and deficits).
- Anterior spinal artery syndrome (leading to paralysis).

Specific Deficits

Foot Drop

"Foot drop" after delivery is a major deficit that arises through various mechanisms, including hereditary neuropathies, disc lesions, positional compression, and regional anesthesia-induced injury. It mandates early investigation and treatment.

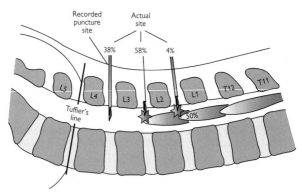

Figure 13.3 Hazard to the spinal cord from spinal needle insertion due to error in estimating the correct intervertebral level (because of variations in anatomical level of the supracristal, or Tuffier's line) and due to variability in the level of termination of the spinal cord. Planned insertion at L$_{3/4}$ was radiologically demonstrated as incorrect in 62% of cases. Reprinted with permission from Bromage PR. Neurologic complications of labor, delivery, and regional anesthesia In: Chestnut DH, *Obstetric Anesthesia 2nd ed.* 1999, Elsevier.

The deficit may involve:

- Complete or partial weakness of ankle and toe plantarflexion or dorsiflexion, and foot inversion or eversion.
- Loss of the Achilles tendon reflex.
- Sensory changes such as hypoesthesia in the lateral calf and foot or a glove-and-stocking distribution associated with plexopathy.

Examination helps determine whether the pathology is proximal (lumbar nerve root, lumbosacral plexus near the pelvic brim, sciatic

Table 13.9 **Manifestations of Traumatic Nerve Root Damage**	
Nerve root sensory change	*Motor weakness*
L$_2$ Upper anterior thigh	Hip flexion
L$_3$ Lower anterior and medial thigh	Hip adduction
L$_4$ Lateral thigh, knee and leg	Knee extension
L$_5$ Lateral leg and dorsum of foot	Ankle dorsiflexion
S$_1$ Outer border of foot	Ankle plantar flexion

nerve) or distal (lateral popliteal nerve at the head of the fibula or under peroneus longus). For example:

- Sensory change in the thigh and abnormal gluteal function suggest a plexus injury versus a sciatic nerve injury distal to the take-off of the gluteal nerve branches.
- Weakness of knee flexion suggests injury proximal to the sciatic division into the lateral popliteal (common peroneal) and tibial nerves.
- Painless sensory change confined to the dorsum of the foot, with normal foot inversion and ankle jerk, suggests a lateral popliteal nerve injury.

Subsequent electromyography may demonstrate denervation potentials in muscles supplied by the sciatic nerve (e.g., biceps femoris and semitendinosis). Management involves physiotherapy, orthotic assistance, and neurological review.

Femoral Neuropathy

Femoral neuropathy was once common (3% of births) due to:

- Prolonged labor and delivery (pressure on the L_2–L_4 nerve by the fetal head).
- Instrumental delivery with forceps.
- Nerve entrapment within the pelvis associated with excessive hip abduction and external rotation.

  It is now very uncommon, and recognized by features including:

- Diminished knee tendon reflex.
- Weakness of knee extension and hip flexion, which impairs walking and makes rising from squatting or stepping up stairs impossible.
- Sensory loss in the anterior thigh and anteromedial leg.
- If the obturator nerve is also involved, hip adduction is impaired and sensory loss occurs over the medial thigh.

Other Deficits

Neurological deficits which require urgent review and investigation are:

- Bilateral lower limb weakness.
- Bilateral leg pain or sensory loss.
- Impaired bladder or bowel function (atonic bladder and fecal incontinence due to loss of anal reflexes).
- Unexpectedly prolonged motor block after regional anesthesia, or the reappearance of lower limb weakness after return of normal function.

- Signs of a mass lesion (spinal or epidural hematoma or abscess).
- Signs of spinal cord injury.
  - Cauda equina syndrome with pain, dysesthesias and diffuse neurological changes from low cord injury or sacral nerve root damage.
  - Etiologies including disc prolapse, drug toxicity or spinal canal stenosis with compression or ischemia.

These signs mandate immediate imaging, because establishing a diagnosis may allow early decompression of a space-occupying mass, or steroid administration to reduce swelling, thus maximizing the chance of neurological recovery.

Thrombosis and Pulmonary Embolism

Although thromboembolism is a complication of pregnancy, surgery or anesthesia, the anesthesiologist is often involved in both prevention and treatment. Thromboembolism is five times more frequent during pregnancy and the puerperium (rate 1–2 per 1,000) because of physiological changes that increase venous distension, venous obstruction in the pelvis, and blood coagulation (significant increases in the concentration of most clotting factors and fibrinogen and decreased fibrinolytic activity; see Chapter 2).

Pregnant women at highest risk of a thromboembolic event are those with:

- Inherited thrombophilias or antiphospholipid syndrome (see Chapter 10).
- A previous thromboembolic event (2.5% risk of recurrence during pregnancy), especially multiple events.
- A combination of factors that place them in a moderate to high risk category.
- Extended bed rest (prevalence 15 per 1,000 versus normal pregnancy 1–2 per 1,000).

Other risk factors include:

- Older age (> 35 years).
- High multiparity.
- Obesity.
- Fluid and electrolyte disturbance.
- Emergency surgery (double the risk of elective).

- Postpartum hemorrhage or blood transfusion.
- Postpartum infection.

Approximately half the cases of thromboembolism in pregnancy occur before delivery, although pulmonary embolism is more common post-partum. After cesarean delivery it is rare (0.4 per 1000), but this represents a six- to sevenfold increase in relative risk compared with vaginal delivery.

The prescription of prophylactic drugs to prevent deep vein thrombosis (DVT) and pulmonary embolism after cesarean delivery often falls within the domain of the anesthesiologist. Policies vary, but most hospitals have clinical practice guidelines (Table 13.10). Elective cesarean delivery alone, without other risk factors, is not considered by most units as a sufficient risk to justify heparin thromboprophylaxis, but protocols vary.

The safe management of the anticoagulated pregnant woman, or women on DVT prophylaxis peripartum or perioperatively, and who are scheduled for regional anesthesia, is a major issue (see Chapter 10).

Diagnosis and Presentation

DVT can usually be diagnosed by compression ultrasound or contrast venography, but magnetic resonance imaging (MRI) may be necessary

Table 13.10 Example of a Prophylactic Regimen Against Thromboembolism After Cesarean Delivery
Low risk
Knee-high leg compression stockings until fully mobile
Intraoperative pneumatic calf compression
Early postoperative mobilization
Moderate or high risk
Knee-high leg compression stockings until fully mobile
Intraoperative (and possibly postoperative) pneumatic calf compression
Early postoperative mobilization
Subcutaneous low molecular weight heparin, e.g., enoxaparin 40 mg or dalteparin 5000 IU daily until fully mobile • start at least 4 hours after surgery and give at the same time each day • wait 12 hours after a dose before removing an epidural catheter • wait 2–4 hours after epidural catheter removal before redosing

to detect iliac vein thrombosis. Post-thrombotic syndrome causes long-term morbidity.

Pulmonary embolism (PE) occurs in approximately 1 in 2,000 pregnancies, and is fatal in up to 15% (two-thirds of patients die within 30 minutes to 2 hours of presentation).

PE is a leading cause of maternal death (often ranking in the top two direct causes in developed countries).

The features of pulmonary embolism include:

- Sudden onset of chest pain.
- Dyspnea, hypoxemia and cyanosis.
- Dizziness or cardiovascular collapse.
- ECG or echocardiographic evidence of tachycardia with acute right ventricular strain or ischemia.
- Pulmonary clot on spiral CT pulmonary angiography (imaging of choice), or suggested by ventilation-perfusion scan (the ionizing radiation from which is safe in all trimesters).

Management

Management options vary with the location of the thrombosis, the severity of illness, and the facilities available.

- Therapeutic dosing with either low molecular weight heparin (LMWH; e.g., enoxaparin 1 mg/kg b.d) or intravenous unfractionated heparin (UFH) may be necessary. In less severe cases, twice daily dose-adjusted subcutaneous UFH (higher heparin doses are required during pregnancy because of increased renal clearance) is sometimes used. Heparin may need to be continued until delivery or 6 weeks postpartum to prevent further clot formation, although oral warfarin is another option after delivery.
- Thrombolysis with tissue plasminogen activator (TPA) has been used in patients in extremis (but massive blood loss is a major concern, especially within 24 hours of surgery).
- After recent delivery or surgery, clot fragmentation with a radiologically inserted pigtail or similar catheter, or surgical embolectomy, may be necessary in severe cases.
- In the presence of massive lower limb or pelvic thrombus, or if contraindications to anticoagulation exist, insertion of an infrarenal inferior vena cava filter may be indicated.
- Supportive therapy with vasopressors and inotropes is required if there has been hemodynamic collapse.

Medicolegal Considerations

Ethics in Obstetric Anesthesia

The four essential principles of Western culture bioethics are respect for:

- Autonomy (freedom of self-determination).
- Beneficence ("do good").
- Non-maleficence ("first do no harm").
- Justice (the needs of other individuals and/or society).

Other ethical approaches are also used in various parts of the world, including virtue ethics, Islamic and Confucian ethics, and feminist bioethics. These may place more emphasis on spirituality, family, community, authority, or social hierarchy.

The obstetric anesthesiologist faces many potential ethical issues. Each of us has our own beliefs and biases, and although ethical and moral dilemmas challenge us, they also enrich our professional and personal development and lives.

On a daily basis, the obstetric anesthesiologist may have to confront a number of ethical issues. For example:

- How is informed consent for epidural analgesia in labor obtained in a distressed woman, or in one who has advance directives that are now being contradicted?
- What are the rights of the mother versus those of the child?
- How is patient identification avoided in morbidity reporting, and should permission be sought from the patient prior to publication of case reports?
- When can valid consent for participation in a trial of labor epidural analgesia be obtained, or when is use of a drug for a non-approved indication "experimental"?

Informed Consent

This is such an important facet of professional life, having both ethical and legal implications, that many institutions now provide guidelines about obtaining consent for anesthesia. To make an informed choice, the pregnant woman must have decision-making capacity, and:

- Adequate disclosure (of information that the person would consider of significance to aid their understanding so that they may come to a decision).

- Comprehension (which also implies time for discussion and understanding of the benefits, risks, and alternative options).
- A voluntary choice (persuasion with balanced reasoning is acceptable, but manipulation or insistence without consent is not, and may lead to the charge of battery).

Patient Autonomy

In bioethics and law, the principle of respecting patient autonomy is very strong and one with which we must generally comply. This reinforces the concept that the woman has control of her body and can make choices. To make these choices, adequate disclosure of information is required, although most women want reassurance and explanation rather than detailed knowledge. How the law views how much and what information is provided ("reasonable" disclosure) varies across jurisdictions, and the detail considered appropriate depends on the individual's prior knowledge, expectations, and concerns. For example, it is not possible to obtain informed consent by general disclosure of a list of risks, so discussion should always be tailored to the individual situation and patient. Clearly, antenatal education can contribute to the process but may be lacking.

An example of when respect for autonomy comes in to play is the case of a patient who refuses treatment that might be life-saving. Those of the Jehovah's Witness faith who refuse blood transfusion have every right to do so. Advance directives and frank discussion prior to an event such as a massive obstetric hemorrhage will clarify consent with regard to management. However, decisions must be made voluntarily, free from external constraints or coercion, so discussion in the absence of other parties is important. In special circumstances, respect for autonomy can be justifiably infringed and in some obstetric emergencies the wishes of the patient are unknown.

An obstetric dilemma arises when the wishes of the mother may not be in the best interests of the fetus—for example, when a woman refuses cesarean delivery despite the life of the fetus being at significant risk if delay occurs. Although in most countries the rights of the unborn child are generally held secondary to those of the mother, these ethics are debated and the legal position varies. In England, Canada, and Australia, for example, the mother's rights (or wishes) prevail in law, and it is not permissible to enforce invasive medical procedures. In contrast, in some states of the United States the law is less clear, and women have been forced by court order to have a cesarean rather than vaginal delivery for the sake of their baby.

Groups such as the American College of Obstetricians and Gynecologists and the American Academy of Pediatricians publish advice on such matters, but counsel from knowledgeable and experienced parties, administrative and legal, should be sought.

Capacity to Consent

To provide informed consent, the person must have the capacity to do so, which involves their values and the capacity to understand, communicate, and reason. Even women in labor and in extreme pain, or under the influence of various drugs, usually retain the capacity to consent. Whether this represents informed consent is debatable, but in the context of a woman incapacitated by pain and expressing the desire for intervention, many would argue that there is a duty to relieve pain, at least until evidence of patient refusal to accept the intervention appears. Rarely, in the case of mental illness or very young age, capacity may be lacking. In most Western countries, many pregnant "minors" (less than 16 or 18 years of age, depending on the law) are considered to have sufficient understanding and independence to make their own decisions, rather than their parents assuming this right. The detail of the consent process in these settings where capacity may be in doubt, or where capacity is evident but women exert their right to refuse information, can be challenging, and the correct ethical, moral, or legal approach in individual cases is frequently debated.

Beneficence

In an emergency such as preparation for general anesthesia, where a life (usually of the baby) is at high risk if there is a delay, the ethical principle of beneficence (the duty of work for the good of the patient) often applies. The anesthesiologist should provide the woman (and partner if present) with as much information as is practical, prioritizing the detail to the time available, and in the case of life-threatening urgency assume consent based on physical and verbal cooperation.

Consent for Research

Research is vital to advancements in care and safety, but consent to participate in research is by nature only partially voluntary because it usually falls within the context of illness or pain and is influenced by the doctor–patient relationship. Thus, when conducting research in pregnant women, certain principles should apply.

• The research is designed and conducted to the highest ethical standards (guidelines specific to obstetric anesthesia research are available, e.g., from the U.K. Obstetric Anaesthetists' Association).

- The welfare of the mother and baby always takes priority over research objectives.
- Trial information and consent should preferably occur well before entry into the study (e.g., when pain is minimal, in the case of studies of analgesia during labor).
- Ideally, the consent process should be witnessed by an independent practitioner.
- If there is any doubt about competence, the person should not be recruited.
- Drugs used outside their approved indications or in unlicensed formulation should be discussed. Explanations as to why "off-label" drug use is essential to best practice, as well as research, are appropriate.

Protection of Privacy

Obstetric medicine has a long history of conducting enquiries into maternal mortality and morbidity, and of using individual case details to illustrate and educate. Anesthesiology is no different in using the publication of case reports or case series for teaching and education, and these are worthy activities. To limit concerns about breach of privacy:

- Many journals now require confirmation that the patient whose case is reported has consented to this information entering a public domain.
- In countries such as Australia and parts of the United States, the clinical detail provided in mortality reports has been limited in recent years because of confidentiality issues.

The handling of patient information in medical reports differs between organizations and legal systems. Relevant legislation must consider the benefits and harms with a view to striking a balance between patient autonomy and confidentiality, and societal and individual benefits.

Avoiding Medical Litigation

In many countries, society has become increasingly litigious, such that every obstetric anesthesiologist is faced with the prospect of alleged medical malpractice. The personal burden of responding to and defending a claim is emotionally draining, and irrespective of the outcome of a claim, substantial legal fees are likely for the professional indemnity organization, health care organization, health service, or hospital.

To prove a claim of medical malpractice in countries with a legal system derived from English law, the claimant must prove there was an obligation (by the anesthesiologist) to provide care of a certain minimal quality (the standard of care). Further, the claimant must show:

- That the duty was breached (violation of the standard of care).
- That the acts caused the damages claimed.
- That the damages (physical or emotional) are present.

Examples of Types of Claim

Claims against obstetric anesthesiologists, which constitute 10%–15% of the U.S. perioperative Closed Claims and 50% of those in the U.K., tend to fall under three categories:

- Claims for personal injury as a result of a complication of a regional anesthetic or analgesic technique (e.g., nerve injury, headache).
- Claims for injury as a result of general anesthesia or delay in providing anesthesia (neonatal brain damage, but also maternal death, respiratory events, and injury).
- Claims for suffering and distress as a result of pain experienced during surgery under regional anesthesia.

In addition, in relation to regional anesthesia and analgesia:

- Claims of nerve damage are now the most common (although in most cases the etiology is not related to anesthesia).
- Claims related to local anesthetic toxicity are now rare.
- Claims of complications secondary to a high block from an undetected intrathecal catheter are increasing.
- Claims for spinal cord injury are increasing.

It is important to note that significant neurological deficits post-delivery need close evaluation by an experienced neurologist, because they can often be defended successfully. Many are due to obstetric palsies, exacerbations of preexisting disorders, or underlying conditions. Claims of inadequate regional anesthesia and unrelieved surgical pain during cesarean delivery are more likely to be upheld, so avoiding litigation by attention to patient management at the time is vital (see Chapter 4). In many cases of newborn death or brain injury, poor communication between the obstetrician and anesthesiologist is a factor that leads to subsequent delay.

Claims for "minor" issues are now also more likely, and payments for successful claims larger than for non-obstetric anesthesia litigation. Factors relevant to patient satisfaction with care include unrealistic

Table 13.11 Strategies to Minimize Litigation
Maximal interaction with the patient (many of whom are awake during their procedure)   – in principle, the more thoroughly and empathetically their concerns are addressed the less likely is litigation
Talk to and listen to the patient and family when a complication occurs   – discussion should be frank, without either admission of guilt or apportioning of blame
Consult with other specialists (who may determine that causation with your care cannot be established)

Document thoroughly
  – accurate, detailed and contemporaneous record keeping provides strong supporting evidence of what was done, as opposed to what was said to have been done
  – write a detailed factual narrative at the time of an "event" that might lead to litigation

Inform and obtain help from your medical protection society, insurer or risk management group if you are concerned about an event or notified of a claim

expectations, and poor patient–physician rapport, resulting in inadequate communication with the patient.

Protection against Litigation

Means of attempting to protect oneself against, or increasing the chance of successful defense against, a malpractice suit, are shown in Table 13.11.

Further Reading

1. Candido KD, Stevens RA. Post-dural puncture headache: pathophysiology, prevention and treatment. *Best Prac Res Clin Anaesthesiol.* 2003;17:451-469.
2. Turnbull DK, Shepherd DB. Post-dural puncture headache: pathogenesis, prevention and treatment. *Br J Anaesth.* 2003;91:5:718-729.
3. Paech M. Epidural blood patch – myths and legends. *Can J Anesth.* 2005;52:6 Annual Meeting Supplement R1-R5.
4. Grewal S, Hocking G, Wildsmith JAW. Epidural abscesses. *Br J Anaesth.* 2006;96:292-302.
5. Horlocker TT. What's a nice patient like you doing with a complication like this? Diagnosis, prognosis and prevention of spinal hematoma (editorial). *Can J Anaesth.* 2004;51:527-534.
6. Loo CC, Dahlgren G, Irestedt L. Neurological complications in obstetric regional anaesthesia. *Int J Obstet Anesth.* 2000;9:99-124.
7. Cook TM, Counsell D, Wildsmith JAW on behalf of The Royal College of Anaesthetists Third National Audit Project. Major complications of central

neuraxial block: report on the Third National Audit Project of the Royal College of Anaesthetists. *Br J Anaesth.* 2009;102:179-190.

8. Stone SE, Morris TA. Pulmonary embolism during and after pregnancy. *Crit Care Med.* 2005;33:S294-S300.

9. Bates SM, Greer IA, Pabinger I, et al. Venous thromboembolism, thrombophilia, antithrombotic therapy, and pregnancy. *Chest.* 2008; 133 (6 Suppl):844S-886S.

10. Yentis SM. Ethical guidance for research in obstetric anaesthesia. *Int J Obstet Anesth.* 2001;10:289-291.

11. Hoehner PJ. Ethical aspects of informed consent in obstetric anesthesia—new challenges and solutions. *J Clin Anesth.* 2003;15:587-560.

Chapter 14

Critical Care of the Obstetric Patient

Michael J. Paech, FANZCA

Resource Allocation and Maternal Morbidity

Severe Morbidity

While most women enjoy an uneventful and uncomplicated labor and delivery, a small percentage of women suffer complications or have coexisting disease requiring a significantly higher level of care. Such women benefit from the resources of an intensive or critical care unit (ICU), or a high-dependency unit (HDU). Women who might otherwise have died or suffered severe morbidity (without luck and/or good care) include those who suffer:

- Serious complications of pregnancy (e.g., hemorrhage, preeclampsia and eclampsia).
- Life-threatening disease or illness exacerbated by pregnancy (e.g., serious cardiac disease).
- Trauma.
- Serious surgical and medical conditions (e.g., vascular events, severe sepsis, complex surgery or life-threatening complications of surgery and anesthesia).

Epidemiology and Service Allocation

Depending on definitions, medical resources, and the availability of units, critical care is needed by 1%–3% of the pregnant population.

In developed countries with sophisticated critical care services, approximately 0.1%–1% of pregnant women are admitted to an ICU.

Reasons for admission include the need for:

• Ventilatory support.
• Inotropic support.
• Sophisticated invasive monitoring.

Less life-threatening cases, for example women with single organ failure, those stepping down from ICU, or those likely to benefit from more intense postoperative or postpartum monitoring or care, are frequently accommodated in an intermediate care setting, such as an HDU. These units were recommended in the U.K. Confidential Enquiries into Maternal Deaths over 20 years ago.

In low resource settings (e.g., developing countries), delay in obtaining care and delay in transfer to a critical care facility markedly increase patient risk, and the death to severe morbidity ratio is much higher (1 in 10–20 rather than 1 in 50–80 in developed countries), because more of these women die.

Despite the presence of multiple complicating illnesses, many pregnant women ultimately requiring critical care do not have significant pre-pregnancy comorbidities. For this reason:

• Mortality rates should ultimately be very low (less than 5%).
• ICU duration of stay is usually short.
• Rapid and full patient recovery are the norm.

At a local level, systems are required to identifying and manage women who are likely to benefit from critical care. About a third to half the pregnant women requiring critical care, and 20% of those requiring intensive care, are identifiable in advance, mainly because of preexisting disease; this typically involves the cardiorespiratory or hematological systems.

Components of maternity-based critical care systems include:

• Antenatal outpatient clinics, sometimes multidisciplinary and often led by anesthesiologists.
• Inpatient anesthesiology referral services.
• A HDU protocol-based referral to an ICU.
• Ready access to an ICU, either on-site or by transfer.

Critical care resources are most often needed in the postpartum period (75% of admissions) because of obstetric emergencies, especially postpartum hemorrhage and complications of severe preeclampsia. Due to the complexity of patient transfer and issues of bed availability, maternity units that are not "stand alone" and that are integrated with other inpatient services are more likely to admit patients to critical care.

Improvement in critical care quality and delivery requires planning and regular review, with the latter used to generate recommendations about resource allocation and implementation of practice guidelines. Attempts to improve the understanding of the incidence and nature of severe maternal morbidity during pregnancy include:

- New national morbidity reporting systems in some countries.
- Population-based cohort studies.
- The establishment of registries to document specific rare conditions.

Recognizing and Assessing the Sick Parturient

Issues and Considerations

While difficult to prove scientifically, it seems intuitive that early recognition of severe pathology is likely to improve the chance of survival and subsequent good health. Changes in training and medical work patterns appear to have reduced the exposure of residents in training and junior doctors to life-threatening illness. This has led to recommendations for simulation training and competency-based accreditation. Only about 7 per 1,000 admissions to an ICU involve pregnant women, so even the exposure of intensivists to this group of patients is very limited.

The assessment of sick pregnant women is challenging, and several factors are important to remember.

- The physiological changes of pregnancy increase reserve but predispose to hypoxemia, aspiration, late hemodynamic collapse, and more thrombotic events (see Chapter 2).
- The physiological changes of pregnancy often alter "normal" laboratory values.
- The anatomical changes of pregnancy impact on airway management and the risk of rapid massive hemorrhage.
- Obesity is more prevalent during pregnancy, and not only increases the risks of a number of medical and obstetric complications, but makes patient assessment, monitoring, and management more difficult (see Chapter 9).

More women with complex medical disease are able to become and are choosing to become pregnant. Deterioration of preexisting medical disease (e.g., cardiac disease) may be subtle and difficult to recognize in some cases, but rapid and catastrophic in others. New cardiorespiratory symptoms during pregnancy may be the result of normal physiological adaptation (increased minute ventilation and respiratory work), but must be taken seriously and investigated because they may reflect:

- Deterioration of mild disease (e.g., asthma)
- Significant respiratory infection
- Severe underlying pathology (e.g., undiagnosed pulmonary hypertension, cardiomyopathy or pulmonary edema)

In general, therapy which was necessary in the pre-pregnancy period will continue to be necessary when the patient becomes pregnant.

- Essential drugs should not be withheld because of fetal concerns.
- Necessary imaging should not be withheld because of fetal concerns, but attempts to limit fetal radiation exposure are appropriate (Chapter 6).

Scoring Systems

Assessing the severity of illness in critically ill obstetric patients can be based on early warning scoring systems, but multiple organ dysfunction syndrome scores have not been specifically validated in pregnancy so have low sensitivity. These scores often overestimate the risk of death, making them unsuitable for admission triage or withdrawal-of-life-support decisions.

The high false positive rates and unnecessary work created by current scoring systems mandates that new scores are modified to take into account different physiological limits, with parameters set for mental response, pulse rate, systolic blood pressure, respiratory rate (probably the most sensitive indicator of well-being), temperature, and urine output.

Consequences of Failing to Recognize Significant Illness

In the 2003–2005 United Kingdom Confidential Enquiries into Maternal and Child Health report, a number of cases of failure to appreciate the severity of illness were highlighted. These included deaths from post-operative respiratory failure of an obese asthmatic woman; from hypovolemia due to concealed hemorrhage in the post-anesthesia care unit; and from anemia and sepsis in a woman being cared for by junior staff in a ward environment.

Such events gave rise to several key recommendations.

- Pregnant women from populations and countries where women experience poorer general health should have a full clinical assessment.

- Clinical staff must learn from critical events and serious untoward incidents. All staff should undergo regular formal training for identification and management of serious medical conditions, the early recognition and management of severely ill women, and impending maternal collapse. Life support skills, including basic and advanced cardiac life support (BCLS and ACLS), should be regularly reinforced.

- A national modified early warning scoring system for all obstetric women should be developed.

The Anesthesiologist's Role in Critical Care

A summary of potential roles is shown in Table 14.1.

Teaching and Training

Although decisions should always be made collaboratively among disciplines, anesthesiologists have a number of core competencies that are required for critical care, so should be involved in the teaching and training of other doctors and nurses. These competencies and skills include:

- Airway management and ventilation.
- Vascular access.
- Hemodynamic monitoring.
- Cardiovascular support.
- Pain management.

In addition, anesthesiology has led the way in medical simulation. In the obstetric unit, simulation training can:

- Hone clinical and nontechnical skills in dealing with emergencies.
- Expose junior staff to emergency drills and management protocols.

Patient Care

Coordinated multidisciplinary care is often required in those with severe preexisting disease or critical illness. Participation of anesthesiologists, maternal–fetal medicine specialists, and obstetric medical specialists, is important as part of a multidisciplinary, multispecialty approach, along with a variety of other health care professionals as

Table 14.1 The Anesthesiologist's Role in Critical Care of the Obstetric Patient

Leadership in creating a culture of safety
- National and state health systems
- Hospital-based governance, including protocols, guidelines, and critical incident monitoring
- ICU/HDU unit administration

Leadership in team-working during crisis management
Antenatal assessment and management of "high risk" women (outpatient and inpatient)

Coordination of training responsibilities involving simulation dealing with:
- Obstetric emergencies
- Inpatient "drills"
- Simulation courses
- Education and training in the recognition of severe illness

Clinical services to sick pregnant women
- Assessment
- Resuscitation and stabilization
- Anesthesia and pain management. Examples include:
  - Exercising judgment in choosing the most suitable method, and expertise in modifying and delivering the anesthetic to suit the circumstances
  - Cesarean delivery should not be done in the ICU unless transfer to an operating room is unsafe or it is a perimortem procedure
  - Use of regional techniques requires understanding of the hemodynamic effects and risks in patients who are anticoagulated, infected, or at risk of bleeding

Perioperative care
- Critical care (HDU/ICU)
  - Respiratory and cardiovascular care and fluid management
- Transfer of critically ill patients to an ICU
- Advanced life support

ICU = intensive care unit; HDU= high-dependency care unit.

appropriate (i.e., cardiologists, surgeons, neonatologists, midwives, and nurses). Anesthesiologists should play a leading role in:

- The antenatal assessment and management of high-risk pregnant women, based on obstetric referral of both inpatients and outpatients.
- Intensive care, and invasive monitoring and supportive care of patients with hemorrhage or hypertension.
- Goal-directed therapy and rapid antibiotic treatment of those with sepsis, then circulatory support and fetal resuscitation *in utero*.
- The transfer of critically ill patients based on the guidelines of relevant organizations, as well as internal hospital protocols

(with antenatal transfer to critical care areas preferable to intrapartum timing of transfer).

Maternal Mortality

Overview and Principal Causes

Maternal deaths are "the tip of the iceberg" in terms of the prevalence of severe maternal morbidity during pregnancy, this being up to 80 times higher (the majority of cases related to obstetric hemorrhage). Documenting severe morbidity is likely to be more beneficial in terms of clinical lessons and evaluation of the quality of maternal care.

Nevertheless, maternal mortality worldwide occurs on a frightening scale (Table 14.2). An estimated 500,000 pregnant women die each year, with over 99% of these deaths in developing countries, especially in sub-Saharan Africa and parts of Asia, where health care resources are inadequate and maternity care appears not to be a priority.

The primary causes of maternal death are:

- obstetric hemorrhage (25% of all maternal deaths, and the second most common cause in the United States)
- the consequences of obstructed labor (failure of descent and cephalopelvic disproportion, or CPD)
- infection

In some developed countries, the majority of maternal deaths are now more often "indirect" (i.e., due to preexisting disease exacerbated by

Table 14.2 **World Health Organization Maternal Mortality Data from Selected Regions**		
Region	*MMR*	*Lifetime risk estimate 1 in...*
Worldwide	400	92
Asia	330	120
Africa	820	26
Oceania	430	62
Developed regions	9	7,300
USA	11	4,800
UK	8	8,200
Australia	4	13,300

MMR = maternal mortality ratio (defined as the number of maternal deaths per 100,000 live births). From: www.who.int/whosis/mme_2005.pdf

pregnancy, or new disease arising during pregnancy but unrelated to obstetric complications) than "direct" (i.e., due to diseases of pregnancy or obstetric conditions; see Table 14.3). In the United States, the most recent data indicate direct deaths still constitute the majority of maternal deaths, though national data collection is not performed.

- Major causes of indirect maternal death are cardiac disease (especially adult congenital heart disease, myocardial infarction and peripartum cardiomyopathy) and suicide.
- Major causes of direct death are thromboembolism, obstetric hemorrhage, amniotic fluid embolism, and complications of hypertensive disease.
- Complications of anesthesia are infrequent causes of maternal death (3%–5% of all deaths in both developed and developing countries).

The failure of health professionals to recognize the signs and symptoms of preeclampsia, and to adequately control maternal blood pressure, has been identified as an issue, as has poor management of major hemorrhage and failure of medical staff, including anesthesiologists, to appreciate the severity of maternal illness (including complications such as pulmonary edema). The difficulties of dealing with morbidly obese pregnant women results in a disproportionate representation of these women in maternal mortality reports from the United States and the U.K.

Table 14.3 Main Causes of Maternal Death in Developed Countries

Indirect
Cardiac disease
Suicide
Infection (e.g., human immunodeficiency virus, viral or bacterial pneumonia)
Cerebrovascular hemorrhage
Direct
Obstetric hemorrhage
Pulmonary thromboembolism
Amniotic fluid embolism syndrome
Preeclampsia and eclampsia
Obstetric infection
Incidental
Trauma
Cancer not specifically influenced by pregnancy

The Anesthesiologist's Role

In many developing countries the lack of specialist anesthesiologists, or even physicians with the most basic knowledge and training in the requisite skills, is concerning. A well-organized anesthesiology service can have significant influence in reducing the number of maternal deaths.

- Countries with high standards for anesthesia service and delivery have exceptionally low anesthesia-related death rates (e.g., estimated 1 in 750,000 births in Australia).
- Anesthesiologists are core providers of safe multidisciplinary management of women with hypertension, and cardiac and other medical diseases.
- Anesthesiologists can assist with compliance with local policies for prophylaxis against infection and thromboembolism.
- Anesthesiologists have life-saving roles in the management of obstetric hemorrhage.

Given the frequency of massive hemorrhage in causing adverse outcomes, this complication of pregnancy is one clearly amenable to outcome improvements by addressing:

- Institution of 24-hour obstetric and anesthesiology coverage.
- Improved availability of health care resources (e.g., blood bank availability, early transfer to tertiary units).
- Wider adoption of improved technologies (e.g., cell salvage, interventional radiology or new blood products).

Reducing Maternal Mortality

Cost-effective resource allocation and clinical governance are likely to represent the best means of minimizing critical incidents and adverse outcomes. The accurate collection of "near miss" and specific morbidity data is being established in many countries, and could have an educational impact similar to that apparent from the U.K. triennial reports.

Taking a broader view, future reductions in maternal mortality in developed countries are likely to be small, although many women who die are economically and socially disadvantaged. In developing countries, improvements in health services are likely to be far more important than the introduction of new therapies or technologies, but will not occur unless political will determines that changes are made.

Further Reading

1. Clutton-Brock T. Critical Care. (Ch. 19) In *The Confidential Enquiry into Maternal & Child Health* (CEMACH). Saving mother's lives: Reviewing maternal deaths to make motherhood safer. 2003-2005. The seventh report of the Confidential Enquiries into Maternal Deaths in the United Kingdom. London: CEMACH, 2007.

2. Critical care in pregnancy. The American College of Obstetricians and Gynecologists (ACOG) Practice Bulletin, Number 100. Available at: http://www.guideline.gov/summary/summary.aspx?doc_id=14179.

3. Baskett TF. Epidemiology of obstetric critical care. *Best Prac Res Clin Obs Gynaecol.* 2008;22:763-774.

4. Williams J, Mozurkewich E, Chilimigras J, et al. Critical care in obstetrics: pregnancy-specific conditions. *Best Prac Res Clin Obs Gynaecol.* 2008;22:825-846.

5. Plaat F, Wray S. Role of the anaesthetist in obstetric critical care. *Best Prac Res Clin Obs Gynaecol.* 2008;22:917-935.

Chapter 15

Neonatal Resuscitation

Emily Baird, MD, PhD
Valerie A. Arkoosh, MD, MPH
Robert D'Angelo, MD

Introduction

Following birth, numerous physiologic changes must rapidly transpire for the fetus to successfully make the transition from fetal to neonatal physiology. Due to the complexity of this process, approximately ten percent of newborns require some assistance to begin breathing, and one percent of newborns require full resuscitation in the delivery room. However, the risk of neonatal distress rises exponentially among newborns weighing less than 1500 grams. Although the need for full neonatal resuscitation is relatively rare, it is essential for all delivery room personnel to understand neonatal adaptations to extrauterine life, recognize the predictors of the need for resuscitation, and have both the provisions and knowledge to respond appropriately.

Pathophysiology

In the fetal circulation, the presence of two cardiac shunts—the foramen ovale and the ductus arteriosus—create a substantial right-to-left shunt, with gas exchange occurring exclusively in the placenta.

The shunt persists due to high pulmonary vascular resistance (PVR) coupled with the low systemic vascular resistance (SVR) created by the placenta. Following delivery, the fetal circulation must promptly transition to the pulmonary and systemic circulations operating in series to avoid fetal death or permanent neurological damage.

Fetal Physiology

- Oxygenated blood from the placenta mixes with venous blood from the lower body in the inferior vena cava (Figure 15.1).
- Blood entering the right atrium from the inferior vena cava is preferentially directed into the left atrium via the foramen ovale.

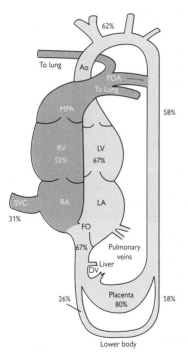

Figure 15.1 Diagrammatic representation of the fetal circulation. *In utero*, pulmonary vascular resistance is high and 90% of right ventricular output flows across the ductus arteriosus. Numbers represent SaO_2 in vessels or chambers.

- Blood in the left atrium flows into the left ventricle and out the ascending aorta, perfusing the upper body.
- Deoxygenated blood returning from the upper body via the superior vena cava enters the right atrium and is preferentially directed into the right ventricle.
- The majority of the blood flow from the right ventricle is shunted across the ductus arteriosus because of high PVR.
- Blood enters the descending aorta from the ductus ateriosus and perfuses the lower body and placenta.

Transition to Neonatal Physiology

- Compression of infant thorax during vaginal delivery prompts the expulsion of fluid from the mouth and upper airways.
- Crying fills the lungs with air, which stimulates the release of surfactant.
- Increased oxygen tension and pulmonary blood flow leads to the release of nitric oxide, and subsequent pulmonary vasodilatation.
- Clamping of the umbilical cord increases SVR as the low-resistance placenta is removed from the circulation.
- The dramatic decrease in PVR and concurrent increase in SVR leads to a substantial reduction in right-to-left shunt across the foramen ovale and ductus arteriosus.
- These changes occur within minutes of delivery, so that neonatal circulation more closely resembles that of an adult rather than a fetus (Figure 15.2).

Pathophysiology of Persistent Pulmonary Hypertension of the Newborn

- The presence of persistent hypoxemia and acidosis increases PVR and promotes patency of the ductus arteriosus.
- Shunting of blood across the ductus arteriosus leads to further decreases in oxygen saturation.
- Prolonged neonatal hypoxemia results in redistribution of blood flow to the heart, brain, and adrenal glands.
- If oxygen demand exceeds supply despite redistribution, a decrease in myocardial contractility and cardiac output ensues.
- Spontaneous ventilatory drive is reduced by both indirect central nervous system depression and direct diaphragmatic depression.

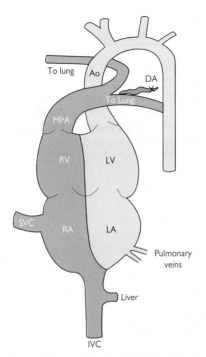

Figure 15.2 Diagram of neonatal (adult-like) circulation. At birth, pulmonary vascular resistance drops dramatically, and the ductus arteriosus constricts; right ventricular output flows primarily through the lungs. Changes in vascular resistance markedly decrease the shunt across the foramen ovale.

Predicting Need for Neonatal Resuscitation

The need for neonatal resuscitation can be predicted in about 80% of cases with the use of antepartum and intrapartum fetal assessment. Antepartum assessment includes evaluation for major fetal anomalies, and identification of maternal factors that may influence fetal well-being (Table 15.1). Intrapartum events often predict the need for neonatal resuscitation (Table 15.2). Assessment must continue throughout labor, as the clinical situation can rapidly change.

Table 15.1 Maternal and Fetal Factors Associated with Need for Resuscitation

Maternal diabetes
Pregnancy-induced hypertension
Chronic hypertension
Previous Rh sensitization
Previous stillbirth
Bleeding in 2nd or 3rd trimester
Maternal infection
Lack of prenatal care
Maternal substance abuse
Known fetal anomalies
Post-term gestation
Preterm gestation
Multiple gestation
Size–dates discrepancy
Polyhydramnios
Oligohydramios
Maternal drug therapy including: reserpine, lithium, magnesium, and adrenergic-blockers

Table 15.2 Intrapartum Events Associated with Need for Resuscitation

Cesarean delivery
Abnormal fetal presentation
Premature labor
Rupture of membranes > 24 hours
Chorioamnionitis
Precipitous labor
Prolonged labor > 24 hours
Prolonged second stage > 3–4 hours
Nonreassuring fetal heart tracing
General anesthesia
Uterine tetany
Meconium-stained amniotic fluid
Prolapsed cord
Placental abruption
Uterine rupture
Difficult instrumental delivery
Maternal systemic narcotics within 4 hours of delivery

Fetal Heart Rate Tracing

Intrapartum fetal heart rate (FHR) monitoring is the first line of fetal assessment. A reassuring FHR tracing is more than 90% accurate in predicting a 5-minute Apgar score of greater than seven. In predicting fetal compromise, however, FHR monitoring has a false positive rate of at least 35%–50%. Even though an abnormal FHR trace may not correlate with a poor long-term prognosis, the presence of an abnormal tracing is highly correlated with the need for neonatal resuscitation in the delivery room. Additionally, it is important to remember that even in the presence of a reassuring FHR trace, nearly 50% of babies born by cesarean delivery will require some active form of resuscitation.

Deceleration Patterns in Fetal Heart Rate Tracings

- Early decelerations are thought to be a normal vagal response to head compression during descent of the fetus.
- Late decelerations are associated with fetal compromise resulting from uteroplacental insufficiency.
- Variable decelerations result from umbilical cord compression, and in their severe form may signify fetal asphyxia.

Preparation for Neonatal Resuscitation

Preparation for neonatal resuscitation is an ongoing activity on all labor and delivery units. A number of tasks including acquisition and maintenance of the proper equipment, education and training of responding personnel, and development of contingency plans for additional personnel if needed must be constantly monitored for completeness. Equipment and medications should be organized together in one location in the delivery room, checked frequently for proper functioning and expiration date, and replenished immediately after use (Table 15.3). At least one person skilled in newborn resuscitation should attend every delivery, and additional personnel should be available when a high-risk delivery is anticipated.

Special Considerations in Preparation for Neonatal Resuscitation

- Laryngeal mask airway (LMA): The size-1 LMA has been used to successfully resuscitate newborns of both normal and low birth weight who required positive pressure ventilation (PPV) at birth.

Table 15.3 Equipment and Medications for Neonatal Resuscitation

- **Suction equipment**
  - Bulb syringe
  - Mechanical suction
  - Suction catheter 5F–10F
  - Meconium aspirator
- **Medications**
  - Epinephrine 1:10,000
  - Volume expander
  - Dextrose 10%
  - Sterile water & normal saline
- **Bag & mask equipment**
  - Neonatal bag with pressure relief valve
  - Face mask (newborn & premature)
  - Oral airways
  - Oxygen with flowmeter and tubing
- **Intubation equipment**
  - Laryngoscope
  - Straight blade #0 and #1
  - Extra bulbs and batteries
  - Endotracheal tube 2.5–4.0 mm
  - Stylet
  - CO_2 detector
- **Miscellaneous**
  - Radiant warmer
  - Stethoscope
  - ECG
  - Adhesive tape
  - Syringes & needles
  - Umbilical artery catheterization tray
  - Umbilical catheters 3.5F, 5F
  - Umbilical tape
  - 3-way stopcocks
  - Feeding tube, 5F

The LMA can be life-saving in neonates with conditions associated with hypoplastic mandible, where mask ventilation and endotracheal intubation have failed.

- End-tidal CO_2 detection: Clinical trials have demonstrated that both infrared absorption and pediatric-size colorimetric disposable devices are significantly more rapid than clinical exam in both confirming endotracheal intubation and detecting esophageal intubation.

Intrapartum Resuscitation

Intrapartum resuscitation is initiated once fetal compromise is identified. Maternal and intrauterine factors that may impair oxygen delivery to the fetus must be identified and corrected immediately.

Possible Causes of Fetal Compromise

- Maternal hypotension or decreased cardiac output secondary to aortocaval compression, epidural-induced sympathectomy, hemorrhage, or cardiac disease.
- Disease states that may interfere with maternal oxygenation, including asthma, pneumonia, and pulmonary edema.
- Conditions compromising fetal blood flow, including umbilical cord prolapse, uterine hyperstimulation, uterine tetany, placental abruption, or uterine rupture.

Recommended Response to Signs of Fetal Compromise

- Administer 100% oxygen by face mask to increase maternal, and thus, fetal oxygenation.
- Position the parturient with left uterine displacement to decrease aortocaval compression.
- Treat maternal hypotension with vasopressors and intravascular fluids (in the absence of pulmonary edema and heart disease).
- Discontinue oxytocin infusion, or administer a tocolytic agent to reduce uterine tone.
- Consider a saline amnioinfusion if umbilical cord compression is suspected.
- Emergent delivery is required in the setting of severe placental abruption or uterine rupture.

Neonatal Resuscitation

The American Heart Association/American Academy of Pediatrics recommends the following protocol for neonatal resuscitation (Table 15.4). During the resuscitation, steps should be implemented to minimize heat loss from the neonate. Depressed, asphyxiated infants often have unstable thermal regulatory systems. Cold stress leads to hypoxemia, hypercarbia, and metabolic acidosis, all of which will promote persistence of the fetal circulation and hinder resuscitation.

Table 15.4 Neonatal Resuscitation Protocol*

- **Evaluate Neonate at Birth for:** Term Gestation, Clear Amniotic Fluid, Breathing/Crying, Good Muscle Tone
  - Yes: Routine care (provide warmth, clear airway, dry, assess color)
  - No: Provide warmth, clear airway, dry, <u>stimulate, reposition</u>
- **At 30 Seconds after Birth:** Evaluate Respirations, Heart Rate, and Color
  - If Breathing, HR > 100 bpm, and Pink:
    - Observational care
  - If Breathing, HR > 100 bpm, and Cyanotic:
    - <u>Administer supplemental oxygen</u>
      - If neonate becomes pink:
        - Observational Care
      - If cyanosis persists:
        - <u>Provide positive pressure ventilation</u>
  - If Apneic or HR < 100 bpm:
    - Provide positive pressure ventilation
- **Once Positive Pressure Ventilation Initiated:**
  - If HR > 100 bpm and pink:
    - Postresuscitation Care
  - If HR < 60 bpm:
    - Continue positive pressure ventilation
    - <u>Begin chest compressions</u>
- **Evaluate at 30 seconds after initiating Positive Pressure Ventilation:**
  - If HR > 60 bpm:
    - Continue positive pressure ventilation
  - If HR < 60 bpm:
    - Continue provide positive pressure ventilation
    - Continue chest compressions
    - <u>Consider epinephrine and/or volume</u>
- **Reevaluate every 30 Seconds, Proceed as Indicated**

*Source: the American Heart Association and American Academy of Pediatrics Neonatal Resuscitation Guidelines.

Resuscitative efforts should be guided by repeated assessment of respirations, heart rate, and color. Neonatal cardiac arrest is generally secondary to respiratory failure producing hypoxemia and tissue acidosis. The net result of these metabolic changes is bradycardia, decreased cardiac contractility, and eventually cardiac arrest.

Overview of Neonatal Resuscitation

- Stimulate and provide warmth to neonate.
- Evaluate respirations, heart rate, and color. Cardiac auscultation with a stethoscope is the most accurate assessment of neonatal heart rate.

- If the neonate is gasping or apneic and/or has a heart rate < 100 bpm, initiate PPV at a rate of 40–60 breaths per minute. Peak inspiratory pressures of 30 to 40 cm H_2O or higher may be required for initial lung expansion, but should be reduced to <25 cm H_2O as soon as possible.

- Chest compressions are indicated for a heart rate < 60 bpm despite adequate ventilation with supplemental oxygen for 30 seconds. Chest compressions should be instituted at a rate of 90 compressions per minute. The recommended ratio between chest compressions and ventilations is 3:1, producing 90 compressions and 30 ventilations each minute. Continue compressions until the spontaneous heart rate is greater than 60 bpm.

- Administer epinephrine and/or volume expanders if the heart rate remains less than 60 bpm after adequate ventilation with oxygen and chest compressions for 30 seconds.

- Consider endotracheal intubation if bag and mask ventilation is ineffective, there is an anticipated need for prolonged mechanical ventilation, or as a route to administer medication.

Medications for Neonatal Resuscitation

A summary of recommended medications, doses, and routes of administration is presented in Table 15.5.

- Intravenous epinephrine is the vasopressor of choice, and can be repeated every 3 to 5 minutes until the heart rate is greater than 60 bpm. Adequate ventilation must be established prior to administration of epinephrine. In the absence of adequate oxygenation, the increase in myocardial oxygen consumption caused by epinephrine can lead to myocardial damage. The efficacy of endotracheal administration of epinephrine has not been evaluated in neonates.

Table 15.5 Medications for Neonatal Resuscitation

Medication	Concentration	Dosage	Route	Rate
Epinephrine	1:10,000	0.01–0.03 mg/kg	IV	Give rapidly
Volume expanders	Normal saline	10 mL/kg	IV	Give over 5 min
	O negative blood	10 mL/kg	IV	Give over 5 min
Dextrose	D10% in water	2 mL/kg	PO	
		8 mg/kg/min	IV	Infusion

- Volume expanders are indicated *only* with evidence of acute blood loss and signs of shock. Volume expansion should occur over 5 to 10 minutes. Rapid volume administration has been associated with intracerebral hemorrhage.
- Naloxone hydrochloride is no longer recommended during the initial neonatal resuscitation. It can be administered to neonates with intrauterine opioid exposure after ventilation and heart rate have been restored. It should be avoided in neonates with narcotic-addicted mothers, as this can precipitate acute withdrawal and seizures.
- Sodium bicarbonate is no longer recommended during the initial neonatal resuscitation due to lack of data supporting efficacy.
- Dextrose should be given if the glucose level is < 40 to 45 mg/dl. Approximately 10% of healthy term neonates may have transient hypoglycemia. Neonates born of diabetic mothers, or mothers who received large amounts of intravenous dextrose, are at increased risk.

Management of Meconium

A major shift in thinking has occurred over the last five years concerning the management of meconium. Current recommendations include the following:

- In the presence of meconium, routine intrapartum oropharyngeal and nasopharyngeal suctioning is *not* recommended.
- An infant with strong respiratory efforts, good muscle tone, and heart rate does *not* require endotracheal intubation and suctioning.
- Tracheal suctioning is recommended only if there is meconium-stained fluid *and* the baby is depressed.

Use of Oxygen in Neonatal Resuscitation

The scientific basis for the use of 100% oxygen to resuscitate newborns has never been established. Evidence is growing from both human clinical trials in term infants and animal models that resuscitation with oxygen may be detrimental to some infants. Recent studies have demonstrated that oxygen saturation in healthy, term newborns are quite low during the first minute of age, ranging from 43% to 77%. At 3, 5, and 10 minutes after birth, preductal mean values were 83%, 89%, and 94%, respectively. Exposure to high concentrations of oxygen during resuscitation appears to promote the formation of excessive reactive oxygen intermediates in neonatal tissue, producing injury. A recent meta-analysis including randomized or pseudo-randomized trials of neonatal resuscitation with room air (n=881) versus 100% oxygen (n=856) found the following:

- Overall neonatal mortality was 8.0% versus 13.0% in the room air versus 100% oxygen groups, respectively (OR 0.57, 95% CI 0.42–0.78).
- Apgar scores at 5 minutes and heart rate at 90 seconds were significantly higher in the room air group.
- Time to first spontaneous breath was significantly shorter in the group resuscitated with room air.
- Obviously, this data must be balanced with concerns about tissue damage from prolonged asphyxia.

Current Recommendations Regarding Oxygen for Neonatal Resuscitation

- Resuscitation may be initiated with room air or 100% oxygen.
- 100% oxygen should be used in resuscitation if there is no improvement in the neonate within 90 seconds after birth.

Neonatal Assessment

Apgar scores provide a measure of neonatal well-being (Table 15.6). The 1-minute score correlates with survival, whereas the 5-minute score is related to neurological outcome. If the 5-minute score is less than 7, additional scores should be obtained every five minutes until 20 minutes have passed or until two successive scores are greater than or equal to 7. Survival is unlikely if the Apgar score is 0 at ≥ 10 minutes of age. Current guidelines now suggest that after 10 minutes of continuous and adequate resuscitative efforts, discontinuation of resuscitation may be justified if there are no signs of life.

Table 15.6 Apgar Scoring System			
Sign	0	1	2
Heart Rate	Absent	< 100 bpm	> 100 bpm
Respiratory Rate	Absent	Slow, irregular	Crying
Muscle Tone	Flaccid	Some flexion of extremities	Active motion
Reflex irritability	No response	Grimace	Vigorous cry
Color	Blue and pale	Blue extremities	Completely pink

Summary

The first few minutes following birth are characterized by profound adaptive changes in the neonatal circulatory and respiratory systems. Failure to successfully transition from fetal to adult physiology can result in a downward spiral culminating in permanent neurologic injury or neonatal death. Although the need for full neonatal resuscitation is relatively rare, it is essential that personnel are always available to aid in this transition when necessary. To avoid poor outcomes, practitioners must understand the neonatal adaptations to extrauterine life, recognize risk factors for fetal compromise, and have both the supplies and training to respond appropriately.

Further Reading

1. American Heart Association AAoP. 2005 American Heart Association (AHA) guidelines for cardiopulmonary resuscitation (CPR) and emergency cardiovascular care (ECC) of pediatric and neonatal patients: Neonatal resuscitation guidelines. *Pediatrics.* 2006;117:e1029-1038.

2. Morgan GE, Mikhail MS, Murray MJ. Maternal & fetal physiology & anesthesia. *Clinical Anesthesiology, 4th Edition.* 2006;884-887.

3. Lakshminrusimha S, Steinhorn RH: Pulmonary vascular biology during neonatal transition. *Clin Perinatol.* 1999;26:601-619.

4. Posen R, Friedlich P, Chan L, *et al.* Relationship between fetal monitoring and resuscitative needs: fetal distress versus routine cesarean deliveries. *Journal of Perinatology.* 2000;20:101-104.

5. Guay J. Fetal monitoring and neonatal resuscitation: what the anaesthetist should know. *Can J Anaesth.* 1991;38:R83-88.

6. Trevisanuto D, Micaglio M, Pitton M, *et al.* Laryngeal mask airway: is the management of neonates requiring positive pressure ventilation at birth changing? *Resuscitation.* 2004;62:151-157.

7. Barber CA, Wyckoff MH. Use and efficacy of endotracheal versus intravenous epinephrine during neonatal cardiopulmonary resuscitation in the delivery room. *Pediatrics.* 2006;118:1028-1034.

8. Halliday HL. Endotracheal intubation at birth for preventing morbidity and mortality in vigorous, meconium-stained infants born at term. *The Cochrane Database of Systematic Reviews.* 2000;2.

9. Higgins RD, Bancalari E, Willinger M, *et al.* Executive summary of the workshop on oxygen in neonatal therapies: Controversies and opportunities for research. *Pediatrics.* 2007;119:790-796.

10. Kamlin C, O'Donnell C, Davis P, *et al.* Oxygen saturation in healthy infants immediately after birth. *J Pediatr.* 2006;148:585-589.

Index

Note: Page references followed by 'f' and 't' denote figures and tables, respectively.